Church and People in the Medieval West, 900–1200

The Medieval World

Series Editor: Julia Smith, The University of Glasgow

Alfred the Great
Richard Abels

Christian-Jewish Relations, 1000–1300
Anna Sapir Abulafia

The Western Mediterranean Kingdoms
David Abulafia

The Fourth Crusade
Michael Angold

The Cathars
Malcolm Barber

The Godwins
Frank Barlow

Phillip Augustus
Jim Bradbury

Violence in Medieval Europe
Warren Brown

Medieval Canon Law
J.A. Brundage

Crime in Medieval Europe
Trevor Dean

Charles I of Anjou
Jean Dunbabin

The Age of Charles Martel
Paul Fouracre

Margery Kempe
A.E. Goodman

Edward the Black Prince
David Green

Church and People in the Medieval West, 900–1200
Sarah Hamilton

Bastard Feudalism
M. Hicks

The Formation of English Common Law
John Hudson

The Mongols and the West
Peter Jackson

Europe's Barbarians, AD 200–600
Edward James

Cnut
K. Lawson

The Age of Robert Guiscard
Graham Loud

The English Church, 940–1154
H.R. Loyn

Justinian
John Moorhead

Ambrose
John Moorhead

The Devil's World
Andrew P. Roach

The Reign of Richard Lionheart
Ralph Turner/Richard Heiser

The Welsh Princes
Roger Turvey

English Noblewomen in the Late Middle Ages
J. Ward

Church and People in the Medieval West, 900–1200

Sarah Hamilton

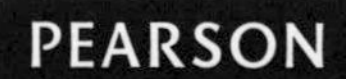

Harlow, England • London • New York • Boston • San Francisco • Toronto • Sydney • Auckland • Singapore • Hong Kong
Tokyo • Seoul • Taipei • New Delhi • Cape Town • São Paulo • Mexico City • Madrid • Amsterdam • Munich • Paris • Milan

PEARSON EDUCATION LIMITED
Edinburgh Gate
Harlow CM20 2JE
Tel: +44 (0)1279 623623
Website: www.pearson.com/uk

First published 2013 (print and electronic)

ISBN: 978-0-582-77280-9 (print)
978-0-273-78678-8 (eText)

British Library Cataloguing-in-Publication Data
A catalogue record for the print edition is available from the British Library

Library of Congress Cataloging-in-Publication Data
A catalog record for the print edition is available from the Library of Congress

10 9 8 7 6 5 4 3 2 1
17 16 15 14 13

Print edition typeset in 10/14pt ITC Galliard Std by 35
Print edition printed and bound in Malaysia (CTP-PJB)

NOTE THAT ANY PAGE CROSS REFERENCES REFER TO THE PRINT EDITION

Contents

Abbreviations

AASS	*Acta Sanctorum quotquot toto orbe coluntur*, ed. J. Bollandus *et al.* (Antwerp and Brussels, 1634–).
Burchard	Burchard, *Decretum*, *PL* 140.
CCCM	Corpus Christianorum Continuatio Mediaevalis
C&S	*Councils and Synods with Other Documents Relating to the English Church* I: *871–1204*, 2 vols, ed. D. Whitelock, M. Brett and C. N. L. Brooke (Oxford, 1981).
EETS	*Early English Text Society*
EME	*Early Medieval Europe*
Mansi, *Concilia*	J. D. Mansi, ed., *Sacrorum conciliorum nova et amplissima collectio*, 59 vols (Venice, 1759–98; repr. Graz, 1960).
MGH	*Monumenta Germaniae Historica*
NCMH	*New Cambridge Medieval History*
Regino	Regino of Prüm, *Libri duo de synodalibus causis et disciplinis ecclesiasticis*, ed. F. W. H. Wasserschleben, rev. and ed. W. Hartmann, *Das Sendhandbuch des Regino von Prüm* (Darmstadt, 2004).
PL	*Patrologia cursus completus, series latina*, ed. J.-P. Migne (Paris, 1844–64).
PRG	*Le Pontifical Romano-Germanique du dixième siècle*, ed. C. Vogel and R. Elze, 3 vols (Vatican City, 1963, 1972).
TRHS	*Transactions of the Royal Historical Society*
ODNB	H. C. G. Matthew and B. Harrison, eds, *Oxford Dictionary of National Biography: From the Earliest Times to the Year 2000* (Oxford, 2004).
RB	*The Rule of Benedict: A Guide to Christian Living*, ed. and trans. G. Holzherr (Dublin, 1994).
RC	J. Bertram, *The Chrodegang Rules: The Rules for the Common Life of the Secular Clergy from the Eighth and Ninth Centuries: Critical Texts with Translations and Commentary* (Aldershot, 2005).

Acknowledgments

It is a pleasure to acknowledge all the help I have been given during the writing of this book; all the faults which remain are, of course, my responsibility. The award of a Postdoctoral Fellowship by the British Academy allowed me to begin the research for this book, and the award of a residential fellowship by Gladstone's Library at St Deiniol's Hawarden helped provide me with space to think at a crucial point. I should also like to thank the staff of the British Library, the London Library, the National Library of Scotland, the Vatican Library, the Warburg Institute, and the University of Exeter library. The comments and questions of all my students at Exeter, particularly those in my third-year Special Subject, have helped shape this book. I have benefited immeasurably from discussing specific aspects with various colleagues, several of whom read chapters in draft, in particular Julia Crick, Helen Gittos, Jinty Nelson, Susan Reynolds, Catherine Rider, Alex Walsham, Ian Forrest and Sethina Watson and all the members of the 'Social Church' research group. I should like to thank John Arnold especially for reading the entire text in draft, and also the anonymous reader whose critical comments helped to sharpen my thinking. I have been extremely fortunate to have had such a supportive academic editor in Julia Smith; her encouragement throughout the process and her pertinent and constructive comments on the initial draft ensured its completion. Thanks too to Mari Shullaw at Pearson both for her extreme forbearance as an editor and for all her advice and support. The support of family and friends has been invaluable, especially that of Matthew and Carol Cragoe; Alice Hamilton and Steven Carden; Anke Holdenried; Naomi Howell; Ruth and Steven Smyth-Bonfield; and Cordelia Warr. My father Bernard Hamilton discussed some of the ideas with me and read several of the chapters in draft. But my greatest debt is to Stephen who has had to live with this book for far too long: this book is dedicated to him as thanks for everything.

Teignmouth, September 2012

Publisher's acknowledgments

We are grateful to the following for permission to reproduce copyright material:

Extracts on pages 259, 261, 264 and 328 from Sheingorn, P. (trans.), *The Book of Sainte Foy* (University of Pennsylvania Press, 1995). Reprinted with permission of the University of Pennsylvania Press.

In some instances we have been unable to trace the owners of copyright material, and we would appreciate any information that would enable us to do so.

chapter 1

Introduction

Rejoice, O Mother Church! Exult in glory!
The risen Saviour shines upon you.
Let this place resound with joy,
echoing the mighty song of all God's people![1]

Since the seventh century this verse has been sung at the beginning of the liturgical celebrations for Easter as part of the Exultet hymn. It avows that the Church is made up of all God's people, and that they all participate in the celebration of Easter, the most important feast in the Christian calendar. But at the same time as the text calls on everyone to celebrate Christ's resurrection, we need to note that the singing of this hymn was reserved to a single member of the clergy, the deacon. On the one hand, clergy recognised that the laity played an important part in the rites of the Church, and on the other they preserved a monopoly over their conduct. It articulates one of the paradoxes of the Church's relationship with the laity, which was at once all embracing and exclusive. It thus makes a fitting start to a text in which I explore the various ways in which the institutional Church related to the peoples of Western Europe in the years between *c.*900 and *c.*1200. In doing so I will seek to reinterpret the ways in which Christianity was experienced by ordinary men and women, and to redefine the nature of the relationships between members of the clergy and the laity across three hundred years.

The focus on these three centuries is a reflection of the fundamental significance historians of western society attribute to the central Middle

Ages.[2] The religious developments which are the subject of this text took place in a world of changing political, social and economic circumstances. The differences between the Latin world of the early tenth century and that of the early thirteenth century are marked. The collapse of the ninth-century Carolingian polity in which members of a single family ruled much of Western Europe was followed by one in which authority in many areas became more localised. Some scholars, particularly those who work on the regions which are now France and Italy, believe a further socio-political change, the 'feudal transformation', took place in the late tenth and early eleventh centuries as the authority of the monarch became weakened and usurped by local lords with much smaller spheres of influence.[3] Royal law courts ceased to be held in the localities, and instead the jurisdiction of local lords held sway. Local lords took the opportunity to increase the taxes and other dues demanded of their tenants, and the less powerful lost the opportunity to appeal to a higher authority against such demands; consequently a diminution in the rights and incomes of the less well-off accompanied these changes amongst the ruling elite. The poor and less powerful became even poorer and less powerful. The picture is somewhat different elsewhere in Europe. In the Germanic lands of east Frankia royal power continued to be strong throughout the tenth and eleventh centuries, but overlay that of very powerful regional lords. Although the Carolingians never directly ruled the kingdoms which came, in the course of the tenth century, to make up England, its Church and people had come within their sphere of influence, with exchanges of texts and personnel as well as political alliances. Here too royal power grew over the course of the tenth and eleventh centuries at the same time as that of local lords. In the late eleventh and twelfth centuries a growth in the powers of royal and papal governments at the expense of local secular and ecclesiastical autonomies followed these developments. Demographic and economic change accompanied this socio-political transformation: populations grew, the number of towns mushroomed, the level of trade increased, and the amount of land under cultivation, both within and on the periphery of the heartlands of ninth-century Europe, expanded. Peoples moved out from the Carolingian and Anglo-Saxon kingdoms of early medieval Christian Europe in modern day France, northern Italy, the Low Countries, Switzerland, much of Germany and Austria, and England into the newly Christianised areas to the east, in Bohemia, Hungary and Poland, to the north in Scandinavia, and to the south in Spain, Sicily and Palestine; at the same time the peoples living in those areas adopted the culture of the heartlands. All these areas came under the nominal control of the Church of Rome. It is this wider area which comprises the medieval west of this text's title. Its main focus, however, will centre on developments in Europe's heartlands, in France, Germany, Italy and England, and on placing them in their broader context.

Of the great religious and ecclesiastical changes unfolding between the end of the ninth and the beginning of the thirteenth centuries, three in particular are worth highlighting here. They are the papal reform movement, the growth in monastic foundations, and the explosion in the popularity of pilgrimage and the cult of the saints. The first factor, and one of the most famous, if contentious, features of the central Middle Ages is the radical renegotiation of the relationship between secular and spiritual authority sought by the ecclesiastical reformers of the eleventh century, the so-called 'Gregorian' (after Pope Gregory VII (1073–85)) or papal reforms. Churchmen sought the independence of ecclesiastical personnel and institutions from lay authority, accompanied by attempts to define the clergy as a group separated from the laity with their own codes of dress and behaviour as well as law. This ideological revolution has conventionally been set against wider socio-political developments. Some scholars interpret it as the result of the growth in the authority of both secular and ecclesiastical rulers, kings and popes, whilst others view it as a consequence of the wider social transformation which resulted in an increased emphasis upon defining the different roles played by nobility and peasants, men and women, clerics and lay people.[4]

Secondly, the establishment of a very large number of new religious institutions transformed the European landscape.[5] These new ecclesiastical establishments are a product of demographic and political change which altered how and where peasants lived, leading to the establishment of new villages, changes in the location of centres of power, the emergence of powerful local lords, and the establishment of new centres of authority. Numerous local churches were founded in rural settlements, next to manor houses, and in the burgeoning towns; numerous abbeys were established in both existing settlements, and in areas newly opened up to cultivation; new cathedrals were set up to reflect changes in lordship and settlement patterns and the opening up of new areas on the periphery of Europe. Many of these buildings were built or rebuilt in stone, and some still survive today. They are a testament to the investment made by, and demanded of, Christians living at the time; their very existence is a product of the increase in overall wealth.

Finally, against this background of a greater economic prosperity increasing numbers of the laity, drawn from all social levels, began to develop and explore their own religious autonomy within a Christian framework.[6] There are increasing numbers of records of ordinary Christians flocking to the shrines of individual saints, travelling to local and more distant shrines in search of intercession. The cult of the saints had long played an important role in Christian life, but new movements also accompanied this growth of lay piety. This period saw the evolution of the idea of crusading, that is, travelling to fight on behalf of Christianity for the atonement of personal sins. At the same time the adoption of a way of life based on that of Christ's apostles became increasingly popular. Imitating the life of Christ's apostles as described in the New Testament, men (and occasionally women) chose to follow a life of voluntary poverty whilst living in community, but with a strong emphasis on Christian mission and charity: preaching, and looking after the sick and vulnerable in hospitals. Some scholars have linked the widespread support for those following the apostolic life to the increasing wealth of society in this period: prosperity generated widespread anxiety about salvation and antipathy towards the dominant values of this world.[7] Recognising the continual interplay between ecclesiastical and religious change, on the one hand, and social and political transformation on the other, is one of the most important developments in recent scholarship, and will be a central premise of this text.

Both the start and end dates of this study represent significant moments when various of these factors came together at what are regarded as key changes in the secular and spiritual spheres. It begins around 900 with the implosion of the Carolingian polity of the ninth century.[8] The Carolingians' rule had been marked by a great concern with Christian education, and had produced a considerable body of writings intended to ensure that the practices of both the clergy and the laity conformed to the Christian teachings of the Bible and the Church Fathers. The evidence of surviving episcopal legislation and liturgical and legal collections shows how they set out to train local priests in Christian doctrine and the correct delivery of Christian rites, and admonished them to educate and minister to their own lay flocks so that they lived their lives according to a Christian framework.[9] The Carolingians' successors in tenth- and eleventh-century Europe inherited this bold programme to educate all those living under their rule in Christian doctrine and practice. In this text I will explore the afterlife of the Carolingians' pastoral ambitions. One of the questions I will consider is how far the churchmen of the tenth and eleventh centuries took up and used the writings of their ninth-century predecessors. How influential were these ideals, composed in a time when rulers and churchmen worked together to promote pastoral care, in the more politically fragmented worlds of the tenth and eleventh centuries?

The text ends in the early thirteenth century with the Fourth Lateran Council held in Rome in November 1215. The most widely attended of all the Church councils held in the medieval west, it is a testament to the successful realisation of the pope's claims to authority over the clergy of the western Church, and the separation of clerical from lay authority. The seventy-one decrees published at its conclusion are thus a product of a very different time to the writings produced by the Carolingian Church, and reflect the growing independence of the Church as a political body.[10] Yet the agenda they set out has much in common with that of ninth-century churchmen. Fourth Lateran prescribed a programme to educate and train local priests, and thus their lay flocks, in Christian discipline and doctrine with the aim of ensuring a minimum level of observance of Christian knowledge and practice amongst all those living in Western Europe. The ways in which local bishops working with the new mendicant clergy, the friars, quickly set out to implement this programme across the medieval west have been described as a pastoral revolution.[11] The investigation of its earlier roots thus draws on, and emerges from, tracing the aftermath of the Carolingian reforms and is another of the central aims of this text.

Moreover, thirteenth-century churchmen, like their ninth-century counterparts, were not particularly ambitious. They were content to try to ensure that Christian practice was followed and the authority of Church doctrine accepted. They were not especially concerned to investigate the extent to which people believed, or did not believe, the tenets of the Christian faith as long as they acknowledged them. Some modern historians have sought to explore the extent of belief, and unbelief, in the medieval world.[12] This text has no such objective. Instead, following the lead given by the sources, its focus is on Christian practice rather than spirituality.

The three centuries which separated the pastoral ambitions of thirteenth-century churchmen from their ninth-century predecessors have not commonly been treated as a whole by ecclesiastical historians.[13] Like their counterparts in the social and political realms, they are often guilty of considering change in rigid 'blocks' and do so at the price of the ability to understand religious transformations across rather longer periods of time. This is particularly true for scholars of the changes within ecclesiastical institutions who have tended to see the period of the Gregorian 'reforms' of the mid-eleventh century as an important and unbridgeable *caesura*. That is, they argue that up to *c*.1000 the world is that of the Carolingians, in which the representatives of Church and state were united in a common endeavour to ensure Christianity was adopted and practised correctly, whereas from *c*.1000 leading churchmen sought to separate the Church from lay authority. The eleventh century therefore becomes either the end point or start point for ecclesiastical history in this period.[14] But this periodization is the product of a teleological approach which views the relationship between the spiritual and secular powers as the central paradigm for understanding ecclesiastical history. This text rejects such teleology and suggests there is much to be gained by approaching the history of this period from a wider perspective.

The dominance of this existing chronological framework can be explained by the fact that up to the mid-twentieth century most scholars studied the development of ecclesiastical institutions, that is, the histories of particular monastic houses, local churches, dioceses, or that of the papacy itself. Such an institutional approach explains why the separation of spiritual from secular authority promoted by the eleventh-century reformers figures so largely in modern accounts: it was an issue of great concern both in the development of particular ecclesiastical establishments and of wider institutional consciousness.[15] This bias towards institutional history led scholars working in the second half of the twentieth century to react against this approach by investigating the popular movements which sprang up in the late eleventh and twelfth centuries, choosing to view them as autonomous from developments amongst the clergy. Historians now acknowledge the importance of these movements' connections with the institutional Church in the eleventh and twelfth centuries but their earlier roots remain neglected.[16] When historians began to investigate the religious history of the laity in this period they therefore did so within the existing chronological framework constructed by earlier historians of ecclesiastical institutions, and this pattern has been perpetuated into the later scholarship.

Work on lay piety is also circumscribed by a second narrative, that of Christianisation. Scholars of the early Middle Ages (up to *c.*900) have mostly focused their attention on the success of the efforts made by churchmen (and women) to evangelise and convert the laity.[17] Their focus has been on the extent of paganism and pagan survivals, and thus on the success of the delivery of pastoral care. In contrast, scholars of the central Middle Ages have ignored pastoral care, preferring to follow their sources which were written by clergy of the eleventh and twelfth centuries who were, in the words of Colin Morris, 'not much interested in ordinary people', but rather in correcting the behaviour of the clerical elite, both secular priests and bishops, and monks.[18] The nature and extent of the laity's involvement with the Church only then becomes the focus of scholarly attention with the emergence of the pastoral concerns of the late twelfth and early thirteenth centuries epitomised by the emergence of a new movement, the evangelising friars, and the Fourth Lateran Council in 1215 which stimulated a renewed interest amongst bishops in lay education and belief. They not only drew up a programme of very basic instruction to ensure a minimum level of observance amongst all Christians but set out to implement it through more effective education of local priests, wide-scale and regular preaching, and detailed guidance on how to hear the confessions of the laity.[19]

These institutional and chronological barriers to the study of religious change means there has been little systematic attempt to consider the ecclesiastical history across the years 900 to 1200; this is a situation which this text seeks to rectify. Turning away from the conventional narratives imposed by earlier periodizations, it seeks a new understanding of change in these formative centuries, through a thematic investigation of religious developments throughout this period. It will argue that there is much to be gained by treating these three hundred years as a coherent period in its own right. Looking across the years 900 to 1200, rather than stopping or starting in the eleventh century, allows us to explore both the continuities and changes across the period.

Rethinking religious change 900–1200

Existing periodizations pose one difficulty to the study of religious change in the central Middle Ages. But the three main prevailing scholarly narratives for change in these centuries also each provide their own challenges. These are, first, the importance of clerical purity and reform as an idea, spreading outwards from monasteries in the tenth century into the secular clergy in the eleventh century; secondly, the idea, which we have already alluded to briefly, that the delivery of pastoral care only came to prominence as a concern of the higher clergy in the late twelfth and early thirteenth centuries, leading to the pastoral revolution generated by Fourth Lateran; and thirdly, that the most important development in this period was the separation of the laity from the clergy, the Church from the State, spiritual from secular power. As we shall see, all three narratives are worth investigating in more detail, in order to reflect upon the problems and consequent challenges they pose for scholars of religious change in this period. We will start with those raised by the use of the word 'reform' to describe religious changes in this period.

Reform

'Reform' as a label is applied indiscriminately by scholars to an enormously broad range of movements in this period. They include the various attempts in the tenth century to return to the purity of monastic rule (the tenth-century reform movement), as well as the changes in the eleventh century lumped together by modern scholars as the papal reform movement or 'Gregorian reform' after Pope Gregory VII, one of its main protagonists. The latter include the attempts by senior clergy to promote the purity of the clergy's lifestyle, removing it from the worldly contamination of marriage and/or sexual relations with women (and men) (nicolaitism) and payment for promotion (simony); to separate ecclesiastical appointments and therefore Church property from lay control (lay investiture); and the popular protests against the corrupt clergy which occurred at the same time. The same label has also been applied to the various movements to return (again) to the purity of the Benedictine Rule or to follow the active life of poverty and preaching of the apostles (the apostolic life or *vita apostolica*) which emerged *c.*1100, that is, the twelfth-century reforms or the medieval reformation.

The very use of the word 'reform' has conditioned historians, influenced by the model of the sixteenth-century Protestant Reformation, to look for ruptures and sudden change affecting the whole of society. But the word reform (in Latin *reformatio* or the verb *reformare*) was not widely employed in this period.[20] *Reformare* tended only to be used to refer to the personal transformation of the individual into the likeness of God; here medieval writers followed the sense in which the word was used in the Latin Vulgate version of the Pauline Epistles.[21] Some central medieval writers utilised it when referring to the reform of individual monastic houses or individual churches, but it was not used in its modern sense of the transformation of the universal Church for the better until the early thirteenth century, and not widely until the fourteenth century.[22] Medieval writers instead chose a different vocabulary to describe the change and improvement of religious institutions. Ninth-century Carolingian writers sought to correct, emend, or admonish negligence, fault and scandal.[23] The tenth-century monastic reformers favoured images of cleansing, removing the filthiness left by neglect under the previous regime.[24] The eleventh-century reformers similarly preferred the language of purity, whilst the twelfth-century reformers often used the language of regrowth and renewal, alongside that of reconstruction.[25]

To describe one, or any, of the movements in this period as a reform movement is therefore anachronistic. Moreover, it is often hard to establish a certain set of features which characterises such medieval reform movements; as Gerd Tellenbach has pointed out with respect to the eleventh-century 'reform' movement, it is virtually impossible to find a way in which the term has been used systematically by modern authors to apply to a consistent set of ideals.[26] This value-laden term, normally used to denote improvement for the better, turns out to obscure the varied results and aspirations of these movements. It also sidelines the importance of the relationship between professional members of the institutions being reformed and the wider Christian population. By adopting an institutional perspective on change – whether it be in abbeys, convents, cathedrals or dioceses – the significance of the laity's role in religious change risks being underplayed.

By choosing to study not the history of reform but rather the rhetoric and reality of the various movements for religious change which occurred in this period, this text has therefore consciously sought to steer a different course from other accounts which focus much more on institutional change. Exploring the various roles played by the laity in the religious changes of these years, especially those which took place within ecclesiastical institutions, and the impact which these developments, in turn, had on their own lives, will allow us to offer a fresh perspective on religious developments in this period.

Pastoral care

But before we do so, we need to examine the second paradigm which underlies much of the scholarship in this period, that is the current grand narrative for the Christianisation of medieval peoples in the central Middle Ages. How and to what extent were people in this period Christian, that is, how far did they understand Christian doctrine and live their lives according to the rites and calendar of the Church? By investigating how interested medieval churchmen were in delivering pastoral care to the laity, in educating local priests in how to administer rites to the laity and preach to them, we can begin to answer the question as to how far members of the laity at every level of society knew the tenets of Christian doctrine, and observed its injunctions.

Early medievalists are keen to investigate the success of the efforts made by churchmen and women to evangelise and convert the laity. The Carolingian rulers of the eighth and ninth centuries, and their advisers, sought to ensure the salvation of all their subjects to such an extent that in 1983 Michael Wallace-Hadrill went so far as to describe their ambitious policies for monitoring and discipline as envisaging a police state. Both the reigns of Charlemagne and Louis the Pious were marked by a concern with correction (*correctio*) and emendation (*emendatio*), that is, a desire to ensure that the practices of both the clergy and laity conformed to the Christian teaching of the Bible and the Church Fathers.[27] The guidance on Christian behaviour and practice issued by various bishops to their diocesan clergy in the form of *capitula* perpetuated these ideas into the late ninth century.[28] Although targeted at parish priests, episcopal *capitula* contained advice on measures to instruct and monitor the behaviour of both priests and their lay congregations. Previous students of pastoral care have ignored the central Middle Ages, focusing either, as we have seen, on the early Middle Ages, that is, the years up to around 900, or on the late twelfth and thirteenth centuries leading to the programme embodied in the decrees issued by the Fourth Lateran Council in 1215. This approach reflects the fact that both the ninth-century and thirteenth-century pastoral reformers generated a considerable number of pastoral texts for use by bishops checking up on clergy, and by clergy in the field. But it is worth noting that ninth-century texts continued to be read and copied in the intervening period, and helped to shape the thought world in which these later works were composed. Bishop Theodulf of Orléans's early ninth-century synodal *capitula*, which were written to help a bishop instruct and check up on knowledge and behaviour of the priests in his diocese, for example, survive in some forty-nine manuscripts, many of them in tenth- and eleventh-century copies.[29] Some 106 manuscripts of one particular type of early medieval penitential designed to administer penance to an individual survive copied between the late eighth and twelfth centuries.[30] These early medieval texts thus survive in comparable numbers to many thirteenth-century confession manuals; like their early medieval counterparts some, like John of Freiburg's *Confessionale*, survive in numerous copies, whilst the circulation of many others was much, much smaller.[31] Diocesan synods offered one opportunity for bishops to monitor the knowledge and equipment of local priests responsible for monitoring pastoral care. Carolingian bishops produced a mass of statutes like those of Bishop Theodulf for such occasions which influenced the composition of similar texts in tenth and eleventh-century Lotharingia, England and northern Italy.[32] In late twelfth-century France synodal statutes testify to the renewed attention paid by some bishops to monitoring the local priests responsible for the delivery of pastoral care.[33] In the thirteenth century this interest was followed by an explosion in the composition of such guidance all over Europe.

Given such evidence, to what extent were medieval churchmen in the central Middle Ages really uninterested in pastoral care? The years 900 to 1200 saw the building and rebuilding of many local churches: is it really safe to presume that leading clerics, unlike their earlier and later counterparts, were not interested in the role performed by the clergy serving them? Actual records of episcopal visitations only survive from the thirteenth century onwards, although the first text to prescribe how such visitations should be conducted in detail survives from the start of our period. Thirteenth-century records, such as that of Archbishop Eudes of Rouen, suggest bishops paid more attention to monitoring and disciplining the behaviour of their parish clergy than that of members of the laity.[34] But Regino of Prüm's early tenth-century account of how a bishop should conduct an episcopal visitation is equally concerned with investigating the behaviour of both the local clergy and their flock. It demonstrates the prevalence of pastoral concerns amongst some of the higher clergy in early tenth-century east Frankia and suggests that it worth delving further into the history of pastoral care in the central Middle Ages.

It is found in a portable guide to church law which Regino of Prüm composed in about 906 at the request of his patron, Archbishop Ratbod of Trier. Regino envisaged that the bishop would take it with him on his tours of his diocese and use it to interrogate both the local priest and a jury of seven of 'the more mature, honest and truthful men' of each parish he visited. He thus included two lengthy questionnaires as guides to the bishop; the first, which includes 96 questions, was directed at the priest, the second, some 89 questions long, at the lay jury. The questions asked of both local priests and their parishioners have much to tell us about the clergy's attitude to the laity, and the roles the laity were expected to play in their local church, at the beginning of the tenth century. Those to be asked of the priest include: did all the faithful come to communion three times a year, at Christmas, Easter and Pentecost? Did he preach to all his flock the need to observe the periods of fasting four times a year? Were tithes paid? Had he taught all his parishioners the Lord's Prayer and the Creed? Had he admonished the married men in his flock as to what times they should abstain from sexual relations with their wives?[35] Through such means the bishops could establish whether the local church was properly equipped, its priest sufficiently well-educated and living a life in accordance with church law, and whether pastoral care was being properly administered. At the same time the text emphasised the bishop's claims to authority over the local clergy.

The questions asked of the laity foresaw all manner of bad behaviour, from murder to sexual misconduct, theft to perjury, magic to pagan superstition, food pollution to incorrect Christian practice.[36] Many sought to establish whether serious offences had been committed: had there been a homicide in this parish when the killer had killed the man either 'from free will or through passion, or because of greed, or by chance, or unwillingly and under orders, or to avenge a relation, what we call a "feud", or in war, or on the orders of a lord, or his servants'. Others seem, from their wording, to be as concerned to prevent violence as to discover sin: 'If any man through hatred has not returned to peace, or sworn never to be reconciled with his brother, because it is contrary to God, this is a sin unto death.' Interestingly, several closely echo the wording and concerns of the questions asked of the priest, and seem designed not only to discipline the laity but to check with a lay jury the answers the priest had given to his own examination on these matters. They focus upon whether everyone within that particular parish is practising Christianity correctly: 'If anyone has not observed the Lenten fast, nor Advent, nor the Major litany nor Rogationtide without permission to abstain being obtained from the bishop', and 'If there is any Christian who has not communicated three times a year, that is at Easter, Pentecost and Christmas, unless he has been removed from communion by the judgement of the bishop or the priest for deadly sins.' The only justification for failure to participate in the Eucharist was excommunication. Had anyone kept back the tithe he owed to God and the saints? Did the godparents instruct their godchildren in the Creed and the Lord's Prayer? The purpose of the bishop's visit was first and foremost to ensure that Christianity was being correctly followed, and correctly administered in that parish, and secondly that episcopal authority and jurisdiction was respected. The jury had to swear a public oath to report any act which they know to have been committed and which fell within the remit of the synod and which 'pertain[ed] to the ministry of the bishop' on pain of damnation.

But some questions envisage a system in which the parish community policed itself to ensure conformity. The bishop should ask if those whose profession took them outside the heart of the community attended church regularly, that is 'if the swineherds and other shepherds come to church on Sunday and hear Mass, and similarly on other feast days'. He should also ask if everyone attended Sunday Mass: 'if there is any man who has worked on the Lord's day or special feasts, and if they all come to matins and to mass and to vespers on these days'. Even if he attended church regularly, a parishioner's conduct might not be considered blameless: the jurors should testify 'if any man, on entering church, is accustomed to recite stories and not to listen diligently to divine worship, and leaves before the mass has finished'. Clearly chatting during, and early departure from the mass were sufficiently commonplace to merit this disapproving mention. But Regino also presumed that there was a system already in place to ensure religious conformity, for the bishop should ask 'If in each parish the *decani* are constituted through the villages', defining *decani* as 'truthful, Godfearing men, who admonish others that they should go to church at matins, mass and vespers, and not work on feast days; and if anyone transgresses these injunctions, that the *decani* immediately report him to the priest and deprive him from luxury and all work'. The reference to *decani* is unique to this text. Modern scholars have therefore debated whether they were early tithe collectors or church wardens. Whatever the case, the text prescribes a system of self-policing within these villages to ensure religious conformity which was in turn subject to episcopal inspection.

Regino's portrait of an episcopal visitation represented an ideal; it is not a description, but rather a vision of how the world should be conjured up by an anxious man writing in very uncertain times. He witnessed and participated in the events which accompanied the disintegration of the Carolingian empire in the late ninth century. He composed his church law collection whilst in exile, having been ejected in 899 from the important Carolingian monastery of Prüm, in Lotharingia, of which he had been elected abbot in 892. He was to remain in exile for the rest of his life as, in the words of Simon Maclean, 'an embittered outsider'.[37] The author of various works, including a *Chronicle* which covered events up to 906, his law collection must be treated as the work of an idealist, looking back to a golden age which had never existed when bishops were able to control and monitor both local priests and local communities, and local communities co-operated to enforce and monitor Christian law. It represents Regino's aspirations for control and regulation in what was in reality an increasingly uncertain world.

But Regino did not make the text of his law collection up. Rather it is the culmination of ninth-century ideas about the importance of promoting and adjusting Christian behaviour to fit with Christian teaching. He drew most of his material from ninth-century sources: the questions to be asked of the priest came from various Frankish (episcopal) *capitula*, whilst many of those to be asked of the laity seem to have been based on early medieval penitentials.[38] The epitome of ninth-century concerns with *correctio*, Regino's text thus represents an important hinge between the concerns of Carolingian ecclesiastical reformers, and those of later reformers, especially those of the eleventh and twelfth centuries. Albeit in an idealised form he transmitted Carolingian ideals for the regular inspection and monitoring of clerical and lay behaviour into a new period, after the demise of the political authority of the Carolingian family, and is in part responsible for ensuring that these ideas were perpetuated into the tenth, eleventh, and twelfth centuries and beyond.

The textual afterlife of Regino's pastoral vision in the succeeding three centuries points to the continuing significance of Carolingian ideals of pastoral care, which is an important theme of this text. Long after the particular circumstances in which Regino had composed his text had passed, it continued to be read and copied. The *Libri duo* itself circulated throughout the German *Reich* of the Ottonian and Salian rulers, surviving in some ten manuscripts and four fragments from the tenth and eleventh centuries. It was also one of the main sources for the most influential canon law collection of the eleventh-century Church, Burchard of Worms' *Decretum* (*c*.1020) which spread quickly and more widely throughout much of the medieval west, surviving in seventy-seven manuscripts with a German, French and Italian provenance.[39] Burchard's compilation, which included a version of Regino's visitation questionnaire, in turn became an important source for some of the cornerstones of twelfth-century canon law, including the writings of Ivo of Chartres (d. 1115x1117).[40] Nor was Regino's a lone voice at the time: other texts were composed by and for bishops in both England and northern Italy in the course of the tenth century which were intended to guide them in how to inspect the standards of their local clergy and which harked back to ninth-century ideals.[41] The ninth-century texts themselves, upon which Regino drew, also continued to be widely copied in the tenth and eleventh centuries. And, as we shall see, their concerns continued to resonate through the central Middle Ages.

The Church's relationship with the laity

Returning to Regino's guide, it highlights the importance attached by one medieval churchman to the responsibility of the laity in policing both their own behaviour and that of the clergy. Given the significance attributed by modern scholars to the eleventh-century campaign to separate the laity from the clergy, we need to investigate further the evidence for the roles which churchmen expected the laity to play in the life and reform of the Church in this period. Was the Church's attitude to the laity and their role in the life of the Church as negative as that suggested by eleventh-century reformist polemic? After all, any attempt by the ecclesiastical authorities to make a distinction between the clergy and the laity came up against the intractable problem of family and community affiliations.

The eleventh and twelfth centuries, as we have seen, are generally understood as moving away from the Carolingian and post-Carolingian worlds of the ninth and tenth centuries, in which secular and ecclesiastical power were viewed as working together, to one in which the clergy sought to liberate themselves from lay control of both appointments to clerical office and of ecclesiastical property, and to emphasize the distinction between the clergy and the laity, and the superiority of the clergy.[42] This shift is understood as being in large part the work of the papal reformers of the second half of the eleventh century. Thus writing in *c.*842 the Carolingian monk and courtier, Walahfrid Strabo (d. 849) systematically compared the ecclesiastical and secular orders of government, concluding:

> *Through the union of both orders and their mutual love one house of God is built, one body of Christ is made by all the members of His Office who contribute fruits for mutual benefit.*[43]

Writing over two centuries later, in 1057, one of the leading papal reformers, Cardinal Humbert of Silva Candida envisaged a world of separation between the two powers rather than co-operation:

> *Just as secular matters are forbidden to the clergy, ecclesiastical matters are forbidden to the laity.*[44]

Where these writers led, modern scholars have followed. Historians of the earlier period have been happy to explore the positive role played by secular rulers and nobles in promoting the Carolingian programme of *correctio*, the success of that policy, and what it meant for 'ordinary' members of the laity.[45] Scholars working on the central Middle Ages, however, divide into those who investigate the history of clerical reform, largely from the point of view of the clergy – be they popes, members of the papal *curia* (court), local bishops, or monastic reformers[46] – and those who are interested in the emergence of lay religious autonomy exemplified by movements such as the crusades, saints' cults, and popular heresy.[47] There are of course exceptions, notably historians of monasticism who have fruitfully explored the complex relations between members of the secular elite and their local monastery, and Maureen Miller's study of the complex social developments which underlay the 'reform' of the religious institutions of Verona in this period.[48] Whilst building on earlier work, this text is intended to provide a new perspective on these three centuries, studying ecclesiastical developments in this period through the relationship between Church and people.

The relationship between the ordained clergy and the laity is fundamental to the history of the Church, and yet it is one which, as André Vauchez observed, was subject to 'considerable shifts of emphasis' throughout the Middle Ages.[49] The danger is that such shifts are seen as all-encompassing, as in the schema sketched out above, which was one Vauchez himself subscribed to, viewing these centuries as witnessing a move from the co-operation of the ninth century to the separation of clerical from secular power in the eleventh and twelfth centuries. The dyad of the clergy and the laity certainly became very popular amongst the writers of these centuries, and it is, perhaps, best articulated in the most influential canon law collection of the twelfth century, Gratian's *Decretum*, compiled *c.*1140:

> *There are two kinds of Christians. There is one kind which, being devoted to God's business and given up to contemplation and prayer, should refrain from all activity in worldly affairs. These are the clergy and those devoted to God, that is the* conversi . . . *The shaving of their head shows the putting away of all temporal things. For they should be content with food and clothing and having nothing of their own among themselves, but should have everything in common. There is also another kind of Christian, laymen. For* laos *means 'people'. These are allowed to possess temporal goods, but only to the extent that they make use of them . . . They are allowed to take a wife, to till land, to judge between man and man, to conduct lawsuits, to place oblations upon the altar, to pay tithes, and thus can be saved if they avoid sin by well-doing.*[50]

Although it circulated widely within the circles of eleventh-century Italian reformers, the idea is much older. Gregory the Great (d. 604) distinguished between the clergy and the laity in the *Moralia in Iob*, when he divided the Church into 'the order of preachers' and 'the multitude of hearers'.[51] It is Gregory's idea which seems to underlie this depiction of Mother Church on an Exultet Roll made at the monastery of Monte Cassino in southern Italy in *c.*1087. The personification of *Mater Ecclesia* stands in the middle; on the left-hand side are the clergy (*clerus*), represented by a group of men, some with tonsures, some without; on the right are the *populus* (the people), at the front of whom are a man and woman holding a child. Used in the Easter Vigil, the Exultet Roll contained the text of a hymn of praise sung during the blessing of the Paschal candle by the deacon, who delivered the *Exultet* from the an elevated lectern facing the congregation, unfurling the roll over its railings, so that the pictures were visible to those members of the congregation close enough to see them. This image echoed the words of the hymn quoted at the start of this chapter, calling on all God's people to rejoice at Christ's resurrection. Here the dyad was not a divisive but rather a unifying image, and one with well-established roots.

Whilst *populus* is sometimes used to refer to both the clergy and the laity, it is more often used, as in the image of the Church in the Exultet Roll, to refer to just the laity. Clerical writers used a range of terms to denote the laity: *populus*, *laici*, of course, but also the unlearned and the married.[52] They recognised the lay order to be a broad one: *laicus* (layman) sometimes denoted a person of low status. Thus some tenth-century Burgundian charters distinguished between clerics, nobles, laymen, and peasants. More often it was used in its modern sense to denote those people who were not members of the clergy. The clergy often referred to the laity as 'God's people' and the 'Lord's people'. Thus canons issued at the Council of Trosly (909) emphasised how the *populus Domini* (the Lord's people) had been neglected by the bishops and priests, who had responsibility for them:

> *The Church of God resides in bishops and priests to whom the people of the Lord are entrusted, and is recognised as distinct.*[53]

The *Constitutions* issued by Archbishop Oda of Canterbury (d. 958) in the early 940s exhorted priests that 'they should teach the people of God (*populum Dei*) through good example and holy habit, and inform and instruct [them] in holy doctrine'.[54] Writing in the early twelfth century one of the crusader chroniclers, Robert the Monk, described how one preacher addressed the crusader army as the people of the Lord and servants of God.[55] 'People', as it was used by medieval writers, had a universalising meaning, covering men and women, lords and peasants.

The clerical-lay dyad was not the only model for the Church available to clerical writers. By the beginning of the tenth century medieval writers who wished to conceptualise the Church were able to draw upon a tremendous variety of different models. In addition to the dyad, they could use, as the seventh-century Spanish bishop Isidore of Seville did, a tripartite model to distinguish between clerics, monks and the laity. This threefold distinction remained popular throughout the Middle Ages; it was taken up in the twelfth century, for example, by the Cistercian author Ailred of Rievaulx who divided society into three orders: the natural order, who were married, enjoyed meat, wine and wealth – that is, the laity; the necessary order, whose members 'expel the passions by keeping itself from licit things' – that is, the clergy, and the voluntary order, whose members make a 'willing sacrifice' – that is, monks.[56] Another model, found, amongst other places, in Gregory the Great's *Moralia*, drew a distinction based not on function but sexual practice: '[there are] three divisions of the faithful, in the state of life in the Church, that is those of pastors, of the continent, and of the married'.[57] This threefold model became equally popular, and was taken up in the late tenth century by the Anglo-Saxon homilist, Ælfric of Eynsham, who made its hierarchical aspect more explicit:

> *in God's church are three degrees of chosen men. The lowest degree is of believing laymen, who live in lawful marriage, for the sake of a family of children than of lust. The second degree is of widows, who after lawful matrimony live in purity for the attainment of the heavenly life. The highest degree is of persons of the virgin state who from childhood purely serve God and despise earthly lusts.*[58]

But writers of the central Middle Ages were also perfectly capable of attributing a much more positive and active role to the laity than the standard narratives of the period allow. In another sermon Ælfric interpreted Christ's parable of the talents in which a rich man gave one servant five talents, another two, and another one, and the one who received five made another five, and the one who had received two made another two, but the one who received only one went and hid it in the ground, and therefore made nothing.[59] Surprisingly Ælfric interpreted the good servant who received five talents, and made a further five, as an unlearned/lay (*læwed*) man:

> *for some lay men are so constituted, that, with stimulation from the realm above, they give good example to other faithful, and ever teach rightly what they may know by the outer senses, though they cannot comprehend the inward deepness of God's doctrine; and when in their fleshly lusts they are temperate, and in worldly desires not too greedy, and also, through awe of God, preserve themselves from other vices, then also will they direct other men by the righteousness of their lives, and gain to God some man or more.*[60]

The servant who received and made two talents he interpreted as the conscientious clergy, and the servant who hid his talent in the ground, as a member of the slothful clergy. Ælfric's text was based mainly on Gregory the Great's sermon on the same parable; however, whilst Gregory had targeted his sermon at the clergy, and interpreted the various talents representing possession of inner and outer understanding, Ælfric pushed Gregory's text to identify explicitly the first servant with the laity or unlearned; the second servant with the learned, and the third servant with those who abuse their sense for things of the flesh. When the third servant is made to give his talent to the first servant by the master, the clergyman is therefore interpreted as giving the layman the inner understanding which he had previously lacked.[61] In Ælfric's view, therefore, laymen could, if they lived correctly, play a central and important part in the work of the Church. Recent work suggests that Ælfric directed his series of homilies to the clergy of the diocese of Sherborne, in southern England, for use in their preaching: his message was presented to the laity themselves.[62]

Ælfric's view was not unique. The *Visio Tnugdali*, the tale of the vision of an Irish nobleman recorded by a twelfth-century Bavarian monk, recalls how Tnugdal saw in heaven, on a level with monks, men and women under a tree, each crowned with a golden crown, with a golden sceptre in his hand and he was told by his guiding angel:

> *this tree is the allegory of the holy Church and the men and women who are under it are the builders and the defenders of the holy churches. They have striven to build or defend churches and, for the favours which they bestowed on holy churches, they have been welcomed into their religious confraternities, and through the admonitions of the religious, they left the secular condition and restrained themselves from carnal desires which wage war against the soul. They lead sober, righteous and godly lives in this present world, awaiting the blessed hope, which, as you see, has not failed them.*[63]

The laity mentioned in the *Visio Tnugdal* are clearly members of the elite, those lords and princes able to endow materially churches. The author nevertheless shares the ambivalent attitude towards the laity of other clerical writers in this period. On the one hand they are seen as the lowest of the hierarchy, on the other as those who are the most significant members of the Church, and the ones who had the most potential.[64] There was thus widespread recognition that the laity constituted a crucial and important part of the Church, and had a significant role to play in its development.

This view went back to the Gospels where crowds of ordinary people had an important role to play in supporting, and promoting, Christ's message. The crowds (*turbae*) which were fed with five loaves and two fishes, which listened to Christ's Sermon on the Mount, and which witnessed Christ's entry into Jerusalem the week before his crucifixion, were interpreted in scriptural exegesis as prefiguring the faithful of the Church itself.[65] Such an interpretation also underlies the positive view attributed to crowds in many central medieval accounts, and this textual precedent, as much as social change, helps to explain the role which crowds were portrayed as playing in the religious life of the Church in these three centuries.[66] Such reports must, however, be approached with caution, signalling as they do clerical rhetorical tradition rather than social reality. But it is worth remembering that this tradition contained positive as well as negative elements.

Viewing, as we must, the laity through the lenses of clerical writers, it is as well to remember therefore that the Christian people of the medieval west actually constituted a far more variegated body than that reported in many accounts. The bias of much of the surviving evidence for clerical–lay relationships is towards those at the higher end of the social spectrum, those able to afford to patronise the Church, and who were thought worth remembering by it. This text's focus is therefore, largely, on the experiences of the lay and clerical elite, but wherever the sources allow it also investigates those of people towards the lower end of the social spectrum.

Reinterpreting the relationship between Church and people

Narratives of change are prone to error, but they are also necessary: we need them in order to make sense of seemingly unrelated changes across long periods of time and we reject them at our peril. But they can, as we have seen is the case with those for reform, pastoral care, and the relationship between spiritual and secular authority, also limit our understanding. This text does not seek to substitute yet another grand narrative but rather to suggest that rejection of the conventional periodization which structures most work on this period offers an opportunity to view the religious developments from a new perspective: that of the varying and multi-faceted relationship between the Church and people.

Adopting such an approach cuts across the conventional internal barriers erected by scholars of medieval religious history in this period, who tend to study specific institutions or religious movements, and joins up developments currently spread across a series of separate sub-fields in the scholarship: work on the development of parishes, monastic reform, clerical reform, the delivery of pastoral care, saints' cults, pilgrimage and other forms of lay devotion, and its flipside, heresy. By examining the developments in the ecclesiastical institutions which made up the Church in this period through their relationship with the laity, I hope to bring a more integrated approach to the study of religion in western Christendom in this period.

This text is in three parts. The first part investigates the relations of members of the laity with ecclesiastical institutions and personnel, that is, with local churches, the secular clergy (including bishops), monasteries and canons, and considers their role in the successive changes which these institutions underwent in these centuries. The second part explores the evidence for the laity's experience of Christianity, both that offered by the routine rites and services of the official 'Church', and that of the more autonomous movements which have been viewed as so typical of the later end of the period but many of which have earlier roots: confraternities, saints' cults, long-distance pilgrimage and the crusades. The last part attempts to combine these two approaches by looking at how churchmen reacted to challenges to their authority from the laity. In particular it considers what many churchmen perceived as an increasing threat from heresy: how and why were laymen and women condemned as heretics? To what extent did the charge of heresy result from increasing lay religious autonomy, or was it rather a consequence of the growing awareness of a separate clerical identity, and the consequent desire of clergymen to assert their authority in the face of challenges to it? To conclude we investigate the decrees of the Fourth Lateran Council: how far do they represent the culmination of the religious history of the preceding three centuries?

The dyad of Church and people constituted a powerful rhetorical trope, but it was also a reality. By studying the role the laity played in the changes taking place in the Church in this period, and the impact which the Church had on lay lives this text offers a fundamental reappraisal of what the Christian religion meant in the everyday lives of believers in this period.

Notes and references

1 'Lætetur et mater Ecclesia, tanti luminis adornata fulgoribus: et magnis populorum vocibus hæc aula resultet.' Literally: 'Let mother Church rejoice, wearing the radiance of this great light; let this temple echo with the great voice of the people'. Adaptation of translation in *The Missal in Latin and English Being the Text of the Missale Romanum with English Rubrics and a New Translation* (London, 1949), p. 398.

2 E.g. Richard Southern's classic study of the eleventh and twelfth centuries: *The Making of the Middle Ages* (London, 1953), and the revisionist study of Western European expansion in the eleventh, twelfth and thirteenth centuries by his pupil, Robert Barlett, *The Making of Europe: Conquest, Colonisation and Cultural Change 950–1350* (London, 1993); both works, however, fail to investigate the tenth century in depth.

3 For a summary of this view see J.-P. Poly and E. Bournazel, *La mutation féodale, Xe–XIIe siècles* (Paris, 1980), trans. C. Higgitt as *The Feudal Transformation, 900–1200* (New York, 1991), and the ongoing critique by D. Barthelémy now available as idem, *The Serf, the Knight and the Historian*, transl. Graham Robert Edwards (Ithaca, NY, 2009) which also includes references to the wider literature.

4 Older accounts privilege political explanations, e.g. A. Fliche, *La Réforme grégorienne et la Reconquête chrétienne (1057–1125)* (Paris, 1950). For more nuanced social interpretations, see those offered by R. I. Moore, *The First European Revolution c.970–1215* (Oxford, 2000) and the synthesis by K. G. Cushing, *Reform and the Papacy in the Eleventh Century: Spirituality and Social Change* (Manchester, 2005) which seeks to reconcile the two approaches.

5 See Chapters 2 and 4 below.

6 A. Vauchez, *The Laity in the Middle Ages: Religious Beliefs and Devotional Practices*, ed. and trans. D. E. Bornstein (Notre Dame, IN, 1993), 27–50.

7 M.-D. Chenu, 'The Evangelical Awakening', in his *Nature, Man and Society in the Twelfth Century: Essays on New Theological Perspectives in the Latin West*, trans. J. Taylor and L. K. Little (Chicago, 1968), 239–69; L. K. Little, *Religious Poverty and the Profit Economy in Medieval Europe* (London, 1978).

8 S. MacLean, *Kingship and Politics in the Later Ninth Century: Charles the Fat and the End of the Carolingian Empire* (Cambridge, 2003).

9 R. McKitterick, *The Frankish Church and the Carolingian Reforms, 789–895* (London, 1977); C. van Rhijn, *Shepherds of the Lord: Priests and Episcopal Statutes in the Carolingian Period* (Turnhout, 2007).

10 *The Decrees of the Ecumenical Councils*, ed. N. P. Tanner, 2 vols (London, 1990), I, 227–71.

11 P. Michaud-Quantin, 'Les methodes de la pastorale du XIIIe au XVe siècle', *Miscellanea Medievalia* 7 (1970), 76–91; A. Vauchez, ed., *Faire croire: modalités de la diffusion et de la réception des messages religieux du XIIe au XVe siècle*, Collection de l'École française de Rome 51 (Rome, 1981); R. N. Swanson, *Religion and Devotion in Europe c.1215–c.1515* (Cambridge, 1995).

12 E.g. J. H. Arnold, *Belief and Unbelief in Medieval Europe* (London, 2005); A. Vauchez, *La spiritualité de moyen-âge occidental VIII–XII siècles* (Paris, 1975), English trans. by C. Friedlander as *The Spirituality of the Medieval West: The Eighth to the Twelfth Century* (Kalamazoo, MI, 1993).

13 Indeed very few works treat the years 900 to 1200 as a whole; one recent exception is J. C. Crick and E. van Houts, eds, *A Social History of England, 900–1200* (Cambridge, 2011).

14 See for example the recent volumes in the Cambridge History of Christianity which break around 1100: T. F. X. Noble and J. M. H. Smith, eds, *The Cambridge History of Christianity III: Early Medieval Christianities c.600–c.1100* (Cambridge, 2008); M. Rubin and W. Simon, eds, *The Cambridge History of Christianity IV: Christianity in Western Europe c.1100–1500* (Cambridge, 2009).

15 For recent introductions to a vast literature, see Cushing, *Reform and the Papacy*; C. Morris, *The Papal Monarchy: The Western Church from 1050 to 1250* (Oxford, 1989); G. Tellenbach, trans. T. Reuter, *The Church in Western Europe from the Tenth to the Early Twelfth Century* (Cambridge, 1993); B. Bolton, *The Medieval Reformation* (London, 1983); G. Constable, *The Reformation of the Twelfth Century* (Cambridge, 1996); U.-R. Blumenthal, *The Investiture Controversy: Church and Monarchy from the Ninth to the Twelfth Century* (Philadelphia, 1991).

16 E.g. M. Bull, *Knightly Piety and the Lay Response to the First Crusade: The Limousin and Gascony c.970–c.1130* (Oxford, 1993); S. Yarrow, *Saints and their Communities: Miracle Stories in Twelfth-Century England* (Oxford, 2006); R. I. Moore, *The Origins of European Dissent* (London, 1977).

17 J. Chélini, *L'Aube du moyen age: naissance de la chrétienté occidentale, 2nd edn* (Paris, 1997); and the revisionist stance of J. M. H. Smith, 'Religion and Lay Society', in R. McKitterick, ed., *New Cambridge Medieval History c.700–c.900* (Cambridge, 1995), 654–78. See also V. I. J. Flint, *The Rise of Magic in Early Medieval Europe* (Oxford, 1993); K. Jolly, *Popular Religion in Late Saxon England: Elf Charms in Context* (Chapel Hill, NC, 1996).

18 Morris, *Papal Monarchy*, 489; see also Bolton, *Medieval Reformation*; Constable, *Reformation of the Twelfth Century*; Tellenbach, *The Church in Western Europe*.

19 Swanson, *Religion and Devotion in Europe*; S. Watson and N. Tanner, 'Least of the Laity: The Minimum Requirements for a Medieval Christian', *Journal of Medieval History* 32:4 (2006), 395–423.

20 For what follows I am heavily indebted to the work of J. Barrow, 'Ideas and Applications of Reform', in Noble and Smith, eds, *The Cambridge History of Christianity III*, 345–62; eadem, 'The Ideology of the Tenth-century English Benedictine "Reform"', in P. Skinner, ed., *Challenging the Boundaries of Medieval History: The Legacy of Timothy Reuter* (Turnhout, 2009), 141–54.

21 G. B. Ladner, *The Idea of Reform: Its Impact on Christian Thought and Action in the Age of the Fathers* (Cambridge, MA, 1959).

22 In addition to works cited in nn. 20 and 21 see G. B. Ladner, 'Gregory the Great and Gregory VII: A Comparison of their Concepts of Renewal', *Viator* 4 (1973), 1–31.

23 J. M. H. Smith, '"Emending Evil Ways and Praising God's Omnipotence": Einhard and the Uses of Roman Martyrs', in K. Mills and A. Grafton, eds, *Conversion in Late Antiquity and the Early Middle Ages: Seeing and Believing* (Rochester, NY, 2003), 189–223; M. de Jong, *The Penitential State. Authority and Atonement in the Age of Louis the Pious, 814–840* (Cambridge, 2009).

24 Barrow, 'Ideas'.

25 G. Constable, 'Renewal and Reform in Religious Life: Concepts and Realities', in R. Benson and G. Constable with C. D. Lanham, eds, *Renaissance and Renewal in the Twelfth Century* (Oxford, 1982), 37–67.

26 Tellenbach, *The Church in Western Europe*, 157–84.

27 J. M. Wallace-Hadrill, The *Frankish Church* (Oxford, 1983), 299; Smith, '"Emending Evil Ways and Praising God's Omnipotence"'; de Jong, *The Penitential State*.

28 van Rhijn, *Shepherds of the Lord*.

29 *MGH Capitula Episcoporum I*, ed. P. Brommer (Hannover, 1984), 75–99.

30 R. Meens, 'The Frequency and Nature of Early Medieval Penance', in P. Biller and A. J. Minnis, eds, *Handling Sin: Confession in the Middle Ages* (Woodbridge, 1998), 35–61.

31 Personal communication from Catherine Rider.

32 Ruotger of Trier (d. 931), *MGH Capitula Episcoporum I*, ed. P. Brommer (Hannover, 1984), 57–70; Rather of Verona, *Synodica*, *Die Briefe des Bischofs Rather von Verona*, ed. F. Weigle, *MGH Die Briefe der deutschen Kaiserzeit* 1 (Weimar, 1949), 124–37; *The Complete Works of Rather of Verona*, trans. P. L. D. Reid (Binghamton, NY, 1991), 444–52; Wulfstan, 'Canons of Edgar', *C&S* I, 313–38.

33 E.g. Roger of Cambrai, *Precepta Synodalia*, ed. J. Avril, 'Les *Precepta synodalia* de Roger de Cambrai', *Bulletin of Medieval Canon Law*, New series 2 (1972), 7–15; O. Pontal, *Les statuts synodaux*, Typologie des sources du moyen âge 11 (Turnhout, 1975).

34 E.g. *The Register of Eudes of Rouen*, trans. S. M. Brown and ed. J. F. O'Sullivan (New York, 1964); see also N. Coulet, *Les Visites pastorales*, Typologie des sources du moyen âge occidental 23 (Turnhout, 1977).

35 Regino, I, q. 60, 58, 50, 55, 61 p. 32.

36 Regino II. 1–5, pp. 234–50.

37 *History and Politics in Late Carolingian and Ottonian Europe: The Chronicle of Regino of Prüm and Adalbert of Magdeburg*, trans. and annotated by S. MacLean (Manchester, 2009), 1–8, quotation at p. 6.

38 On sources for priest's questionnaire, see Regino, 24, n. 7; on Regino's debt to the questionnaire found in one line of transmission for the *Paenitentiale mixtum Pseudo-Bedae-Egberti*, see R. Haggenmüller, 'Zur Rezeption der Beda und Egbert zugeschriebenen Bussbücher', in H. Mordek, ed., *Aus Archiven und Bibliotheken. Festschrift für Raymund Kottje zum 65. Geburtstag* (Frankfurt a. M., 1992), 149–69; L. Körntgen, *Studien zu den Quellen der frühmittelalterlichen Bussbücher* (Sigmaringen, 1993), 237–43; idem, 'Canon Law and the Practice of Penance: Burchard of Worms's Penitential', *EME* 14 (2006), 103–17 at pp. 109–10.

39 L. Kéry, *Canonical Collections of the Early Middle Ages (c.400–1140). A Bibliographical Guide to the Manuscripts and Literature*, History of Medieval Canon Law 1 (Washington, DC, 1999), 133–55; G. Austin, *Shaping Church Law Around the Year 1000: The Decretum of Burchard of Worms* (Ashgate, 2009), 24–27, 39–41.

40 Ibid. 239; Burchard, I. 90–94, *PL* 140, 572–79.

41 E.g. Atto of Vercelli, *Capitulare*, *MGH Capitula Episcoporum III*, ed. R. Pokorny (Hannover, 1995), 243–304; Rather of Verona, *Synodica*, *Die Briefe des Bischofs Rather von Verona*, ed. F. Weigle, MGH Die Briefe der deutschen Kaiserzeit I (Weimar, 1949), 124–37; *Aelfric's Pastoral Letter for Wulfsige III, Bishop of Sherborne*, no. 40, *C&S* I.i, 191–226.

42 Vauchez, 'The Laity in the Feudal Church' in Idem, *The Laity*, 39–44.

43 Walahfrid Strabo, *Libellus de exordiis et incrementis quarundam in observationibus ecclesiasticis rerum*, ed. V. Krause, MGH Capit. II (Hannover, 1897), cited in Alice L. Harting-Correa, Walahfrid Strabo, *Libellus de exordiis et incrementis quarundam in observationibus ecclesiasticis rerum. A Translation and Liturgical Commentary* (Leiden, 1996), 194.

44 Humbert of Silva Candida, *Libri III Adversus Simoniacos*, III.9, ed. F. Thaner, MGH Libelli de Lite I, 208.

45 The literature is vast: see especially H. H. Anton, *Fürstenspiegel und Herrscherethos in der Karolingerzeit* (Bonn, 1968); Chélini, *L'Aube du moyen âge*; McKitterick, *The Frankish Church*; Smith, 'Religion and Lay Society'; A. Angenendt, *Geschichte der Religiosität im Mittelalter* (Darmstadt, 1997).

46 E.g. Cushing, *Reform and the Papacy*; Morris, *The Papal Monarchy*; Tellenbach, *The Church in Western Europe.*

47 Bull, *Knightly Piety*; Yarrow, *Saints and their Communities*, Moore, *Origins.*

48 E.g. Bull, *Knightly Piety*; E. Jamroziak and J. Burton, eds, *Religious and Laity in Western Europe 1000–1400: Interaction, Negotiation and Power* (Turnhout, 2006); M. C. Miller, *The Formation of a Medieval Church. Ecclesiastical Change in Verona, 950–1150* (Ithaca, NY, 1993).

49 Vauchez, 'The Laity in the Feudal Church' in Idem, *The Laity*, 39.

50 Gratian, *Decretum*, Pars II. C. XII.q.I, c. 7 (*Decretum Gratiani* available at Bayerische Staatsbibliothek Münchener DigitalisierungZentrum Digitale Bibliothek http://geschichte.digitale-sammlungen.de/decretum-gratiani/online/angebot, accessed 19th August 2012); translated Morris, *Papal Monarchy*, 318.

51 Gregory the Great, *Moralia in Job*, I.14, *PL* 75, 535: 'In septem ergo filiis ordo praedicantium, in tribus vero filiabus multitudo significatur auditorum'.

52 For helpful discussion, see G. Constable, *Three Studies in Medieval Religious and Social Thought* (Cambridge, 1995), 251–323.

53 Council of Trosly, c. 5, *PL* 132, 686.

54 c. 4, *PL* 133, 948.

55 *Historia Hierosolymitana*, VII.1, *Recueil des Historiens des Croisades*, 16 vols, Academie des Inscriptions et Belles Lettres (Paris, 1841–1906), Historiens Occidentaux, vol. III, pp. 771–882.

56 Constable, *Three Studies*, 299–300, citing Ailred's *Speculum caritatis.*

57 I.14, *PL* 75, 535.

58 'Dominica II. Post Aepiphania Domini', trans. in B. Thorpe, *The Homilies of the Anglo-Saxon Church. The First Part containing the Sermones Catholici or Homilies of Ælfric in the original Anglo-Saxon, with an English Version*, 2 vols (London, 1846; repr. New York, 1971), II, 71.

59 Matthew 25. 14–30.

60 In Natale Unius Confessoris', in Thorpe, *Homilies*, II, 551.

61 M. Godden, *Ælfric's Catholic Homilies: Introduction, Commentary and Glossary*, EETS SS 18 (2000), 647–54.

62 J. Wilcox, 'Ælfric in Dorset and the Landscape of Pastoral Care', in F. Tinti, ed., *Pastoral Care in Late Anglo-Saxon England* (Woodbridge, 2005), 52–62.

63 c. 21, *Visio Tnugdali*, *The Vision of Tnugdal*, ed. and trans. J.-M. Picard, with introduction by Y. de Pontfarcy (Dublin, 1989), 151.

64 See Constable's comments about the 'rising status' of laity in eleventh and twelfth centuries: *Three Studies*, 310–11.

65 Mid-Lent Sunday, trans. Thorpe, *Homilies*, I, 185; The Third Sunday after the Lord's Epiphany, ibid. I, 121; G. Dickson, 'Medieval Christian Crowds and the Origins of Crowd Psychology', *Revue d'histoire ecclésiastique* 95 (2000), 54–75.

66 Contra R. I. Moore's famous, if nuanced, observation that 'one of the most obvious novelties of the eleventh century . . . the appearance of the crowd on the stage of public events': 'Family, Community and Cult on the Eve of the Gregorian Reform', *TRHS* 5th ser. 30 (1980), 49–69 at p. 49. I hope to consider depictions of the crowd in the central Middle Ages in more detail elsewhere.

part 1

Churches, churchmen and people

chapter 2

Local churches and their communities

When the bishop goes around his diocese, the archdeacon or archpriest ought to go ahead of him by one or two days to each of the parishes which he will visit, and calling the people together, ought to announce the visit of their pastor, and so that they all do not forget to come to the synod on the set day, and using the authority of the holy canons, to admonish them all, and to announce threateningly that if anyone fails to attend except because of grave necessity, he shall be expelled from the Christian community.[1]

In his idealised portrait of how an episcopal visitation should be conducted the early tenth-century Frankish monk, Regino of Prüm, envisages the parish as the centre of religious life for the local community. The jurors from the community are required, amongst other things, to testify before the bishop as to how far every member of the community regularly attends church, observes the Lenten and Advent fasts, takes regular communion, conducts funerals in a Christian fashion, pays their tithes, and fulfils their obligations as godparents.[2] Regino's vision is very reminiscent of the life of the late medieval parish church which by providing pastoral care for the majority of the population in Western Europe became the focus for their religious and social lives.[3] In the later Middle Ages the majority of lay people baptised their children in their local church, celebrated the feasts of the church year there together, held funeral rites for, and remembered, members of their family after their death. Those living within the parish boundaries maintained and supported their local church through the payment of tithes and other charges. The parish thus signified both a unit of territory and the community which it served, and both were often, but by no means always, co-terminus with the boundaries and membership of the local village. Regino's vision is, as we have already seen in the previous chapter an idealised one. It is not evidence for the actual experience of early tenth-century Christians, nor can be it presumed to anticipate straightforwardly that of their late medieval counterparts. But by highlighting the importance of ideals of parochial community to one influential tenth-century churchman and his readers, it demonstrates the significance of the most obvious and fundamental religious change to occur in this period: the proliferation of local churches serving individual lay communities across Europe.

This change in ecclesiastical provision is therefore the focus of this chapter. It investigates the processes by which laymen and women working individually and together with each other and churchmen established a network of local churches throughout western Christendom. Although often beginning much earlier, these developments gathered pace from the tenth century onwards so that in most regions the parish network which had emerged by 1200 remained almost wholly unchanged until the nineteenth century. This growth in the sheer number of local churches had profound implications for the religious lives of ordinary men and women who for the first time came under the closer jurisdiction of their local priest, and who could now be expected to live Christian lives, structured by ecclesiastical teachings and rites. Their emergence is not, however, the result of top-down decision making by the ecclesiastical hierarchy, but rather of the myriad decisions and anxieties of mostly lay individuals acting either alone or in small groups. These new buildings represented lay individuals' investment in their own spiritual afterlives, as well as being the product of other more secular concerns.

Examining the extent and nature of lay agency in this important change, this chapter will investigate the evidence for the growth in the number of such churches and for the extensive rebuilding of existing ones in these years. It is in four parts. In order to understand the laity's role in the expansion of these networks it is first necessary to consider how the ways in which pastoral care was delivered to the laity changed in this period. How far did the process and timescale by which such networks of local churches were established vary considerably across Latin Christendom? Secondly, it investigates the evidence for the establishment of new churches in this period and the extent to which their erection reflects changes in population, settlement or lordship. The third section investigates the evidence for who built churches, their motives for doing so, and the significance of where they chose to build them – was it at the centre of the settlement or rather proximate to particular points of secular authority within the area? Is local church building, in other words, merely an extension of other, more secular ambitions by lay lords? Or are more complex forces at work in this movement? The fourth and final section therefore investigates how churches were maintained and by whom, and the implications of this for understanding the role these local churches came to play in the religious lives of the local communities they served.

Changes in the organisation of pastoral care

What changes took place in the delivery of pastoral care and when did they occur? Modern historians of local churches and pastoral care often tend to treat developments in their own area of study as paradigmatic and fail to recognise the extent of variation across Latin Christendom. The model which prevails in much of the scholarship is based mainly on Frankish and English evidence, and suggests that in the early Middle Ages, *c.*400–*c.*800, the delivery of pastoral care had been organised in two tiers.[4] Under this system a team of clergy, based in a 'mother' church, had responsibility for delivering pastoral care to the people living in a large area, albeit one smaller than a diocese. Whilst people could worship in various local chapels (*oratoria*, *ecclesiae*, *capellae*), which were subordinate to the 'mother church', the clergy of the 'mother church' retained jurisdiction over key pastoral services, that is, baptism, burial, and the Mass, and derived their income from the entire area for which they were responsible. The clergy of the mother church either served the various *ecclesiae* or retained authority over the clergy of the subordinate churches. Thus churches founded as a result of local initiatives, often (but as we shall see, not always) by the local lord, remained subordinate to the mother church.

The efforts of the Frankish reformers in the late eighth and ninth centuries are, under this paradigm, held to be responsible for the shift to a one-tier system, in which the priest of the local church assumed responsibility for administering the full range of pastoral services to his parishioners, including baptism, and burial. Both Carolingian capitularies and councils envisaged a system of autonomous local churches, each endowed with land by local communities, and supported by the tithes of their parishioners.[5] Tithes were a proportion of the produce of members of that community, usually (but not always) a tenth, which is the meaning of the Latin term for tithe, *decima*. Instead of being served by a team of clergy based in an often distant settlement, the new local churches were located in the communities which financed them; local clergy administered pastoral rites to their parishioners, including those for entry into, and exit from, life easily at hand. The territories and responsibilities of mother churches became consequently reduced and transferred to the new parish churches.

But more localised studies suggest that this shift, from two tiers to one, was a long and more drawn-out process, which occurred across the medieval west over the entire course of our period (900–1200), moving at different rates in different regions. Processes which began in the eighth and ninth centuries in west Frankia were not always completed until the twelfth century, and in some areas, including parts of west Frankia, may have begun rather later than suggested by the traditionalist model outlined above.[6] Regino of Prüm's description of an episcopal visitation seems, in fact, to envisage a two-tier system: as we saw in Chapter 1, he describes how Godfearing men, described as *decani*, from the manor or village (*villa*) should go through all the settlements (*villae*) admonishing everyone to attend church, and reporting to the priest those who do not attend and do not refrain from working on feast days. Regino envisages the parish as being composed of several settlements, *villae*, and also refers to 'the priests *[note the plural]* who must show service to the bishop in that place'. In other words Regino, writing in the diocese of Trier in the early tenth-century system, describes a mother church structure for the delivery of pastoral care along the lines of that followed at the time in northern Italy and England, both areas which witnessed a somewhat later shift to a single-tier system.[7] In England this change seems to have begun in the mid-tenth century, with parishes emerging perhaps as late as the eleventh and twelfth centuries, and the switch did not take place fully in northern Italy at all; there the mother churches and their territories, known as *pievi*, generally retained their rights over baptism into the later Middle Ages, although local churches began to take responsibility for burial rites in the years 900–

1200.[8] Even in England the process had not been completed by the end of the twelfth century: in various places, such as Leominster in Herefordshire and Bakewell in Derbyshire the practice of mother churches retaining jurisdiction over the pastoral services and chapels of a relatively large area survived into the thirteenth century and beyond.[9] A similar pattern holds true when we turn to those areas of Europe which only converted to Christianity in the tenth and eleventh centuries: evidence from Silesia suggests that whilst Christianisation only came to eastern Europe in the tenth century these areas too underwent a similar transition, from two tiers to one, over the course of the next three centuries, as did those in Scandinavia.[10]

Although a gradual and drawn-out process, the evolution of a specific vocabulary to designate the financial rights and thus the territory of a local church points to its eventual success. The most resonant word is that used by Regino, *parochia*, which is translated above as parish. Derived from the Greek, *parochia* originally designated a foreign resident in a Greek city, but came to be used by early Christian authors to denote the Church's residence in the temporal world. Early medieval Latin writers used *parochia* to refer specifically to a bishop's diocese; they used *ecclesia* to denote a local church. By the ninth century the terminology had become confused, reflecting the gradual nature of the development of the parish as an institution.[11] Starting in late ninth-century west Frankia, *parochia* begins to be used in records to denote both a local church and its financial rights. For example, a study of the province of Narbonne in the Languedoc found the first use of *parochia* in the sense of meaning both a local church's financial rights and the area under its control in 898 in the record of a council held in the church of S. Maria at Portus when the clergy, together with a small number of pious laymen, of the province of Narbonne met to hear a dispute between the patrons of two local churches. Adalfredus, the priest of St John the Baptist of Cocon, came with Pharald, the lay patron of his church; they claimed that at the foundation of the church at Cocon, the bishop had recognised the parish of this church as coterminous with the villa of Cocon, that is the territory and its tithes, but that in 891 Abbo, the bishop of Maguelone, had arbitrarily taken part of these revenues to support his recent foundation at Saint-Andouqe. These rights are described as 'the parish of this church in the villa of Cocon and in all its territory'. The council decided in favour of the earlier, lay foundation, and ordered Bishop Abbo to restore the land and to compensate the church at Cocon for the loss of the previous seven years' income from that land.[12] Previous to these texts, Languedocian documents had referred to a *villa* with its church (either *ecclesia* or *capella*) rather than to a church with its *parochia*. The province of Narbonne does not seem especially precocious in this regard; clergy in the early tenth-century Mâconnais and Limoges also began to use *parochia* to denote both the revenues and endowment of a church.[13] These examples are all from the southern and western Frankia and too much should not be made of this linguistic change. They are not, by themselves, evidence for more than changes in diplomatic formulas. In northern and central Italy, for example, a rural church with a baptistery was known from the eighth century onwards as *plebs* or *pieve*, and in Tuscany the word *parochia* is not used to denote a local church supported by tithes until 1118.[14] Norman charters refer to the *parochiae* of local churches from the 1020s onwards, but the term is seemingly only introduced into England at the beginning of the twelfth century.[15] In tenth-century and early eleventh-century England a variety of vernacular terms served instead – *hyrness* (lordship), *folgoþe* (authority), *þeowdom* (service), *scriftscir* (absolution district), and *ciricsocn* (literally church-seeking, that is, those who attend a church for worship or for lordship). This variety suggests either an institution still in a state of flux, or, as John Blair has hypothesised, the conservatism of the English clerical hierarchy which refused to acknowledge that local village churches might have their own 'parishes'.[16] In any case it is worth noting that with the exception of *scriftscir* these terms focus on lordship rather than the church's spatial authority. *Parochia* nevertheless became over the course of the tenth, eleventh and twelfth centuries the most popular term in use in northern Europe to designate both the territory and revenues pertaining to a rural church, and thus the people who owed such revenues. Although the process began earlier under the Carolingians the emergence in tenth-century west Frankia and twelfth-century England and Italy of the use of *parochia* to designate both a local church and the territory from which it drew its revenue, and over whose inhabitants it had authority, reflects an important step in the emergence of the parish.

Church building 900–1200

What is the evidence for an expansion in church building in this period? This change in terminology occurred at the same time as a substantial increase in the number of churches established. Various Latin writers observed a massive building and rebuilding programme taking place in their particular region in the course of the eleventh and twelfth centuries. William of Malmesbury (d. 1143) wrote in early twelfth-century England:

> *You may now see in every village, town and city, churches and monasteries rising in a new style of architecture.*[17]

Alongside the construction of abbeys and cathedrals, local churches were rebuilt and new ones established. This process, many clerical writers observed, owed much to the laity. Rodulfus Glaber famously noted that:

> *just before the third year after the millennium, throughout the whole world, but most especially in Italy and Gaul, men began to reconstruct churches, although for the most part the existing ones were properly built and not in the least unworthy. But it seemed as though each Christian community was aiming to surpass all others in splendour of construction. It was as if the whole world were shaking itself free, shrugging off the burden of the past, and cladding itself everywhere in a white mantle of churches. Almost all the episcopal churches (*ecclesiae*) and those of monasteries dedicated to various saints, and little village chapels (*oratoria*) were rebuilt better than before by the faithful.*[18]

Half a century later Goscelin of Saint-Bertin reported how Herman, bishop of Ramsbury, told Pope Leo IX in 1050 of how England was 'being filled everywhere with churches which daily were being added anew in new places; about the distribution of innumerable ornaments and bells in oratories; about the most ample liberality of kings and rich men for the inheritance of Christ.'[19]

Scholars have learnt to be wary of such hyperbole. Their authors included each of these accounts in order to make a point within their wider work. Rodulphus Glaber, for example, began his *Histories* in order to record the events which happened around the first millennium of Christ's Incarnation; Book III, from which this description comes, deals with what happened just after 1000, which Glaber portrayed as a time of renewal and rebirth, exemplified by this widespread rebuilding programme. But the physical evidence of surviving churches suggests that the years 900 to 1200 witnessed a considerable investment in local churches. Local architectural and archaeological studies from across Europe demonstrate how a physical reality underlies these excited descriptions of the great building and rebuilding of the eleventh and twelfth centuries.[20] Archaeology reveals that what appear to be new buildings might actually be rebuildings: excavations at Barton-on-Humber in Lincolnshire, Raunds Furnell in Northamptonshire, and Rivenhall in Essex, for example, suggest that on these sites a larger stone building replaced a smaller, probably tenth-century, church.[21] A local study in Italy has revealed that even where there is earlier documentary evidence for a church, the earliest architectural evidence for church buildings is only eleventh-century.[22] As well as the buildings themselves, the presence of Norman fonts in many later medieval English churches today testifies to this earlier building programme in England.[23]

What such activity meant for individual settlements becomes clearer if we start to compare the evidence for this rise in the number and therefore density of local churches between different regions. The timing of this growth varied from place to place, yet the scale of the increase in different regions is often very similar. As conversion only began in the tenth century it came late to eastern Europe: in central Silesia the number of parish churches doubled in the twelfth and thirteenth centuries.[24] But dioceses in Italy, where Christianity had been established over 500 years earlier, witnessed a similar increase a century earlier. In the diocese of Verona in northern Italy, for example, the number of churches more than doubled between 1000 and 1150, and most of this growth took place in the countryside as a consequence of the development of new settlements in previously under-populated areas. In the early Middle Ages churches had huddled around the old Roman roads, the river and the lake; in the century and a half following 1000 new churches were established together with new settlements on newly drained lands in the plains and clearings in the upland valleys. Many of these new churches possessed pastoral rites: 38 per cent of those established in the countryside were *pievi* and more than 50 per cent of those established in Verona and its immediate environs had similar status. At the same time older churches were rebuilt to house larger congregations.

These changes in ecclesiastical provision in this north Italian diocese reflect not just demographic and economic growth, nor are they entirely the result of lay piety, but rather a result of the diversity of political power during these 150 years. The decline in church foundations from the twelfth century onwards has been attributed to both a decline in the establishment of new settlements, and to the increased authority of the city commune over the urban area leading institutions to become more effectively litigious in protecting their revenues than they had been able to be in the preceding period during a time of weaker and overlapping jurisdictions.[25] Elsewhere in Italy changes in political power also impacted on local church provision. In the Lazio in central Italy, Pierre Toubert's research suggests that the process of *incastellamento*, that is, the movement of settlements into fortified villages, *castelli*, led to the disappearance of the large public *pievi* as the focus for communal piety (although the *pievi* continued to retain their baptismal rights), and the emergence of smaller, recognisably parish churches in *castelli* in the century and a half or so from 950.[26] Further south, in the principality of Capua, the evidence for *pievi* is poorer, and evidence for rural *pievi* with baptismal rights only emerges in the latter part of the twelfth century with the revival of strong lordship.[27]

Growth took place earlier than the eleventh century in parts of west Frankia. In the Limousin, Michel Aubrun has estimated the existence of some one thousand churches by the eleventh century, that is one church for every five or six square kilometres. Of these he identified some five hundred as having been created in the ninth century, and only two hundred new places of worship as being built in the eleventh and twelfth centuries; he thus suggested that these new churches did not modify in any profound way the parish map established by the Carolingians in the ninth century.[28] In the Ardèche, however, Charles-Laurent Salch and Danielle Fèvre identified only twenty churches from the ninth century, but eighty-three from the tenth and eleventh centuries. Almost all of these new churches were built by laymen. As Salch and Fèvre noted, their establishment coincided with the building of castles, although the churches outnumber the number of known castles by almost two to one; they therefore suggested that many of these new churches may have been built as symbols of lordship over the local area. In order to overcome biases in the evidence, they also recorded the number of known churches against the number of known settlements, *villae*, in each century: one church is mentioned for every three *villae* known from documentation in the ninth-century Ardèche, and one for every 2.5 *villae* in the tenth and eleventh centuries.[29] Sometimes private churches were promoted to parish status, sometimes mother churches were moved from the *villa* to the new castle, and sometimes new parishes were built on newly cleared land. The development of the network of local churches in this area resulted from both increased population *and* changing settlement *and* changing power structures.

Contrasting with this picture of gradual growth presented in these studies from west Frankia, studies of England suggest a pattern more akin to that in Italy: both regions saw an apparent explosion in the number of local churches across the years 900 to 1200. Scholars of England agree that these three centuries witnessed the foundation of a large number of parish churches and that there were around 6000–7000 churches in England by 1100. They differ, however, as to when the main period of growth took place. Richard Morris believes that the tenth century was crucial to the establishment of local churches, and that the better documented foundations in the fifty years after the Norman Conquest merely represent 'a final infilling of the parochial map'. John Blair, on the other hand, argues that this process took much longer and was not completed until the early twelfth century.[30] Both agree that most local churches were built and rebuilt in the period of 'great rebuilding', 1050–1150.

Taken together, the fragmentary documentary, archaeological and architectural record suggests that these three centuries witnessed a considerable investment in local churches and a considerable growth in the number of churches across the medieval west.

Lay investment in local churches

Who built these churches, where, and why did they build them? Most local churches, were probably built at the initiatives of local lords. Such churches are often referred to as *Eigenkirchen*, proprietary churches.[31] Landowners built proprietary churches on their lands, chose their clergy, and took possession of the church's revenues. Bishops consequently made repeated attempts to assert authority over these proprietary churches; whilst recognising the lord's right to choose the priest, bishops reserved the rights to approve the priest or release him from his office, and to define the area of the parish.[32] Scholars generally view the motives for such lordly investment as primarily social and economic: lords anxious to benefit from the tithe payments due to the church also used the ownership of that church to promote their lordship over the local area. As we have already seen, one study of the Ardèche has demonstrated that the building of churches outnumbered the building of castles by two to one in the tenth and eleventh centuries, suggesting that these new churches acted as symbols of lordship in the landscape, much as castles did later. In eleventh-century eastern England, church building sometimes accompanied speculative building: according to the Domesday Book, Colswein built thirty-six houses with two churches in Lincoln, presumably for profit.[33]

As the majority of the surviving evidence is biased towards that for possession of economic rights, the lay erection of churches is thus naturally viewed as a consequence of lordship and concern with financial rights. This view of church building as primarily an extension of lordship in large part echoes the concerns of eleventh- and twelfth-century reformers, anxious to recover clerical control over ecclesiastical institutions, as it was expressed in both conciliar proceedings and the trail of charter evidence over local disputes, when what was at issue was the possession of these revenues. Tithes became central to the rationale for the transfer of churches from lay to religious ownership once reformist critiques made lay ownership less tenable. In the twelfth century in England, for example, lordship over the parish church began to be transferred to monasteries; and from the 1170s monasteries appointed themselves rectors, appropriating the revenue from tithes and other dues for their own use, less a small vicarage for the priest serving the church. Ownership of tithes from existing parishes increasingly governed negotiations for the establishment of new ones as they were carved out of the territory of existing churches, with a consequent loss of income.

But there are other indications that local churches were viewed as more than just economic entities. In both England and west Frankia ownership of a church seems to have been a sign of noble status.[34] In the Ardèche, as we saw above, local churches marked lordship rather than more secular buildings.[35] The building of churches in *castelli* in the Lazio resulted from the actions of lords and consequent shifting settlement patterns.[36] But lords had other motives as well, as is implied by the inscription on a sundial over the south door of the church at Kirkdale in Yorkshire which records that Orm, the son of Gamal, bought the church (*minster*) when it was in ruins and rebuilt it from the ground.[37] In a largely illiterate society, this inscription advertising Orm's piety and largesse was not included for the local peasantry, who made up most of the congregation, but rather for a clerical, and probably also a celestial, audience.[38] Orm wished to be remembered in their prayers. He was not unusual, for local churches and chapels were often founded as family mausoleums. This at least seems to be the implication of charters limiting burial rights to the founding family; other members of the congregation had to travel to the burial ground of the old mother church. Earl Odda built a small church, dedicated to the Holy Trinity, in memory of his brother Ælfric (d. 1053), on his manor at Deerhurst, which was also the site of the minster church of St Mary's.[39] The chapel acted as a family mausoleum, and indicates Odda's grief for, and concern about, the fate of his brother's soul, but the building itself also displayed Odda's lordship in that area. Odda's actions were part of a more widespread trend amongst the eleventh-century nobility who actively supported, endowed and rebuilt their local churches for a variety of purposes which combined piety with lordship.[40]

Sometimes these new churches seem to have been erected purely for the convenience of their founders: in twelfth-century Poland a noble built a church on his own lands, and attracted condemnation for using it for a family wedding 'almost immediately after the consecration'.[41] Throughout Europe churches are found often located close to lords' seats. In the archdeaconry of Colchester, for example, nineteen out of twenty-nine Anglo-Saxon churches are located beside secular halls.[42] Church building accompanied castle building in the eleventh and twelfth centuries. Sometimes lords carved out a new parish from the old one in order to support a parish within their castle fortifications.[43] There are also several examples from the tenth, eleventh and twelfth centuries of lords transferring the site of the local church from its earlier site, in the local community, to their new castle, to suit their convenience.[44] That such arrangements had an impact on the local community is clear from the following example. At the parish of Châtillon en Berry (central France), established as a result of lordly initiative in the mid-twelfth century, all the inhabitants below the status of knight had to attend the pre-existing church at Toiselay at least nine times a year: at Christmas, on St Stephen's day (Boxing Day), the feast of the Purification of the Virgin (2nd February), Palm Sunday, Easter, the Ascension and Pentecost, and for the feasts of All Saints (1st November) and All Souls (2nd November).[45] This requirement that they should celebrate the major feast days of the church calendar away from their own church must have had an impact on the religious lives of the members of this particular community. The legacy of the older two-tier system thus survived here, as elsewhere, in the financial arrangements made by members of the elite to create new churches, as established churches sought to protect their income, but this example also, perhaps, reveals something of the family interests and motives of their founders.

It would be wrong to generalise about a founder's motives. The early twelfth-century *Life* of Bishop Wulfstan II of Worcester (d. 1095) implies that for some eleventh-century Anglo-Saxon noblemen their emotional investment in their church went far beyond the economic and was such that they were prepared to go to considerable lengths to get the right man to consecrate it. A rich Buckinghamshire man, Swertlin, built a church at Wycombe at his own expense, but was anxious to have it consecrated by a man he regarded as holy, Wulfstan, bishop of Worcester. As the church lay in the diocese of Lincoln, the author of Wulfstan's life records that Swertlin anxiously sought, and received, approval from the bishop of Lincoln to allow Wulfstan to dedicate the church in his place. The dedication ceremony, we are told, was followed by a sermon, and confirmation of those children present, ending with a meal at Swertlin's house close by.[46] It mattered to Swertlin to invite a holy man to dedicate his church. Later in the *Life* another nobleman, Sæwig, invites Wulfstan to dedicate the church at his *villa* at Ratcliffe-on-Soar outside Nottingham, because 'in his piety he was anxious to have it dedicated by the holy man', and therefore successfully applies for a licence for the church to be dedicated by a bishop from outside the diocese.[47] Both these accounts of church dedications, like others, suggest that these were important events in the locality: crowds turned out to witness the ceremony and hear the bishop's sermons. The roads were packed as the crowds converged on Ratcliffe.[48] At the consecration of another church, Longney in Gloucestershire, there was not enough room for the people.[49] In large part this may be hagiographical hyperbole, and the author of the *Life* probably included the reference to episcopal licence to show Wulfstan to be a good, orthodox and law-abiding reforming bishop. He is portrayed as an exemplary one who also took the opportunity on such occasions not only to preach the word of God, but to promote peacemaking, as well as to confirm children and release penitents from their penance.[50]

In eastern Europe the foundation of local churches also happened largely as a result of secular lords' initiatives. As in the west, they seem to have been motivated by a combination of reasons: financial, pious, that is, to create a centre for family memory, and social, that is, the desire to display lordly status on a religious stage.[51] As throughout Christendom, these churches were not merely convenient; they were important adjuncts to lordly authority. Private chapels by excluding normal people acted as a marker of status. Parish churches located next to the manor or inside a castle provided a setting through which the lord could display his superiority before both the local community and visitors.[52] The proximity of his own dwelling to a holy place acted as a further mark of status. Finally, by serving as burial places for lordly families, these churches acted as focuses for their memory.[53]

The east reflected the more general pattern in northern Europe, where it was typical for churches to be established on a single person's inheritance, but in southern Europe – southern France, southern Italy and Spain – where primogeniture was less common the evidence suggests that consortia of wider family groups, or groups of like-minded lesser nobility sometimes acted together to found parish churches.[54] In 1092, for example, Bernard of Marens, with his brother Berinirus, Arduin of Marens, Sanche of Marens and his brothers gave to the cathedral church of Saint-Sernin in Toulouse, three churches, with their tithes, on condition that a new church was built in a place called Courlens. Over the next seven years the tithes from these churches should finance the construction of the new church, excepting the archbishop's quarter share which was not remitted. Once the church at Courlens had been built the canons of Saint-Sernin should receive a quarter of the tithes, half the offerings and the proceedings of all the burial rights, and the clerics installed in the new church should get half the tithes and offerings. The donors also gave the land on which the new church was to be built, which was to be free and exempt from all charges.[55] This prosperous noble family acted together to found the new church.

But throughout the core regions of the Latin West there is evidence that local lay communities sometimes established churches at their own initiative, not that of their lord or lords. In twelfth-century England, for example, inclement weather and topographic barriers led the inhabitants of Whistley in Berkshire to secede from the parish of Sonning, which was three miles away and across a river. They founded a new church in their own settlement, on the grounds that winter rains often made the ford impassable, making it impossible for them to attend church at Sonning.[56] In this case the lord of Whistley reached agreement with the abbot of Abingdon and the lord of Sonning: the new church could have its own priest, and all oblations could be kept for the use of the church, but half a mark must be paid annually out of the income of the new church to the bishop of Salisbury and lord of Sonning, and they agreed that 'the church of Sonning should have all the dues which it used to receive from the villa of Whistley in the time of King Edward'.[57] In Burgundy the destruction of the church of Sologny in a flood led the villagers to refuse to pay the tithe to the monastic patron of the church until the church had been rebuilt on a safer site.[58] In Provence the women from one village offered the local chapel to the monks of Lérins on condition that they were assured of regular divine service within their community.[59] In the Languedocian archdiocese of Narbonne there are five examples of local inhabitants demanding the consecration of a church for their use.[60] In the Loire the canons of Saint-Hilaire of Poitiers received from the inhabitants of St Hilaire des Loges a pledge that they would contribute both money and labour to the building of their church. Described as *homines rusticani*, peasants, the text cites some fifty names, together with the sum they pledged, which ranged from ten sous in thirteen cases, to twelve deniers in others.[61] The peasants also agreed a rate of four cows, or five sous, for their burial. Thus we know that amongst those who pledged to build the church were Mainard the merchant, Odolric and Engalbert, both cobblers, and Ademar the weaver, although no profession is given for the majority of names listed. Similar arrangements survive from twelfth-century Lotharingia where the men from the village of Senon obtained the abbot of Gorze's permission to build and equip their own church, on condition that it belong to the monastery on whose lands it was built, and twelfth-century Tuscany when a group of fifteen households agreed to build a chapel at Barbaricini, in the diocese of Pisa, with the support of their lord, the local abbot, and retained joint rights, with the abbot, to appoint the chaplain.[62]

There is less detailed but equally suggestive evidence from eleventh-century eastern England that members of rural communities sought to ensure they received adequate pastoral care. A study of some fifty-nine Lincolnshire churches built in the eleventh and twelfth centuries found that twenty-one (31 per cent) were built on a green, or common grazing land, that is public space within the *villa*, surrounded by planned rows of properties. Their location suggests a level of 'public' involvement in the process of church building, especially as it coincides with settlements known to have had a high number of sokemen (freemen) and a non-resident lord. It has therefore been suggested that these churches were built by leading landowners in the community in conjunction with an absentee lord.[63] In

East Anglia several examples of groups of freemen founding churches are documented. St Mary, Thorney in Suffolk is on the edge of the graveyard of St Peter's, Stowmarket, and according to the Domesday Book entry for Stowmarket four brothers built St Mary, Thorney because the mother church was no longer large enough to accommodate the congregation:

> *There was in the time of King Edward a church with 1 carucate of free land. But Hugh de Montfort has 23 acres of that carucate and claims it as belonging to a certain chapel which 4 brothers, free men under Hugh, built on land of their own hard by the cemetery of the mother church. And they were inhabitants of the parish of the mother church (and built this chapel) because it could not take in the whole of the parish. The mother church had always a moiety of the burial fees, and had by purchase the fourth part of the alms which might be made. And whether or not this chapel was consecrated the Hundred doth not know. In this carucate of the church there were 5 bordars and 1 villein. Then as now two ploughs.*[64]

The reference to the mother church being too small to accommodate the whole parish has the ring of truth: in eleventh-century Winchester, for example, one church excavated was only 13 × 16 feet.[65] Elsewhere in Suffolk there are other examples of freemen patronising their local church: nine freemen gave the church at Stonham, Suffolk twenty acres for the salvation of their souls; whilst ownership of the church at Wantisden, Suffolk was divided between twenty-five freemen: twenty-two freemen owned half of it, two owned a quarter of it, and the last quarter was owned by one freeman.[66] Such arrangements led to a disassociation between landholding and church building and explain why, in such co-operative arrangements, new churches were built on established holy sites, such as a pre-existing graveyard, or on common land, rather than on land owned by only one member of the group.[67] Such arrangements are not unique to the areas of Europe where Christianity had been long established. In Norway, where Christianity arrived only in the tenth and eleventh centuries, king and nobles built the earliest churches on their own estates, but from the twelfth century onwards the *thing* congregations and settlement districts built their own churches, and took responsibility for administering the tithe and electing the priest, as well as providing furnishings, ornaments and bells.[68] There is evidence in Andorra and Catalonia as well of communal church foundations.[69] These examples suggest that church building was never solely the prerogative of lords: local communities were often prepared to make sacrifices in order to ensure they got their own church where they wanted it.

Disputes about tithes sometimes provide evidence of the continuing active involvement of the lay congregation in the affairs of their local church. In the 1150s a dispute between Stone Priory and the two priests of the church of Swinnerton in Staffordshire as to whether Swinnerton was a dependent 'chapel' of the priory's church at Stone came before the bishop of Coventry, Walter Durdent, who asked the archdeacon of Stafford, Elias, to settle it. Elias held a court of clergy and laity at Stone at which the two priests acknowledged the dependent status of their church, and, with the assent of the lord of Swinnerton, restored it to the priory; the priests remained in possession although they had to pay two shillings annually to the church at Stone in recognition of their dependent status.[70] The presence of the unspecified laity suggests, on the one hand, that lip-service was paid to written and practical legal norms, but also, perhaps, that it was not only the lord's assent which was needed for the resolution of this dispute, and that the status of their local church mattered to the congregation of Swinnerton: after all it might affect where they paid their tithes, and dues, where they were baptised and buried, in future. Such disputes can easily be dismissed as property disputes, or as examples of ecclesiastical government in action, in this case the archdeacon acting as the bishop's deputy, but we should not forget their wider resonances for the local community whose religious life took place in this church.

Most of the examples considered up to now have been rural but the pattern of local church provision within towns also varied considerably. Some towns had very many churches, albeit perhaps sometimes rather small ones; Lincoln, for example, had between thirty-two and thirty-seven churches by 1110, and fifty by the end of the twelfth century, Norwich forty-six, London had about a hundred in the late twelfth century, whilst Poitiers and Bourges each had between twenty and thirty churches.[71] But whilst in eastern England and western France such churches were often independent of each other, in most of Europe, that is western England, Italy, the Low Countries, Burgundy, the Rhineland and Bavaria, it was common for all the churches within a town to be subordinate to one parish. In Würzburg parochial worship remained within the cathedral as well, whilst Paderborn possessed a single parish church separate from the cathedral.[72] The proliferation of churches in some towns, but not others, as in the countryside, almost certainly reflects the absence of powerful religious institutions able to prevent churches being created at the expense of their existing rights.[73] Evidence for such intervention is to be found in 1092, for example, when 'the most ancient persons' from three counties met in Worcester cathedral and decided that the city of Worcester should contain only one parish, the cathedral church, 'even though it had other and ancient churches'.[74] The organisation of local churches within a town often also depended on whether individual churches came with burial rights: subordinate churches were built on street corners or in the middle of the street where burial was not a consideration.[75] In other cities, as in villages, graveyards were often used as sites for markets, and, at least in Brittany, became the nucleus for later towns.[76]

In those towns where churches proliferated, various different explanations have been given for the motives of their founders and the geography of their distribution. Studies of urban geography have offered three explanations for the origins of urban parishes: those originating on the property of their founder, those originating in local communities of townsfolk which are marked by having crossroads at their centre, and those where the nearest church has become the parish for those dwellings.[77] Some urban churches clearly are the result of lordly initiative; for example, Earl Siward built a church dedicated to St Olaf just outside the gate of York in 1055 in which he was buried.[78] Others, however, are the result of freemen's investment: for example three men, Grim, Æse, and another built the church of St Mary, Castlegate, in York in the late tenth or early eleventh century.[79] The Domesday survey records that the church of Holy Trinity in Norwich was held by twelve burgesses in the time of King Edward the Confessor.[80] The dedicatory inscription on the tower of St Mary-le-Wigford in Lincoln names one Eirtig as patron; it has been suggested that he was probably only one member of a group of burgesses who joined together to establish a church for their local community.[81] In towns, as in the countryside, the origin of local parishes owes a great deal to the actions of local communities as well as local lords, sometimes working together, and sometimes independent of each other. There is thus a good deal of evidence to suggest that laymen and women initiated the foundation of many local churches motivated by pious concerns.

Relations with the local community

How were local churches maintained and by whom? In later medieval England the assigning of financial responsibility for the maintenance of substantial parts of the church fabric to the laity helped create a sense of collective responsibility amongst the lay community, and led to distinctive forms of lay piety focused on the local church. The transfer of such obligations also led to the emergence of the office of churchwarden charged with ensuring they were fulfilled.[82] There are, as we shall see, tantalising hints in the central medieval evidence that churchwardens had earlier roots, and there are also suggestions that even where lay men and women had not built their local church, they took pride in it, and felt a level of responsibility for it. The incidental mention of the existence of a custodian (*aedituus*) of the southern English church which housed the relics of St Lewinna in an eleventh-century Flemish text may be an early reference to a churchwarden.[83] We should also remember that Regino's vision of the duties of the *decani* overlaps with those assigned to churchwardens in the later Middle Ages. Although formal responsibility for the maintenance of naves of churches did not pass to the local community until the thirteenth century, there is earlier evidence which suggests that in some cases parishioners were concerned about the ownership and maintenance of their church.[84] In 1086 the burgesses of Lincoln protested that lordship over one of their churches had been unjustly transferred to the abbot of Peterborough when the previous lord's heir became a monk at Peterborough, arguing that 'neither Garewine nor his son nor anyone else could grant their possessions outside the city or outside the patronage of the king's consent'.[85] A complex case, with other claimants to the lordship, it nevertheless suggests a desire to keep ownership of the church within the local community. Others expressed their loyalty to their church through concern for its decoration. In the diocese of Brussels, for example, a humble peasant, Guido (d. 1012) reportedly decorated the chancel and tomb of the saints of his local church with flowers and branches.[86] When combined, these examples suggest a world in which lay people and lay communities took pride not only in building but maintaining their churches.

This might not always be the case. The requirement that the laity pay tithes for the support of the clergy and the maintenance of the church and its furnishings went back to the fifth century. Legislation from the eighth century onwards sought to enforce payment of tithes, and was regularly repeated at times of religious renewal such as the ninth century in Frankia and the late tenth and early eleventh centuries in England.[87] But at the same time as groups of men and women came together across Europe to erect new churches, in other places the payment of tithes to support the church was widely resented and sometimes served as a stimulus for anti-clericalism. In the early eleventh century the peasant Leutard led a tithe strike in the area around Liège, which sufficiently worried the clerical authorities that the Burgundian monk Rodulphus Glaber mentioned it as one of the disturbing signs surrounding the first Christian millennium.[88] A century later, Guibert of Nogent reported how in Beauvais a peasant tried to poison his local priest by adding a toad to the jar in which the priest kept the communion wine: as the laity had not yet been formally excluded from taking communion in both kinds, the man's action was not a doctrinal protest against a clerical monopoly, but rather an expression of his more general resentment of the priest's authority at a time when the laity were not expected to communicate more than three times a year.[89] Resistance to paying tithes ran up through the strata of society, from the peasantry to the nobility. The monks of Our Lady at Rocamodour, in south-western France recorded in their miracle book (1172 × 1173) the miraculous cure of a young man who rashly dared to enter the church at Rocamodour and approach the altar of Our Lady, despite having been excommunicated by his priest for wrongly claiming his local church's tithes and keeping them for himself.[90] The widespread loathing for tithes supplies the basis for many cautionary tales told within clerical communities throughout Europe. In late twelfth-century England Walter Map recounted the tale of how, one night, a Northumbrian knight was sitting alone after dinner when the spirit of his long-dead father appeared before him and asked his son to fetch a priest. Upon the priest being summoned, the spirit announced to him: 'I am that wretch whom you long ago excommunicated unnamed, with many more, for unrighteous withholding of tithes, but the common prayers of the church and the alms of the faithful have, by God's grace, so helped me that I am permitted to ask for absolution', which the priest granted, and the spirit returned to his grave.[91] Payment of tithes no doubt focused resentment on the local church, at the same time as the evidence suggests that parishioners assumed responsibility for the establishment of local parishes.

But payment of tithes may, in fact, have helped to focus people's loyalties on their local church, just as responsibility for the fabric of the nave did in the later Middle Ages. The men of one Cornish settlement, when summoned to a twelfth-century inquiry into some lost rights of the minster at Lanow, explained that they had chosen to attend and pay their tithes to a neighbouring church because of a feud with men from other communities under the minster's jurisdiction. Fearing for their lives, they had unilaterally chosen to move jurisdictions. Such actions may be rare – most clergy were much more vigilant in preserving their rights – but they serve as a reminder of how payment of tithes linked ordinary men and women to their local church.'[92]

The secular life of local communities also focused on the church. Manumission from slavery might be performed at the altar. Local churches often provided the setting for court hearings, and certainly for trials by ordeal. On occasion they even served as prisons. The continual repetition in conciliar proceedings of the prohibition on using churches as granaries and stables suggests that they must, at least sometimes, have been put to such uses.[93] They also acted as a focus for legal sanctuary.[94] From at least the tenth century, parish cemeteries were regularly consecrated, and in the period before 1200 church graveyards became the focus for a good deal of non-religious activity because their consecration rendered them as what Barbara Rosenwein has described as 'a kind of attack-free population zone'.[95] They thus became the setting for markets in Brittany, England and Catalonia.[96] Markets had the potential to be volatile and violent occasions, uniting disparate members of the community: the sacred ground of the local church's graveyard provided a suitably neutral setting. Local community relations might not always be amiable but the local church was central to the ways in which they were conducted.

Conclusions

The evidence about the origins of parish churches and their relations with the communities they served is complex and difficult to interpret. Much of church law, both prescriptive and documentary, treats the local church as a bundle of legal and economic rights rather than as a centre for the delivery of pastoral care. Charters record clergymen anxious to define the tithes and fees belonging to a particular church, and to defend its authority to levy them from the people living in a particular area against poaching by neighbouring clergy or greedy secular lords. Such records deal with institutions already in existence. There are unfortunately very few records for most parish church foundations: it is usually the case that we only have evidence about the foundation of new churches where their establishment infringed on the rights of an older one. Thus unlike monastic endowments, the problems of the documentation mean we lack evidence for the motives of the majority of founders and patrons of local churches. It is difficult to get beyond the concern with legal and economic rights in the surviving evidence – what Martin Brett has described as the 'scaffolding of the church' – to study the relations between the clergy and the laity.[97]

Yet, as we have seen, it is far from impossible. It is as well to remember that this scaffolding was, in large part, erected by, and at the wishes of, individual members of the laity. The establishment of a network of local churches throughout Europe was not the result of ecclesiastical initiative but rather was driven by the concerns of local lords, and other members of local communities working together, by individual lay men and women's desires for a family mausoleum, and by their desires to have an easily accessible church, be it in their castle, or village, rather than a distant one. Local lords and lay communities worked separately and in parallel: churches could be established as an extension of a lord's claim to lordship over an area, but might also be founded by communities of freemen anxious to have a church in their own community. Status and piety are therefore inextricably combined as reasons for the widening of the network of local churches in this period. The implications of this emerging network of local churches for both those who administered them and those served by them is the subject of the rest of this book.

Notes and references

1 Regino, II.1, 234.

2 See Chapter 1.

3 On the late medieval parish see, amongst other works, E. Duffy, *The Stripping of the Altars: Traditional Religion in England c.1400–c.1580* (New Haven, CT, 1992); K. French, *The People of the Parish: Community Life in a Late Medieval Diocese* (Philadelphia, 2001); B. Kümin, *The Shaping of a Community: The Rise and Reformation of the English Parish c.1400–1560* (Aldershot, 1996); K. French, G. G. Gibbs and B. A. Kümin, eds, *The Parish in English Life 1400–1600* (Manchester, 1997).

4 J. Blair, 'Secular Minster Churches in Domesday Book', in P. H. Sawyer, ed., *Domesday Book: A Reassessment* (London, 1985), 104–42; idem, 'Local Churches in Domesday Book and Before', in J. C. Holt, ed., *Domesday Studies* (Woodbridge, 1987), 265–78; idem, 'Minster Churches in the Landscape', in D. Hooke, ed., *Anglo-Saxon Settlements* (Oxford, 1988), 35–58; idem, ed., *Minsters and Parish Churches: the Local Church in Transition, 950–1200* (Oxford, 1988); idem, *Church*. See critique of Blair's thesis by Y. Hen, 'Review Article: Liturgy and Religious Culture in Late Anglo-Saxon England', *Early Medieval Europe* 17 (2009), 329–42. For an earlier critique, see the debate which ran in *Early Medieval Europe* in the mid-1990s: E. Cambridge and D. Rollason, 'Debate: The Pastoral Organization of the Anglo-Saxon Church: A Review of the "Minster Hypothesis"', *Early Medieval Europe* 4 (1995), 87–104; J. Blair, 'Debate: Ecclesiastical Organization and Pastoral Care in Anglo-Saxon England', *Early Medieval Europe* 4 (1995), 193–212; D. M. Palliser, 'Review Article: The "Minster Hypothesis": A Case Study', *Early Medieval Europe* 5 (1996), 207–14.

5 J. J. Contreni outlines the legislation in 'From Polis to Parish' in T. F. X. Noble and J. J. Contreni, eds, *Religion, Culture and Society in the Middle Ages: Studies in Honour of Richard E. Sullivan* (Kalamazoo, MI, 1987), 155–64.

6 S. Reynolds, *Kingdoms and Communities in Western Europe 900–1300* (Oxford, 1984), 81–90.

7 Regino, II. 5. 69, 248 (*decani*); ibid. II. 5. 1: 'Deinde, adscitis secum presbyteris, qui illo in loco servitium debent exhibere episcopo', 234.

8 For England, see Blair, *Church*, 368–425; for Italy, see C. E. Boyd, *Tithes and Parishes in Medieval Italy: the Historical Roots of a Modern Problem* (Ithaca, NY, 1952), 154–64; C. Violante, 'Sistemi organizzativi della cura d'anime in Italia tra Medioevo e Rinascimento: Discorso introduttivo', *Pievi e parrochie in Italia nel basso Medioevo (sec. XIII–XV)*, (2 vols, Rome, 1984), I, 3–41.

9 E.g. B. Kemp, 'Some Aspects of the *Parochia* of Leominster in the Twelfth Century', in Blair, ed., *Minsters and Parish Churches*, 83–95.

10 P. Gorecki, *Parishes, Tithes and Society in Earlier Medieval Poland ca. 1100–1250*, Transactions for the American Philosophical Society 83.2 (Philadelphia, 1993); S. Brink, 'The Formation of the Scandinavian Parish, with Some Remarks Regarding the English Impact on the Process', in J. Hill and M. Swan, eds, *The Community, the Family, and the Saint: Patterns of Power in Early Medieval Europe* (Turnhout, 1998), 19–44.

11 P. A. Deleeuw, 'The Changing Face of the Village Parish I: The Parish in the Early Middle Ages', in J. A. Raftis, ed., *Pathways to Medieval Peasants* (Toronto, 1981), 311–322 at pp. 312–15.

12 E. Magnou-Nortier, *La société laïque et l'église dans la province ecclésiastique de Narbonne (zone cispyrénéenne) de la fin du VIIIe à la fin du XIe siècle* (Toulouse, 1974), 423–24, 609–10.

13 J. Avril, 'La "paroisse" dans la France de l'an Mil', in M. Parisse, and X. Barral i Altet, eds, *Le roi de France et son royaume, autour de l'an Mil* (Picard, 1992), 203–18 at 209; J. Semmler, 'Zehntgebot und Pfarrtermination in karolingischer Zeit', in H. Mordek, ed., *Aus Kirche und Reich: Festschrift für Friedrich Kempf* (Sigmaringen, 1983), 33–44.

14 Boyd, *Tithes and Parishes*, 47–74. On Lucca, see L. Nanni, *La Parrocchia studiata nei documenti lucchesi dei secoli viii–xiii* (Rome, 1948).

15 Blair, *Church*, 428, n. 5.

16 Ibid. 427–33. The clerical hierarchy was unwilling to 'concede, either before or for some time after 1066, that ordinary village churches could control anything so formal as a "parish" or "parishioners"', ibid., 432.

17 William of Malmesbury, *Gesta Regum Anglorum*, ed. and trans. R. A. B. Mynors, R. M. Thomson and M. Winterbottom, 2 vols (Oxford, 1998–99), III. 246, 461.

18 Rodulfus Glaber, *Historiarum Libri Quinque*, ed. and trans. J. France (Oxford, 1989), III.13, 114–16.

19 *Historia Translationis Sancti Augustini*, II. 3, *PL* 155, 32, translated by R. Gem, 'The English Parish Church in the Eleventh and Early Twelfth Centuries: A Great Rebuilding?', in J. Blair, ed., *Minsters and Parish Churches: The Local Church in Transition, 950–1200* (Oxford, 1988), 21–30 at p. 21.

20 F. Oswald, L. Schaefer, H. R. Sennhauser, *Vorromanische Kirchenbauten. Katalog der Denkmäler bis zum Ausgang der Ottonen*, 2nd edn (Munich, 1991); H. M. Taylor and J. Taylor, *Anglo-Saxon Architecture*, 3 vols (Cambridge, 1965–78); R. Morris, *Churches in the Landscape* (London, 1989); E. Fernie, *The Architecture of the Anglo-Saxons* (London, 1983); idem, *The Architecture of Norman England* (Oxford, 2000); Gem, 'The English Parish Church: A Great Rebuilding?'; C. F. Davidson, 'Written in Stone: Architecture, Liturgy and the Laity in English Parish Churches, *c.*1125–*c.*1250' (University of London Ph.D. thesis, 1998); Blair, *Church*, 407–22.

21 W. Rodwell and K. Rodwell, 'St Peter's Church, Barton-upon-Humber', *Antiquaries Journal* 62 (1982), 283–315; A. Boddington, *Raunds Furnells: The Anglo-Saxon Church and Churchyard* (London, 1996), 5–15; W. Rodwell and K. Rodwell, *Rivenhall: Investigations of a Villa, Church and Village*, 2 vols, Council for British Archaeology Research Reports 55, 80 (London, 1985–93), 85–96, 130–44; Gem, 'The English Parish Church: A Great Rebuilding?', 23; see Blair, *Church*, 413 for other examples.

22 I. Moretti and R. Stopani, *Chiese Romaniche in Val di Pesa e Val di Greve* (Florence, 1972), cited by D. Bullough, 'The Carolingian Liturgical Experience', in R. N. Swanson, ed., *Continuity and Change In Christian Worship*, Studies in Church History 35 (Woodbridge, 1999), 39, n. 37.

23 Blair, *Church*, 459–63; C. S. Drake, *Romanesque Fonts of Northern Europe and Scandanavia* (Woodbridge, 2001).

24 Gorecki, *Parishes*, 34.

25 M. Miller, *The Formation of a Medieval Church: Ecclesiastical Change in Verona, 950–1150* (Ithaca, NY, 1993), 22–40.

26 Pierre Toubert, *Les structures du Latium medieval: Le Latium méridional et la Sabine du IXe à la fin du XIIe siècle* (Rome, 1973), II, 855–98.

27 G. A. Loud, *Church and Society in the Norman Principality of Capua, 1058–1197* (Oxford, 1985), 220–23.

28 M. Aubrun, *L'ancien diocèse de Limoges des origines au milieu du XIe siècle* (Clermont-Ferrand, 1981).

29 C.-L. Salch and D. Fèvre, 'Réseau paroissial et implantations castrales du IXe au XIIIe siècle en Vivarais', *L'Encadrement religieux des fidèles au Moyen Age et jusqu'au Concile de Trente. Actes du 109e Congrès national des sociétés savants, Dijon, 1984: Section d'histoire médiévale et de philologie* (Paris, 1985), 47–66.

30 Morris, *Churches in the Landscape*, 140–67, esp. 147; Blair, 'Local Churches in Domesday Book and Before', 265–78; idem, *Church*.

31 U. Stutz, 'The Proprietary Church as an Element of Medieval German Ecclesiastical Law', trans. G. Barraclough, *Mediaeval Germany 911–1250* (Oxford, 1938), II. 35–70; P. Imbart de la Tour, *Les origines religieuses de la France: les paroisses rurales du 4e au 11e siècle* (Paris, 1900). See now the masterly revisionist study by S. Wood, *The Proprietary Church in the Medieval West* (Oxford, 2006), especially Part III on lower churches.

32 G. W. O. Addleshaw, *The Development of the Parochial System from Charlemagne (768–814) to Urban II (1088–1099)*, Borthwick Papers 6 (London, 1954), 6–7.

33 Morris, *Churches in the Landscape*, 171.

34 C. 2, II Edgar, *English Historical Documents* I, 395; Addleshaw, *The Development of the Parochial System*, 13.

35 Salch and Fèvre, 'Réseau paroissial'.

36 Toubert, *Les structures du Latium*.

37 L. Watts, P. Rahtz, A. Okasha, S. A. J. Bradley and J. Higgitt, 'Kirkdale – the Inscriptions', *Medieval Archaeology* 41 (1997), 51–99; Blair, *Church*, 358–59.

38 The church is described as a minster in the inscription, and reference is made to a priest, which may suggest that the church was served by a small clerical community: Watts *et al.*, 'Kirkdale – the Inscriptions', 88.

39 A. Williams, 'Thegnly Piety and Ecclesiastical Patronage in the Late Old English Kingdom', in J. Gillingham, ed., *Anglo-Norman Studies 24: Proceedings of the Battle Conference 2001* (Woodbridge, 2002), 1–24 at 15–16.

40 Williams, 'Thegnly Piety'.

41 Gorecki, *Parishes*, 25.

42 R. Morris, *The Church in British Archaeology*, Council for British Archaeology Research Report 47 (London, 1983), 72. Out of a further eighteen possibly Anglo-Saxon churches, thirteen were next to medieval halls or fortifications, ibid.

43 M. Aubrun, *La Paroisse en France, des origines au XV siècle* (Paris, 1986), 212; E. Zadora-Rio, 'Constructions de châteaux et fondation de paroisses en Anjou aux XIe–XIIe siècles', *Archéologie médiévale* 9 (1979), 115–25.

44 For example in the twelfth century at Hanslope in Buckinghamshire the new church became the parish church, and the old church was demoted to the status of a chapel, E. Mason, 'The Role of the English Parishioner 1100–1500', *Journal of Ecclesiastical History* 27 (1976), 17–29 at p. 19. For similar processes in the Lazio, see Toubert, *Les structure du Latium*, II. 855–881.

45 Aubrun, *La Paroisse*, 75.

46 William of Malmesbury, *Vita Wulfstani*, ed. M. Winterbottom and R. M. Thomson, *William of Malmesbury, Saints' Lives* (Oxford, 2002), II. 9, 78–80.

47 Ibid., II. 22, 104–6.

48 Ibid., II. 22, 104.

49 Ibid., II. 17, 94.

50 Ibid., II. 9 (confirmation and preaching), II.15 (penance and preaching and peace making at Gloucester), II.22 (preaching and peace making), 78–80, 88–94, 104–06.

51 Gorecki, *Parishes*, 21–48.

52 As one symbol of display amongst other signs of consumption by new elite: R. Fleming, 'The New Wealth, The New Rich and the New Political Style in Late Anglo-Saxon England', *Anglo-Norman Studies* 23 (2001), 1–22.

53 Wood, *Proprietary Church*, 600.

54 Ibid., 605–06.

55 Aubrun, *La Paroisse*, 211.

56 R. Lennard, *Rural England 1086–1135: A Study of Social and Agrarian Conditions*, Oxford 1959, 297–8.

57 Ibid., 303.

58 Aubrun, *La Paroisse*, 93.

59 Aubrun, *La Paroisse*, 94.

60 Magnou-Nortier, *La société laïque et l'Église dans la province ecclésiastique de Narbonne*, 373.

61 Aubrun, *La Paroisse*, 95, 216.

62 Wood, *Proprietary Church*, 655.

63 D. Stocker and P. Everson, *Summoning St Michael. Early Romanesque Towers in Lincolnshire* (Oxford, 2006), 60–78.

64 Cited by P. Warner, 'Shared Churchyards, Freemen Church-Builders and the Development of Parishes in Eleventh-century East Anglia', *Landscape History* 8 (1986), 39–52 at 41.

65 J. Campbell, 'The Church in Anglo-Saxon Towns', in D. Baker, ed., *The Church in Town and Countryside*, Studies in Church History 16 (1979), 119–35 at 127, citing M. Biddle and J. Keene, 'Winchester in the Eleventh and Twelfth Centuries', in M. Biddle, *Winchester in the Early Middle Ages* (Oxford, 1976), 241–448, 554–556 at 319–25, 498–89.

66 Warner, 'Shared Churchyards', citing F. Barlow, *The English Church 1000–1066: A History of the Later Anglo-Saxon Church* (London, 1979), 193.

67 Warner, 'Shared Churchyards', 50.

68 B. Kümin, 'The English Parish in a European Perspective', in French, Gibbs and Kümin, eds, *The Parish in English Life*, 15–32; Brink, 'The Formation of the Scandinavian parish', 19–44.

69 Wood, *Proprietary Church*, 653; H. Kamen, *The Phoenix and the Flame. Catalonia and the Counter Reformation* (New Haven, 1993), 158.

70 B. Kemp, 'Archdeacons and Parish Churches in England in the Twelfth Century', in G. Garnett and J. Hudson, eds, *Law and Government In Medieval England And Normandy: Essays In Honour of Sir James Holt* (Cambridge, 1994), 341–64 at pp. 343–44.

71 C. N. L. Brooke, 'The Missionary at Home: the Church in the Towns, 1000–1250', in G. J. Cuming, ed., *The Mission of the Church and the Propagation of the Faith*, Studies in Church History 6 (Oxford, 1970), 59–83; Morris, *Churches in the landscape*, 168–69.

72 J. Barrow, 'Urban Cemetery Location in the High Middle Ages', in S. Bassett, ed., *Death in Towns: Urban Responses to the Dying and the Dead, 100–1600* (Leicester, 1992), 78–100.

73 Brooke, 'The Missionary at Home', 76–77; Campbell, 'The Church in Anglo–Saxon Towns', 127.

74 Brooke, 'The Missionary at Home', 64.

75 Ibid., 89.

76 H. Guillotel, 'Du role des cimètieres en Bretagne dans le renouveau du XIe et de la première moitié du xiie siècle', *Memoires de la sociétè d'histoire et d'archéologie de Bretagne* 52 (1972–74), 5–26.

77 N. Baker and R. Holt, 'The Origins of Urban Parish Boundaries', in *The Church in the Medieval Town*, ed. T. R. Slater and G. Rosser (Aldershot, 1998), 209–35.

78 *Anglo-Saxon Chronicle* 'C', 'D', *a.* 1055 cited in Morris, *Churches in the Landscape*, 171.

79 Morris, *Churches in the Landscape*, 171.

80 Williams, 'Thegnly Piety', 7. Seventeen in total of the churches in Norwich recorded in the Domesday Book were held by burgesses.

81 D. A. Stocker, 'Monuments and Merchants: Irregularities in the Distribution of Stone Sculpture in Lincolnshire and Yorkshire in the Tenth Century', in D. Hadley and J. Richards, eds, *Cultures in Contact: Scandinavian Settlement in England in the Ninth and Tenth Centuries* (Turnhout, 2000), 179–212 at 189.

82 Mason, 'The Role of the English Parishioner', 17–29; Duffy, *Stripping*, 132–3.

83 D. Defries, 'The Making of a Minor Saint in Drogo of Saint-Winnoc's *Historia translationis s. Lewinnae*', *Early Medieval Europe* 16 (2008), 423–44 at 426–29; J. Blair, 'Bishopstone, Its Minster and Its Saint: the Evidence of Drogo's *Historia translationis sanctae Lewinnae*', in G. Thomas, *The Later Anglo-Saxon Settlement at Bishopstone: A Downland Manor in the Making*, Council for British Archaeology Research Report 163 (York, 2010), 22–26.

84 C. Davidson Cragoe, 'The Custom of the English Church: Parish Church Maintenance in England before 1300', *Journal of Medieval History* 30 (2010), 20–38.

85 Barlow, *The English Church 1000–1066*, 193; Wood, *Proprietary Church*, 649.

86 Aubrun, *La Paroisse*, 94.

87 Cragoe, 'The Custom of the English Church'.

88 Rodulfus Glaber, *Historiarum libri quinque*, II. 22, 88–91. This case is discussed further in Chapter 9.

89 *Monodiae*, *PL* 156, 954–55; *Self and Society in Medieval France: The Memoirs of Abbot Guibert of Nogent*, trans, J. F. Benton (New York, 1970; repr. Toronto, 1984), III. 18, 217–18.

90 *The Miracles of Our Lady of Rocamadour: Analysis and Translation*, trans. M. Bull (Woodbridge, 1999), I.5, 104–05.

91 Walter Map, *De Nugis Curialium*, II.30, ed. M. R. James, R. A .B. Mynors and C. N. L. Brooke (Oxford, 1983), 206–07.

92 From a seventeenth-century copy of the lost Plympton Priory Cartulary, ed. and trans. by Blair, *Church*, 519–22 at 522.

93 J. Gaudemet, 'La paroisse au moyen âge: état des questions', *Revue d'histoire de l'église de France* 59 (1973), 5–21.

94 J. Charles Cox, *Sanctuaries and Sanctuary Seekers* (London, 1911); for its early medieval history see W. Davies, '"Protected Space" in Britain and Ireland in the Middle Ages', in B. E. Crawford, ed., *Scotland in Dark Age Britain* (Aberdeen, 1996), 1–19; R. Meens, 'Sanctuary, Penance and Dispute Settlement under Charlemagne: The Conflict between Alcuin and Theodulf of Orléans over a Sinful Cleric', *Speculum* 82 (2007), 277–300; for an account of the twelfth-century sanctuary at Hexham, see David Hall, 'The Sanctuary of St Cuthbert', in G. Bonner, D. Rollason and C. Stancliffe, eds, *St Cuthbert, His Cult and His Community to AD 1200* (Woodbridge, 1989), 425–36; on cemeteries as a focus for sanctuary, see Barrow, 'Urban Cemetery Location in the High Middle Ages'.

95 For consecration, see H. Gittos, 'Creating the Sacred: Anglo-Saxon Rites for Consecrating Cemeteries', in S. Lucy and A. Reynolds, eds, *Burial in Early Medieval England and Wales*, Society for Medieval Archaeology Monograph Series 17 (London, 2002), 195–208, where she argues that consecration rites in both England and Frankia originated in the tenth century. B. Rosenwein, *Negotiating Space: Power, Restraint, and Privileges of Immunity in Early Medieval Europe* (Manchester, 1999), 179.

96 Barrow, 'Urban Cemetery Location in the High Middle Ages', 91–4; Guillotel, 'Du role des cimètieres en Bretagne.

97 M. Brett, *The English Church under Henry I* (Oxford, 1975), 233.

chapter 3

Bishops, priests and the wider world: The rhetoric and reality of the 'reforms'

The conduct of a prelate ought so far to transcend the conduct of the people as the life of a shepherd is wont to exalt him above the flock.

Gregory the Great, *Pastoral Care*, II.1[1]

That the bishops should not present a bad example to the people. Bishops and priests ought to manifest and set a good example to the people not only through their words but also their deeds.

Council of Hohenaltheim (916), c. 8[2]

Throughout these three centuries bishops of dioceses all over Europe anxiously tried to ensure that the clergy under their supervision lived pure lives, distinct from their lay counterparts. The dangers of too worldly a lifestyle were not, of course, a source of unease for all bishops at all times, but nevertheless they were a major concern for many of them, especially as regarded that of those members of the clergy responsible for the delivery of pastoral care to the laity. Although in theory bishops had responsibility for both pastoral and monastic clergy within their diocese, in practice their authority over monasteries was often curtailed, and they concentrated their attention on those charged with ministering to the laity – priests, deacons and those in lesser orders.[3] Conciliar proceedings, church law collections, episcopal letters and accounts of bishops' lives all testify to the zeal with which many bishops promoted the idea that those who ministered to the laity should lead lives unsullied by secular demands.

The popularity of clerical reform across this period owes much to its highly practical agenda. Churchmen explained disasters, both natural and manmade, of the sorts which befell Frankia in the early tenth century and England in the eleventh century, as due to widespread disobedience of God's law. Clerical negligence of the law led in turn to lay contempt, and thus Church and people together incurred God's wrath. For example, the official record of the east Frankish Council of Hohenaltheim, held at a time of political instability in 916, stated that the bishops and priests ought to set a good example to the people, not only through their words, but also their deeds. Seven years earlier, in the wake of Viking attacks and famine, the clergy of the archdiocese of Rheims, assembled at the Council of Trosly, had accused the pastoral clergy of abdicating responsibility for the people, of not preaching, and of leading their flock into sin, and sought to introduce remedies to ensure a dignified and zealous clergy.[4] Over a century later Archbishop Wulfstan of Worcester and York raised a similar cry following Viking attacks on England: clerical failures led to more general sinfulness on the part of the laity in their care.[5] Lay transgressions resulted from poor clerical behaviour.

The roots of the idea that those who ministered to the laity should lead exemplary lives, because of their role as moral leaders, lay in Christ's words to His disciples in the Sermon on the Mount: 'You are the salt of the earth', and 'You are the light of the world'.[6] This idea achieved wide circulation through Pope Gregory the Great's (590–604) guide to clerical behaviour, the *Regula pastoralis*. This work was held is such high regard in the ninth century that it became part of the equipment to be given to each bishop at his ordination.[7] Although originally written for bishops, from the early ninth century onwards commentators extended Gregory's ideal of ministry to incorporate the wider priesthood.[8] Gregory described how bishops should act as exemplars to all the members of their flock, both clerical and lay, how they should teach and preach, by word and example, preserve their own purity, be humble, and chide everyone towards the eternal life through ensuring they corrected their behaviour.[9] The early ninth-century bishop of Orléans, Theodulf (d. 821), took up this link between purity and an exemplary life in his guidance to his diocesan clergy:

Whence it is right that you should always be mindful of so great an office, mindful of your consecration, mindful of the holy unction which you have received in your hands, that you do not fall short of the standards set by this office, nor render in vain your consecration, nor pollute with sin the hand anointed with holy oil, but preserving cleanliness of heart and purpose, presenting to the people an example of good living, you should present to those of whom you are in charge guidance to the heavenly kingdom.[10]

Theodulf's statutes were extremely popular in the years 900 to 1200.[11] The overall ideal that the pastoral clergy should lead a pure and exemplary life was, as we shall see, a remarkably static one, one to which episcopal commentators returned again and again.

This idea of clerical purity, cutting oneself off from the demands of the world, owed much to monasticism, but as clergy were expected to live amongst, and interact with, lay society, it brought its own pressures. Commentators identified various markers of clerical status which, taken together, represent a wholesale rejection of the norms of lay society, particularly those of the aristocracy. Clergy should not have sexual relations with women either through marriage or concubinage, nor trade in church offices and property (simony), nor accept or acknowledge the authority of secular lords, nor follow the common aristocratic pursuits of gambling, drinking and hunting. More positively, they expected clerics to adopt distinctive dress and hairstyles and to follow a specific education. Whilst concern about sexual purity remained a constant of reformist critiques between the tenth and twelfth centuries, the degree of interest in other indicators of clerical separation varied across the period, as we shall see.

Clerical reforms thus fit into a familiar narrative of increased separation from the laity through behaviour, education and investiture. Revisiting these changes from the perspective of lay–clerical relations will cast a fresh perspective on these developments and allow us to challenge this view of a single, all-encompassing, clerical reform movement which came to a head under the papal curia in the second half of the eleventh century, and to review the degree to which the expectations and behaviour of the pastoral clergy changed across the years 900 to 1200. This chapter is therefore in two main parts.

In the first part we investigate the rhetoric of clerical reform in more detail. Tracing how the emphasis of episcopal writings on different markers of clerical status changed, across time and place, allows us to identify the extent to which clerical reform and discipline remained a preoccupation of conscientious bishops scattered across Europe throughout the period. Or was it just a consequence of the eleventh-century centrally directed papal reform movement? To what extent did the emphases on different indicators of clerical status vary across the years 900 to 1200? How much did the reformers' idealisation of clerical behaviour owe to earlier legislation? In this section we consider the evidence both for those markers which eleventh-century reformers identified as especially significant – clerical marriage, simony and investiture – but also for those upon which reformers' attention fluctuated across these three centuries: hairstyle, clothing, education. Finally, uncovering the positive as well as negative roles awarded to the laity in reformist rhetoric allows us to reconsider the role of lay agency in changing clerical behaviour.

In the second part we ask how far the reformers really succeeded in transforming the roles played by pastoral clergy in communities across the Latin West. Exploring the evidence for the complex reality of the relations between members of the clergy and the laity, at the level of the episcopate, the local parish, and local communities of clerics, allows us to assess the extent to which changes in emphasis reflect on the one hand the interests of localised reformers, working independently, and on the other the concerns of reforming popes and members of their circle trickling down into local churches. We can investigate, in other words, if papal reformers imposed reform from the top down, working in councils held by the popes themselves and their legates from the mid-eleventh century onwards, or whether the origin and propulsion for clerical reforms lie, in Maureen Miller's words, in the anxiety of lay people about the efficacy of the sacraments and their 'demands . . . that their clergy be held to higher behavioural standards'.[12] Is the increased emphasis on clerical purity part of the growing self-consciousness of the clerical elite as a group set apart from the laity, a movement which Conrad Leyser suggests has its origins in the episcopate of tenth-century Italy?[13] Or is it a reaction to the dynamic and increasingly monetarised economies of Europe, and the laity's consequent moral repugnance directed at a clergy perceived as too tangled up in this world?[14] As we shall see, these may be false alternatives, or rather complementary perspectives on a single phenomenon. Top down and bottom up converged to make the crucial difference of systematic change.

The rhetoric of clerical 'reform'

Distinguishing the clergy from the laity: Expectations and ideals

Each bishop stood at the head of an extensive clerical hierarchy made up of nine grades: doorkeeper, psalmist, lector, exorcist, acolyte, sub-deacon, deacon, priest, and bishop.[15] In practice, bishops sought only to regulate the behaviour of those in the higher echelons: deacon, priest and bishop. As the three aspects of clerical behaviour which most exercised eleventh-century reformers were clerical marriage, simony and lay investiture, we shall begin by considering them in turn.

Clerical behaviour

One of the most important factors which distinguished those at the bottom of the clerical hierarchy from those at the top was the prohibition against clerical marriage and concubinage for those in higher orders. The overt rationale was the demand for purity on the part of those in God's service. C. 14 of Lateran Council IV (1215) enjoined the clergy to 'live chastely and virtuously . . . so that in the sight of Almighty God they may be strong enough to minister with a pure heart and unsullied body'.[16] This passage contain echoes of Bishop Theodulf of Orléans' injunction to his priests four hundred years earlier not to 'render in vain your consecration, nor pollute with sin the hand anointed with holy oil [but preserve] cleanliness of heart and purpose, presenting to the people an example of good living'.[17] But whilst the ninth-century text emphasised how the purity of the priest was essential to his authority as a role model for the 'people' – his flock – Lateran IV stressed instead the importance of purity to the efficacy of the sacramental ministry, perhaps as a result of challenges to sacerdotal authority from the Cathar and Waldensian heresies. Changing circumstances led to changes in emphasis, but both texts owed their essential similarities to a long canonical tradition going back to the fourth and fifth centuries.

Such prohibitions, together with injunctions in favour of an unmarried (celibate) clergy, or at least a sexually inactive and continent one, were a constant of church councils from the early tenth to the early thirteenth centuries. The Council of Trier (927–28) promoted continence and, following Merovingian legislation, it prohibited a priest from allowing a woman to live in his house, and also set out procedures for dealing with priests repeatedly accused of adultery.[18] The canons of the council of the clergy of the East Frankish kingdom held at Augsburg in 952 took up this message, directing, again following late antique church law, that all those clergy in the order of sub-deacon or above involved in a relationship with a woman should be deposed from office, and that no woman should enter the house of a cleric.[19] A reforming English council *c.*969 similarly ordered married clergy to give up their wives on pain of deposition, as did the papal synod of Pavia in 1022, the provincial council of Limoges in 1031, and the reforming council held at Mainz by Pope Leo IX in 1049.[20] The Lateran Council held by Pope Nicholas II in 1059 again condemned clerical marriage, and ordered a boycott of the services of priests who kept concubines.[21] The general tenor of this message in favour of clerical continence continued to be repeated in councils through the later eleventh and twelfth centuries.[22]

Canon law is reiterative and the conciliar decrees drew on canon law but the evidence of more practical texts suggests that enforcement of clerical continence remained an issue for reform-minded bishops throughout the period. In the early tenth century Regino of Prüm instructed a bishop when visiting a local community to ask whether there is any 'suspicion' of any woman being in the priest's house or of his having a wife. The collection also included several canons from earlier church law on the issue.[23] A century later, Bishop Burchard of Worms included Regino's canons in his twenty-book collection of canon law, the *Decretum*.[24] Nor is the reiteration of material confined to canon law. Penitentials were intended to support the bishop and priest in the administration of penance. They record even proximity to a woman as dangerous because it placed a priest in danger: in the view of one tenth-century penitential in Old English: 'A priest who through speech or through glances or scrutiny of a woman pollutes himself and does not want to sin is to fast for 20 days.' The penance should be substantially increased for him 'who with his consent is greatly defiled' to 100 days' fasting.[25] Bishops also used synods to monitor priests' behaviour. One widely circulated checklist of sacerdotal standards from the tenth century, intended to be used by a bishop when addressing his local clergy at a synod, prohibited priests from keeping women in their house, as did the late twelfth-century synodal precepts of Roger de Wawrin, bishop of Cambrai (1179–91).[26] Nor did the issue disappear in the later Middle Ages:

from the thirteenth century onwards medieval visitation records testify to continuing vigilance in this regard.[27]

Simony, the purchase or sale of clerical office, was another long held preoccupation for reform-minded clergy. Named after Simon Magus, who is recorded in Acts (8.18) as trying to buy the gift of the Holy Spirit from the apostle Peter, Pope Gregory I defined it with help from *Isaiah* as the obtaining of clerical office through any kind of remuneration, whether monetary payment or as a reward for service or for flattery.[28] Gregory's own campaign against simony extended into his other writings, especially his letters, and tenth- and eleventh-century authors often cited his sayings.[29] The campaign against simony had not itself been new in the sixth century: councils and synods from the fifth-century council of Chalcedon onwards regularly condemned the practice. The clergy of the tenth and eleventh centuries thus inherited a powerful legacy of texts in the forms of canons, decretals and theological tracts. Simony is not addressed as an issue directly in conciliar canons and episcopal *capitula* from the tenth century. Its absence may be accidental, a reflection of the relative paucity of such texts to survive when compared to the ninth or eleventh centuries, for their provisions reflect a general unease about the sale of other ecclesiastical rites and offices. The east Frankish council of Hohenaltheim (916) enjoined, in the context of criticising those who try to defend communication with excommunicants, that 'we accept the cure of souls from the Lord, not money', whilst that held at Trier in 927–28 forbade charging for services, as did Atto in the *capitula* he composed for the clergy of his diocese, and the authors of the *Admonitio synodalis*.[30] The canons of the Council of Poitiers (*c.*1000) articulated this concern more clearly:

> *A bishop shall not demand gifts for penitence or confirmation. Let no priest receive a gift for penance or for any gift of the Holy Spirit, unless it is freely given.*[31]

Such traces in the textual record represent the continuation of a tradition articulated in the Carolingian episcopal capitularies which forbade taking *munera* (gifts, bribes) hence in effect charging for baptism and burial.[32] They thus reflect both textual traditions and contemporary concerns. But the lack of explicit references to simony *per se* in the tenth century makes it hard to know whether there was, as some historians suggest, a real resurgence of concern about simony only in the eleventh century.[33]

Whatever the apparent lack of interest elsewhere in Europe, in tenth-century Italy two reforming bishops, Rather of Verona and Atto of Vercelli, wrote explicitly about the dangers of simony. Atto, citing Gregory's definition, extended the heresy of simony to cover those involved on both sides of the transaction: the lay princes who sold the bishopric as well as the cleric who bought it, whether through money, flattery, or service. Those who ordained simoniacs polluted the priesthood, and corrupted the people. The ninth-century archbishop, Hincmar of Rheims, had been content to limit the charge of simony to the bishop who obtained cash for ordination; Atto pushed the definition further and saw the contamination of simony spreading and corrupting the whole Church.[34] Bishop Rather viewed simony with similar severity, condemning his fellow clerics for failing to obey canon law, and for continuing, in contravention of canon law, to communicate with those who should be excommunicated for the heresy of simony.[35] Such men contaminated everyone 'since the Lord says, "What the unclean touches will be unclean"'.[36]

There is, therefore, nothing very novel about Pope Leo IX's injunction against the offence of simony at the council of Rheims in 1049. The Rheims canons, like those of tenth-century councils, did not use the word simony but they laid down:

> *That no one should buy or sell sacred orders or ecclesiastical offices or altars; and that if any cleric had bought anything of the sort he should return it to his bishop with suitable satisfaction . . . That no one except the bishop or his representative should presume to exact dues at the entrance of churches. That no one should demand anything as a burial fee or for administering baptism or the Eucharist or for visiting the sick and the dying.*[37]

Leo IX, however, jolted the offence out of the realms of seemingly ineffectual textual condemnation, when he demanded that all those bishops present who were guilty of simony confess their guilt. Whilst most proclaimed their innocence, the Bishop of Langres ran away from the synod in fear and was consequently excommunicated. Bishop Hugh of Nevers made a public confession instead: he declared that his parents had given a lot of money for the bishopric, but he had not known this, and that, fearing for his soul, he would give up his office, if it seemed appropriate to the pope and the assembly, and he matched his words with actions by laying his staff at the pope's feet; Leo then asked him to confirm by oath that the money had been paid without his consent, and then gave him back his office, using a fresh staff. This seemingly novel ritual, of dis- and re-investiture, came about because of the significance that Leo attached to eradicating the practice of simony. It soon caught on, however, and several of Leo's successors, including Alexander II and Gregory VII, used it.[38] It is Leo IX's actions against simoniacal clergy that are new rather than the textual prohibitions of the canons themselves which continued to be repeated at both local and papal councils throughout the late eleventh and twelfth centuries.[39] It is only from the second half of the eleventh century onwards that the accusation of simony became a common theme of high ecclesiastical politics, and thus acquired a reality of its own.

As the story of Hugh of Nevers' resignation and re-investiture makes clear, the ceremonies surrounding entry into episcopal office resonated with meaning. Because bishoprics, as we shall see, acted as important centres of power in the locality, lay authorities sought control over episcopal appointments. Because kings had given lands and rights to bishoprics, the practice of the king investing a new bishop with his temporal properties had become a visible sign of royal authority: the new bishop would swear loyalty to the king and receive from him the insignia of his office that is the pastoral staff and ring. The bishop would then be consecrated by other bishops, but many felt that it was the lay investiture with the symbols of his office which had already made the bishop. Similar ceremonies occurred for entry into abbacies and the priesthood of local churches, as local magnates sought to control appointments to the institutions which they had endowed and which controlled significant resources in their neighbourhood. Whilst eleventh-century writers criticised such practices because they felt they allowed laymen authority over both clergy and ecclesiastical property, lay investiture does not seem to have been an issue in the tenth and early eleventh centuries. Atto of Vercelli criticised the practice whereby lay princes chose bishops, rather than allowing them to be elected by clergy and people, but he allowed the prince to be subsequently consulted, and his consent obtained, prior to the bishop's consecration; he did not, however, mention lay investiture.[40] The west Frankish council of Bourges in 1031 seemingly took action against lay investiture at a lower level, enjoining that laymen should not place priests in office.[41] A member of the papal curia, Cardinal Humbert, raised the issue in his work *Against the Simoniacs* in the 1050s, but the issue only really came into the open at Gregory VII's Lateran Synod, held in November 1078, when amongst the canons is one which states 'That it is forbidden for anyone to receive the investiture of churches from the hands of laymen'.[42] Held at a time of increasing tension in Gregory's relations with King Henry IV, this text needs to be placed in the wider context of a council held, in the words of Gregory's *Register*, for the 'renewal (*restauratione*) of Christendom'; this prohibition is part of what H. E. J. Cowdrey has described as Gregory's policy of the 'moral rearmament of Latin Christendom'.[43] That Gregory attached importance to this measure is clear from the canons of his synod in March 1080 which record how he extended the punitive consequences from churchmen so appointed to also include excommunication of those members of the laity who invested churchmen into their office.[44] Investiture thus became an issue over the course of the eleventh century at both local and papal levels.

Keen to distinguish clergy from their lay counterparts, reformers focused their attention not just on their attitude to women and to office holding, but also on their more general behaviours, reviving ancient prohibitions against drinking, hunting, gambling and bearing weapons. In the words of one text which circulated widely in the tenth and eleventh centuries:

> *Let none of you be drunken or litigious because the Lord's servant ought not to litigate. Let none of you bear arms in sedition, because our arms must be spiritual ones. Let no one indulge in the sport of birds or dogs. Do not drink in taverns.*[45]

The prohibitions against hunting and drinking in taverns and litigation have precedents in the fifth and sixth centuries, whilst that against carrying arms can be found in the ninth century, and continued to be repeated in the twelfth century.[46] Roger de Wawrin, bishop of Cambrai, writing in *c.*1180 forbade priests and ministers of the altar from frequenting taverns, tournaments and ball games on pain of suspension from office. In a nice example of the large gap which often opened up between conciliar aspirations and diocesan attempts to implement them, Roger expanded upon canon 20 of the Third Lateran Council (1178), which merely(!) forbade knights from participating in tournaments, and had not thought it necessary to mention clerical involvement.[47] These prohibitions entered clerical consciousness: when John, abbot of Ford in Somerset, for example, set out to describe the frivolous early life of the twelfth-century hermit Wulfric of

Haselbury he described how 'his priesthood . . . did not prevent him from hunting and hawking, and until his calling he spent his days among men in thrall to worldly vanities'.[48] The occurrence of the same prohibitions in texts intended to educate and instruct churchmen from the early tenth to the late twelfth century suggests these ideas far from being *topoi* are ideals to which conscientious churchmen writing across the period widely subscribed. This review of church law suggests that the eleventh century is by no means unique as a time of clerical reform. But at the same time as many reform-minded clerics espoused and promoted these principles, even more, as we shall see in the second half of this chapter, chose to ignore them.

Clerical appearance

Throughout these three centuries churchmen strove to distinguish clerics not only by their behaviour but also by their appearance, but the emphasis which they put upon different features varied across the period. The tonsure served much the same function as a clerical collar today in marking a clergyman out from other men within society. From the early eleventh century onwards episcopal statutes demanded that all clerics (including monks) should shave their head in a tonsure, and be clean shaven.[49] The canons of the council of Toulouse (1119) went further, imposing excommunication on the 'monk, canon or cleric who would maintain his hair and beard like a layman'.[50]

Reformers also demanded that the clergy differentiate themselves from the laity through their dress. In the words of one widely copied tenth-century text 'Let no one go on the road without a stole; let not one of you wear lay clothes or diverse colours'.[51] The stole served as an acknowledged and public marker of clerical status according to one set of widely circulated canons, originally from late ninth-century East Frankish council of Tribur: a priest should wear distinctive dress whilst travelling because, if he was robbed, wounded or killed when not wearing the stole which marked him out as a priest, then his attacker should make emendation at only one third of the rate he would have to pay if his victim's sacerdotal status had been clear. Steeper punishments for attacks on clerics when compared to members of the laity are a common feature of early medieval church law. These canons also defined lay dress as follows: clerics should not wear lay vestments – a mantel or a coat without a cap – nor precious shoes, nor other new vanities but rather religious and decent habits.[52] Nothing in these canons is particularly new and both Regino of Prüm and Burchard of Worms cited them in their canon law collections, alongside material from a fifth-century collection which directed that clerics dress according to their profession, and eschew decorated shoes and vestments.[53] The issue of clerical dress had not, however, been of great interest to the early ninth-century Carolingian bishops, although the rule for clerical canons approved at the Council of Aachen in 816 specified that, following the writings of the Holy Fathers, they should 'refrain from excessive and ostentatious dress'.[54] Their *capitula* focused instead on sacerdotal purity in the service of the Mass: that sacerdotal vestments should be reserved for the Mass, and thus not become contaminated, and that priests be properly equipped; to this end priests should bring their mass vestments to the synod for inspection. It is thus only really from the end of the ninth century that distinctive clerical dress became a concern.

Tenth-century Italian bishops followed the interests of their late ninth-century Frankish predecessors in attributing greater significance to clerical dress: 'habitus' can mean both dress and behaviour, and therefore criticism of dress carried with it other moral baggage. Rather, bishop of Verona, using the Pauline language of renewal, criticised those of his clergy who 'take off the clothing of God, put on that of the world and do not even shrink from dressing in lay garments' as guilty of a serious fault.[55] Adopting lay dress was for Rather part of a catalogue of vices amongst his clergy, whereby they signalled their neglect for their flock, and failed to act as appropriate examples, indulging instead in secular games, and wanton hunting. It thus facilitated sinful behaviour, and acted as an indicator of it. Atto, bishop of Vercelli also bade his clergy in his *capitula* not to wear secular clothes but rather the sacerdotal tunic.[56] Combined with the legal evidence from reformers in east Frankia these Italian writings suggest tenth-century reformers, like their late ninth-century counterparts, sought to distinguish priests from the laity through their dress.

Concern that pastoral clerics should differentiate themselves from the laity through their dress as well as their more general behaviour runs across the episcopal legislation of later centuries. But it was not consistently expressed. Although the Tribur canons circulated in the eleventh century through Burchard's *Decretum*, the clerical reformers associated with the mid-eleventh-century papal court paid little attention to clerical dress, focusing their attention instead on marriage, simony and lay investiture.[57]

Explicit reminders about the need for distinctive clerical dress emerged again only in late eleventh-century Italy. Amongst a series of canons concerned to separate the clergy from the laity at the Council of Melfi, held in Norman-controlled southern Italy by Pope Urban II in 1089, one states:

> *So that all causes of scandal, all suspicions be removed from the laity, we prohibit clergy henceforth to wear cut clothing (scissis vestibus) and we admonish that they should not dress in ornate garments.*[58]

The reference to cut clothing is unclear but suggests some sort of ostentation; it may refer to garments which had been pinked to give a decorative edge, or perhaps slashed to reveal an undergarment.[59] The issue of dress surfaced next in France in the 1130s: the canons of the Councils of Claremont (1130) and Rheims (1131) formed the basis for c.4 of the Second Lateran Council (1139):

> *bishops as well as clergy take pains to be pleasing to God and to humans in both their interior and exterior comportment. Let them give no offence in the sight of those for whom they ought to be a model and example, by the excess, cut or colour of their clothes, nor with regard to the tonsure, but rather, as is fitting for them, let them exhibit holiness. If, after a warning from the bishops, they are unwilling to change their ways, let them be deprived of their ecclesiastical benefices.*[60]

Taking the age-old theme that the clergy should act as an example for the laity, the bishops assembled in the Lateran palace in 1139 insisted that humble and modest dress constituted an important part of that model. Dress continued to be of interest to reformers in the late twelfth century. Roger de Wawrin, bishop of Cambrai, in his synodal precepts for his clergy, specified that they should wear closed garments and cloaks with a sleeve. In order to serve the altar with honour they should appear as ordained ministers in a habit and tonsure.[61] Abandoning both distinctive dress and haircut were interpreted as an abandonment of the clerical life. In other words although never at the forefront of their concerns, the desire to make sure that the clergy stood out from the laity through their appearance as well as their behaviour constituted an important part of churchmen's efforts to separate the clergy from the laity throughout this period.

But this revival of interest in clerical dress should not be interpreted as a product of changes in pan-European reformist rhetoric, for this rhetoric is only invoked within specific local contexts. Churchmen used clerical dress to indicate their disapproval of a particular group, signalling at the same time their own allegiance to reformist ideals and the path of righteousness. For example, the decision to depict a cleric, distinguishable by his tonsure but dressed identically to laymen, in the late eleventh-century Bayeux Tapestry was probably intended as an explicit critique of the clergy of the Anglo-Saxon Church.[62] Adopting clerical dress signified reforming allegiances in twelfth-century east Frankia as well. Norbert of Xanten's biographer recorded how, in the early twelfth century, Norbert dressed as a layman in silks whilst a cleric in minor orders, living as a sub-deacon at the episcopal court in Cologne; for him clerical dress was a sign of Norbert's ordination to the priesthood and adoption of a more religious life.[63] Norbert went on to found the Praemonstratensian order of canons, an order characterised by their commitment to an active, apostolic life, preaching by example in the world. Wearing clerical dress marked him out from the laity, the unreformed clergy and monks, but at the same time served to indicate his mission to serve as member of a religious order in the world. Such preoccupations with clerical dress thus point to a more complicated reality. The eleventh-century reforms did not generate a sudden interest in clerical dress; rather from the ninth-century onwards churchmen subscribed to, and promoted, the view that clerics should distinguish themselves from both monks and laymen by adopting their own dress code.

Clerical education

Church law expected the clergy to set an example to the laity not only through their way of life, but also through their preaching. This required education. The problem of clerical ignorance is a constant refrain of episcopal legislation from the Carolingian period onwards; untrained, those serving as local priests must be reminded of their duties, and so bishops should use the diocesan synod to check on the level of learning amongst their clergy. In the somewhat defeatist tone of the *Admonitio synodalis*,

> *Let him understand well the prayers of the Mass and the canon, and, if not, at least let him be able to quote them from memory clearly. Let him be able to read the epistle and the gospel well, and would that he could explain its meaning, at least its literal meaning. Let him know how to pronounce the words of the psalms regularly by heart, along with usual*

> *chants. Let him know by heart . . . the sermon of Bishop Athanasius about the creed of the Trinity.He must be able to utter distinctly the exorcisms and prayers for making catechumens, for blessing the water also, and the rest of the [baptismal] prayers over male and female both for individuals and in the plural. Likewise, he must at least know how to say well the order of baptism for helping the sick, and according to the manner canonically reserved for it the order of reconciling and anointing the sick, and the prayers also relating to that necessity. Likewise the order and prayers for making the obsequies of the dead, likewise the exorcisms and benedictions of salt and water he should know by heart. He should know the day and night chants. He should know the lesser computus, that is, the epacts and Easter chronology, and the rest, if possible, and he should have a martyrology and a penitential.*[64]

This extensive checklist of what local priests should know had its origins in the early ninth-century episcopal *capitula* of Bishops Theodulf of Orléans and Haito of Basle, but variants on it circulated in the tenth and early eleventh centuries in Italy, England and Frankia.[65] The focus is on the knowing the words for the liturgy – the priest is expected to memorise a good deal, even if he cannot always understand it; the focus is on practice whilst comparable thirteenth-century prescriptions focus on schemes of knowledge like the seven sins. The widespread copying of prescriptive texts, such as the *Admonitio synodalis*, and other synodal sermons, which occurs in this period indicates that many bishops envisaged the diocesan synod as the place for such instruction.[66] Their practical focus tells us about the limited, but detailed, expectations of priests by their superiors.

The process of clerical education preoccupied bishops as much as agreeing on what knowledge needed to be taught. Some bishops composed, and perhaps even used, examinations of candidates' knowledge prior to ordination.[67] One ninth-century text, for example, asks that good priests should testify that the candidate for ordination is literate, chaste, sober, from a good home, and of good morals. It outlines the duties expected of a priest, and emphasises that he should be chaste and keep the sacrament pure: only the clergy should distribute the Eucharist.[68] The emphasis on purity distances the priest from the laity at the same time as the emphasis on pastoral duties brings them into contact with the laity. The practice continued throughout the period. Bishop Roger of Worcester (1164–79) was portrayed as a model bishop who always examined candidates for the priesthood before their ordination, but there was nothing new about his concern with training.[69]

Education itself might often be a haphazard affair: as Bishop Rather of Verona reminded his clergy at a Lenten synod in 966, ordinands must have been 'educated in letters a little', either 'in our city, or in some monastery, or at the house of some wise man' if they were to be 'suitable for the ecclesiastical dignity'.[70] Rather himself made some provision for the education of his own clergy by setting aside funds for his lesser clergy so they did not have to rush to ordination as priests before they were ready. Other bishops made more systematic efforts to train clergy in cathedral schools. Writing in the early eleventh century, Burchard of Worms described his *Decretum* as 'a little book for the work of our fellow priests', in which he sought to bring together laws from various sources, for 'young boys for study' so that they might 'first be made apt students and afterwards both leaders and teachers of the people, and let them learn in schools what some day they ought to say to those committed to their care'. He warned that they need a comprehensive education, for 'If the blind leads the blind, both fall into the ditch'.[71] The fact that he dedicated the book to the provost of his cathedral, the man in charge of the cathedral school, confirms he envisaged it as having a didactic function. A very substantial work, it is divided into some twenty books, and can only ever have served as a reference work for those with access to the cathedral library. How then was it used to train future priests? The answer, it has been suggested, lies in the questionnaire on penance in Book XIX which summarises the contents of the laws recorded in the preceding eighteen books. Laid out as a series of almost two hundred questions about whether the penitent had committed a particular sin, accompanied by the appropriate penance, it thus served as a sort of *aide-mémoire* for students charged with delivering penance to the laity.[72] The wide scope of this questionnaire, ranging as it does from murder to very specific fertility charms attributed to women via robbery and fornication, is testament to Burchard's ambitions, but is also impractical: could local priests really be expected to master the minutiae of church law in this detail and at the same time to know the prayers and rites for the administration of the other pastoral services besides penance, namely those for baptism, visitation of the sick and burial of the dead, and, most importantly, the Mass? Most eleventh-century reformers clearly thought not: the manuscripts of the *Decretum* remained within the confines of the cathedral and monastic libraries of Europe, and Book XIX only occasionally circulated independently. They represent reformers' aspirations rather than very practical attempts to implement their ideas.

Concern for clerical education is not confined to the cathedral school or diocesan synod. Others took up this challenge to educate the pastoral clergy, as indicated by the survival of much shorter pastoral handbooks, containing everything a local priest needed to know in order to fulfil his ministry. One such codex is now in the Vatican Library; it was probably originally composed for the community of clergy which served the church of SS. XII Apostoli in Rome sometime in the eleventh century. Composed of two different parts which were probably joined together in the second half of the eleventh century, its contents now closely resemble the checklist of knowledge expected of the clergy in the ninth-century *Admonitio synodalis*: the codex supplied the priest with the prayers for the mass, for baptism, for the visitation of the sick, the services for the dead, the blessings for salt and water, a *computus* and Easter table, a martyrology and a penitential. Much less ambitious in scope than Burchard, the author of this very practical guide clearly intended to support and educate those involved in the pastoral ministry by providing a text of routine prayers and services, together with texts for the more occasional, but no less important, things they needed to know, namely the date of Easter, the feasts of the martyrs in the Christian year, and guidance on how to administer penance.[73] Further it contains a didactic poem on the *Vita pastoralis*, which provides a brief guide on the duties and behaviour of the priest: he should guard his sheep carefully, read and study, know the seven canonical hours, and when they should be observed, remember the importance of attending the synod, know the significance of baptism and of the mass and how it is to be celebrated, refrain from accepting money for services, from carrying arms, and from marrying, and know the importance and significance of penance and the rites for the dying. The inclusion of such a mnemonic points to an educative function for the codex: perhaps its compiler intended it for training members of the clergy in pastoral care rather than for direct use itself in the field.[74] It is not unique. Another example of a priest's handbook is now known as the Red Book of Darley. Composed in southern England in *c.*1061, it combines a sacramentary with rites for baptism and the visitation of the sick and burial of the dead. It is just the sort of codex which a parish priest would need for his ministry. The instructions in the pastoral rites are even given in Old English, rather than Latin, and expanded in places on those found in similar Latin rites, making clear, for example, the exact role of godparents in the rite of baptism. These rubrics hint at the book's pedagogic function and suggest it was intended to train pastoral clergy in the delivery of the most important Christian rites, rather than just be used by such a priest in his daily ministry.[75] Its educational purpose perhaps explains why it survived: it was the property of a religious institution, intent on educating priests, rather than an individual priest. Institutional inertia therefore explains why it was kept rather than destroyed after it had ceased to be used. Many local priests may have possessed similar books, but these have not survived; the forces which acted to preserve institutional holdings were not at work in the case of individuals, whose books would be dispersed on their death to be used until no longer relevant, then perhaps sold for their parchment.

Most of these prescriptions to distinguish clerics from the laity through their behaviour, appearance and education are aimed at priests and bishops. The standards set for deacons could be lower, and reformers did not always completely agree as to what they should be. For example the late tenth-century Anglo-Saxon reformer Ælfric of Eynsham enjoined clerical celibacy on bishops, priests *and deacons* whilst his contemporary, Archbishop Wulfstan of Worcester and York, with whom he was in contact, allowed deacons to marry.[76] Such differences notwithstanding, the standards expected of the clergy remained pretty constant across these three centuries. The novelty of the clerical reforms of the later eleventh and twelfth centuries lies not in their ideas, but rather the ambitious scale on which they were promoted. There was little new about the reforming desires expressed by members of the papal curia in the mid-eleventh century, or by reformers in the later twelfth century; rather, individual reforming bishops at local levels can be found throughout the period. Furthermore, the frequent reiteration of these ideas is testimony not just to the conservatism of the higher clergy but to the fact that each generation of clergy would need to be taught them anew. In asking them to live up to them, the reformers sought to create a very clear alternative model of life, far removed from the normal social behaviour and appearance expected of secular men.[77] Many failed to live up to these standards, choosing instead to behave and dress like their lay counterparts. Their continual failure to live up to these high standards is not particularly surprising, but it had implications for the depiction of the laity in reformist rhetoric as well.

The laity's roles

The construction of this clerical ideal, based upon purity, inevitably required a counter image: that of the laity. The pure clergy are defined by what they are not as much as by what they are: they are not to marry, cohabit with concubines, or to be contaminated by contact with money or service to a secular lord, or to hunt, drink in taverns or wear elaborate and worldly dress. They should reject the normal indicators of secular manhood and instead offer to the people 'an example of good living', in Theodulf's words. By following Christ's injunction to exemplify his precepts, they should imitate him; their distinctive tonsure represented Christ's crown of thorns.[78] The laity thus provided the counter ideal against which the clergy should be compared.

At the same time the laity often features in reformist texts as a body which judges the behaviour of the clergy and finds it wanting. Such references must be treated with care: the laity in such texts often represent clerical aspirations rather than the actual demands of secular men and women. For example, Bishop Rather of Verona, writing to a fellow bishop in 963, suggested that the laity would distrust a pastor who obtained his office through simony:

> *For when those of the secular number who are not utterly uneducated hear that on the second day of Pentecost Jesus said to His disciples (that is both those who then were his disciples and those today who do not hate His discipline, that is His teaching, correction and commandments): 'He who does not enter the sheepfold by the door but comes in by another way, that man is a thief and a robber' (John 10.1), they are not unaware that the Truth cannot lie and also that it follows that he who is a thief cannot also be a shepherd; and they understand that the sheepfold is the Church, in that it contains those sheep who will be set up at the right hand in judgement . . . that the shepherd is the lawful bishop, and that the thief is the false bishop . . . What do they care about the blessing of one whom they know to be accursed, since Gregory [the Great] says that the blessing is turned into a curse for him who is promoted so as to become a heretic?*[79]

Rather went on to condemn his fellow clerics for ignoring canon law which excommunicated simoniacs, arguing that the laity will feel justified in making light of episcopal excommunication and absolution if they see the clergy ignoring the law. His portrait of the laity here is totally unrealistic: he expects them to have some knowledge of Scripture, and to be able to go beyond its literal sense to interpret it within an exegetical framework. He is using them as figures to express his own critique of the behaviour of their pastors, and to explain its effects on episcopal authority. The laity thus served as a rhetorical device to substantiate Rather's wider argument about the consequences of clerical simony and negligence.

But not all mentions of lay criticism can be dismissed as rhetorical, for lay nobles had long been showing in very practical terms their enthusiasm for clerical 'reform'. From the beginning of our period there is evidence of members of the laity taking action against individual impure priests. Bishop Mancio of Châlons-sur-Marne (895–910) wrote to Fulk, the archbishop of Rheims (883–900) to report that Angelric, the priest of the church of St Lupus in the villa of Wasnau had confessed, in the course of a diocesan synod, that he had been betrothed to one of his parishioners, Grimma, with the consent of her relations, but when he came to marry her some 'good, pious and faithful men' had opposed this most wretched act. Bishop Mancio himself was undecided as to what to do, and had temporarily suspended Angelric whilst he asked his superior for advice on what action he should take, sending the priest himself as letter-bearer. The group who objected are described as 'homines', (lay)men, not 'clerici'.[80] It is not, however, clear whether they objected to Angelric and Grimma's marriage because of an abstract preference for clerical celibacy, as indicated by the reference to their piety and faithfulness, or whether they merely used the language of clerical purity to object to a union they feared would disrupt power structures within their village. Certainly, as we shall see, there are plenty of examples where priests' wives were accepted by the local community. At the same time as commentators emphasised the importance of purity to service at the altar, celibacy elevated priests above the mundane ties of kinship, allowing them to act as independent peacemakers and mediators within the community: marriage may have signalled a taking of sides, leading those left out of the new alliance to object.

A very different community in which widespread lay concern for clerical purity was also invoked by one party anxious to criticise another was mid-eleventh-century Milan.[81] Here the expression of lay concern and the outcome were very different. At this time a thriving economic centre, Milan represents a rather different world to that of the late ninth-century north

French countryside. The subject of dispute in Milan was clear: in the words of one writer, Andreas of Strumi:

> *At that time the clerical order was led astray into many errors that scarcely one amongst it could be found who followed the right way. For some gave themselves over to hunting with dogs and falcons, others kept inns and managed estates, others proved to be usurers; almost all lived a disgraceful life either with wives or public prostitutes.*[82]

A member of a reformist monastic order, the Vallombrosans, which was heavily involved in campaigning for clerical reform in Florence, Andreas wrote his account of events in Milan some twenty years after they occurred, in *c.*1075, in order to defend not only the Milanese reformers against criticism from the old guard but also to defend the Vallombrosans' general vision for active reform.[83] Nevertheless the parallels between the lifestyle Andreas attributed to the Milanese clergy and the prohibitions on clerical behaviour in ecclesiastical legislation of the time are striking. The reformers subscribed to what were already widely accepted standards for clerical behaviour. Andreas describes how his subject, Ariald, one of the reformers' leaders, pointed out the impurity of the established Milanese clergy and their failure to live up to Christ's exemplary ideal, and called on the laity to refuse to attend the churches and services of sinful clergy:

> *Consider* your priests *who are more rich in worldly goods, more illustrious in building towers and houses, more puffed up with honours, and more beautiful in their soft, choice garments: these are considered more blessed. Indeed these, as you know, openly take wives just like laymen, pursue debauchery just like the most wicked laymen, and to top off this impiety, they are more powerful for being less weighed down with earthly labour, since, of course, they are living off what was given to God. Christ, on the contrary, sought and desired such purity in his ministers that he condemned the evil of debauchery not only in their works, but also in their hearts, saying 'he who shall have looked lustfully at woman has already copulated with her in his heart' (Matt. 5.23). Look into your hearts, dearest ones, look and learn to embrace the true and reject the false.'*[84]

Ariald's message appealed for direct action by members of the laity. He spoke in Gregorian terms of three orders in the church: the preachers, who should exhort the faithful; the continent, who should pray constantly; and the married, who should work with their hands and support religion through almsgiving. He is reported to have preached that action in support of reform was a religious duty, and that inaction against simony, for example, implies acceptance, and therefore guilt by association: the laity should not merely boycott the services of sinful clergy, but rather prevent them from serving at the altar. They should therefore actually fight as well as give alms to repel and destroy simony.[85] One example of such direct action is recorded. Ariald is reported to have set up a community of clerics living the common life in a church donated by its lay proprietor who, heeding the critique against simony, took direct action and removed the previous incumbent who had acquired the office through payment.[86]

When the rhetoric of lay criticism was realised in such a concrete fashion as this, it was very difficult for those on the side of established authority to accept it. Opposition to the reformers was resilient and violent.[87] Two of their leaders were murdered: the cleric Ariald in 1066 and the knight, Erlembald, in 1075. Two clerics, and chroniclers, of the church of Milan, Arnulph and Landulph, wrote accounts critical of the reformers and their activities. Whilst supportive of the need for reform, Arnulph was particularly scornful of the role played in the movement by the lay knight Erlembald and his links to the Roman papal curia which generally supported the movement's attempts to reform the Milanese clergy. The Milanese higher clergy, and their supporters, preferred to look to their fourth-century bishop, Ambrose, as a source of authority for their own customs rather than St Peter and his successors, the popes in Rome. Arnulph commented on Erlembald's links to Rome:

> *Teachers should mind the judgement which Paul uttered absolutely:* If someone preaches another Gospel than the one which you have received, let him be anathema. *When we say these things, however, we are not opposing you, O Roman lords, since our teacher Ambrose says:* I wish to follow the Roman Church in all things. *Truly we believe with you and renounce all heresies with you, but it seems valid to us that a doctor of the Church should display an ecclesiastical right rather than an uneducated layman (*idiota laicus*).*[88]

Arnulph did not oppose the message of reform, which he attributed to the pope in Rome who had in 1061 appointed Erlembald his representative in

Milan, but rather felt that it should come from within the local clergy and not be forced on them by the laity.

Whilst Bishop Mancio's letter hints at tensions within the small village community of Wasnau, Ariald's reforms hint at wider conflicts within a large and diverse city. At both the micro level of a late ninth-century west Frankish village and the macro level of a bustling city in the eleventh century, with its ancient and self-consciously Ambrosian church, tensions within the community were articulated through calls for clerical purity.[89] Ariald may well have been a deacon in the very Church of Milan which he criticised, whilst the movement's lay leaders, the brothers Landulph and Erlembald, seem to have come from a leading noble family within the city. The origins of the conflict came not from outside, but rather from within Milan and perhaps originated in competition for leases of church property at a time of increasing prosperity, for the reforming party seem to have attracted eclectic support from all classes within Milanese society.[90] In both cases, however, the ideals of clerical purity had become part of the wider politics of a community.

Clerical writers never interpreted sinful behaviour on the part of the clergy as a solely clerical matter; treating the services of simoniac and incontinent clergy as contaminated, they inevitably drew the lay 'other' in as possible judges. The accounts of how the eleventh-century reforming clergy called on the laity to take action against the impure clergy need to be read in this rhetorical tradition. The clergy assembled at the council of Limoges/Bourges in 1031, for example, actively courted the laity, calling for lay collaboration in their efforts to promote clerical celibacy: no one should marry the daughter or widow of a priest, or give his daughter to marry a priest, deacon or sub-deacon.[91] Gregory VII called in 1075 on the dukes of Suabia and Carinthia to boycott the 'ministrations of those [they] know either to have been promoted simoniacally or ordained or [who are guilty of] fornication'.[92] Rather than reading these two examples as evidence for the cause being opened up to include the laity, in recording particular efforts to persuade the laity to subscribe to the enforcement of clerical reform, their authors testify to widespread lay disinterest in the cause.

It was not, however, totally lost. As the cases from Wasnau and Milan suggest, the laity are never merely rhetorical figures in reformist tracts but rather they could sometimes act to implement reform. Just as rhetoric specified that the clergy act as pastors of their lay flock, so the laity were expected to monitor the behaviour of their clergy and ensure their separation from the lay world. Yet when they did so, their reformist message often met with resistance and criticism, and clerics all too often regarded the boycotting of the services of unworthy priests as the heresy of donatism. For example two twelfth-century penitentials from southern Italy included canons forbidding the rebaptism of children who had been baptised already by heretics or schismatics, and stating that the worthiness of the priest, even when a heretic, does not affect the validity of the Eucharist. These canons are not commonly found in other penitentials, and seem to have been included to meet a widespread concern about the validity of the ministry of impure clergy amongst the lay congregations of southern and central Italy, perhaps as a result of events in the north half a century earlier.[93] Whilst the twin threads of normative and descriptive evidence suggest that the laity were expected to, and did, play an important role in the reform of the clergy, it clearly remained a contentious one throughout this period.

The reality of the clergy's relations with the laity

Investigating the extent to which the reformist ideals and language considered above were realised in the lives of individual bishops and priests during this period is an equally problematic endeavour. Various questions need to be borne in mind before making such an attempt. What was the nature of relations between the individual members of the pastoral clergy and members of their lay congregations, and when and where did these change across the period? How far did the pastoral clergy really become more clearly distinguished as a group within society, separated by both lifestyle and appearance from their lay counterparts? Or did they instead remain constrained by the expectations of their birth families and structures of lordship within the overall structures of the secular world? Whilst it is impossible to answer all three questions with any degree of certainty for all areas of the medieval west across three centuries, nevertheless the evidence for the lives of both bishops and local priests in these periods, starting with that for the episcopate, suggests that the impact which these aspirations had on the lives of churchmen varied as much according to local circumstance as to Europe-wide changes over time.

Bishops

Throughout these three centuries the office of bishop constituted an important one, both at the level of noble power within a locality and at the level of the royal court. Theoretically responsible for both the local churches and monasteries within his diocese, the bishop usually controlled significant resources, in the form of both lands and rights. He also possessed considerable intangible, ideological capital, in the form of the authority he theoretically exercised over his diocesan clergy: the bishop alone could bless the chrism, essential to both baptism and the rites for the dying, he alone could consecrate new churches, and ordain people into holy orders.[94] Although such episcopal rights were vulnerable to the grants of immunity from them made to monastic institutions, and dioceses varied considerably in size and wealth between different regions, the episcopate nevertheless remained a powerful institution throughout the Latin West in this period.[95]

In the appalled eyes of mid-eleventh-century reformers, like their tenth-century predecessors, the lives of the secular clergy, epitomised by those of their bishops, remained mired in the secular world. Clerics routinely made a gift (of land or money) to obtain office (simony), married or cohabited with women, were tempted to make their office hereditary, to transfer church property to members of their own family, and were appointed or invested into office by laymen. Hence the concern by reformers that bishops should be elected by the clergy and 'people', that is the elite, of the diocese, in line with canon law, rather than being chosen by individual noblemen or rulers. Hence their concern to separate the lives of the pastoral clergy from those of their congregations and to safeguard church property.

Yet investigation of the family backgrounds of bishops reveals the great extent to which their lives remained entrenched within those of the social and political elite across the period 900 to 1200. The tangible benefits to aristocratic families were clear. It has been estimated, for example, that almost a quarter of the land leased out during the pontificate of the reforming tenth-century bishop of Worcester, Oswald (961–92) went to his relations, that is his brother, nephew and nieces.[96] Many bishops, in theory elected by their church, in fact owed their office to their relations. The most prominent cases concern members of the royal family. Otto I of Germany, for example, appointed his brother Bruno to the metropolitan see of Cologne in 953, his son, William, to that of Mainz in 954, and his cousins to the sees of Trier, Verdun, and Utrecht.[97] This practice did not end with the late eleventh-century papacy's efforts to promote free canonical elections: Roger, bishop of Worcester (1164–79) was the son of the earl of Gloucester and grandson of King Henry I; Otto, bishop of Freising (1137–58) was related to four rulers of Germany, being the grandson of Henry IV, the nephew of Henry V, half-brother of Conrad III, and uncle of Frederick I Barbarossa.[98] But the practice was not confined to the royal family. In east Frankia Carlrichard Brühl has estimated that 93 per cent of eleventh- and twelfth-century bishops whose origins are known came from the higher nobility, of whom perhaps 23 per cent were members of the royal family.[99] A study of Neustrian bishops between 950 and 1050 demonstrates that appointments to these sees almost always came from powerful noble families, and that some families might control the see for several generations.[100] Adhemar of Chabannes described as a matter of course how in south-west France on the death of Ebalus, count of Poitou and duke of Aquitaine (d. 935), 'one of his sons became the count, the other the bishop' of Limoges.[101] The practice continued into the later period: the eleventh-century archbishops Hugh and Arnoul of Tours both came from the same family, that of the viscounts of Châteaudun.[102] In Burgundy, of eighteen bishops elected to the see of Auxerre between 950 and 1250 only two came from outside the region.[103] Sees might often remain under the control of the same family for several generations. Five successive eleventh-century bishops of Worms, including Burchard, the compiler of the *Decretum*, came from the same family, albeit in Hesse rather than the area immediately around Worms.[104] Members from two branches of the same family occupied the see of Metz between 929 and 965, and again between 984 and 1089.[105] It is no surprise, therefore, to discover that noble birth was regarded as a *sine qua non* of episcopal office throughout this period; unsuccessful rivals accused their opponents of being of low birth whilst the early twelfth-century canon lawyer, Bishop Ivo of Chartres (1090–1115) even went so far as to defend one bishop against the accusation that his election was invalid on the grounds that he was both well-born and legally elected.[106]

Some local studies from northern France suggest that from the late eleventh century onwards bishops began to come from a slightly lower social stratum. The papal reformers' efforts to ensure the conduct of episcopal elections according to church law meant that the cathedral chapter began to play a much stronger role in them, with the result that the control of particular sees passed from the hands of the comital dynasties, who had appointed family members to them in the tenth and eleventh centuries, into those of lesser nobles in the twelfth century. Families whose authority became confined much more locally to the area, and, indeed, largely derived from their association with the see, then came to dominate particular bishoprics. For example, the families of the lords of Quierzy and of Bazoches, who were related to each other by marriage, held the see of Soissons for much of the twelfth and thirteenth centuries.[107] This particular chronology only works for northern France. Before the mid-eleventh-century papal reforms in tenth- and eleventh-century England the great secular magnates preferred to focus their attention on the wealth of monasteries, leaving control of bishoprics to lesser nobles. The late eleventh-century bishop of Worcester, Wulfstan II, for example, came from a family who were tenants of the church of Worcester in south-east Warwickshire: his father was a priest, then a monk, whilst one of his brothers became a monk at Worcester.[108] Whereas in northern France bishoprics' wealth made the focus for magnates' ambitions in the tenth and eleventh centuries, in England at the same time monasteries were the target, and the relatively poorer bishoprics came under the control of the lesser nobility. Different distributions of local power and wealth, in other words, determined who became bishop, and who constituted the political players behind his appointment. Such trends are not as influenced by broader ecclesiastical changes as one might, at first, suppose.

Clerical relations as much as lay ones determined successful election to a bishopric. Those who argue that bishops came to be drawn from a lower social class in the twelfth century also argue simultaneously for the increasing role of nepotism in determining promotion to higher clerical and episcopal office. But clerical dynasties can be found throughout this period. Families commonly tried to keep sees within the family. The *Life* of Burchard, Bishop of Worms (d. 1025), written shortly after its subject's death, recounts how Burchard eventually succeeded his brother Franco as bishop of Worms. Otto III appointed Franco bishop in 999. Whilst on Lenten retreat with the emperor in a cave near San Clemente in Rome, Franco extracted a promise from him that his brother should succeed him. On Franco's death the emperor did not immediately remember his promise: he appointed not one but two different candidates, but both died soon afterwards, before the emperor remembered and appointed Burchard to a long and productive pontificate.[109] Fraternal succession is presented here as legitimate and predestined. It is a not uncommon pattern. The brothers Heribert (1022–42) and Gezemann (d. 1042) succeeded each other as bishops of Eichstätt, as did brothers Warmann (1026–34) and Eppo/Eberhard (1034–46) to the see of Constance.[110] The pattern of nephew succeeding an uncle is perhaps more widespread and continued throughout the period. The tenth-century English reformer Dunstan, abbot of Glastonbury and archbishop of Canterbury (959–88) was probably the nephew of Athelm, archbishop of Canterbury, and a relation of Ælfheah, bishop of Winchester.[111] In eleventh-century Flanders, Lietbert, bishop of Cambrai (d. 1076) grew up in the household of his predecessor and uncle, Bishop Gerard (d. 1051).[112] In twelfth-century Italy, Bishop Ubald of Gubbio (d. 1160) succeeded his uncle, Bishop Johannes Grammaticus, in 1128.[113] We know about these examples because of the *Lives* written to commemorate their subjects: their authors not only recorded these examples of nepotism but remembered and celebrated the spiritual authority which consequently accrued to the family alongside the lands. These particular sees became centres for family memory as well as authority.

The mechanisms by which families sought to keep their hold on ecclesiastical office did not change across these three centuries. It was normal for uncles to exercise influence on behalf of their nephews to ensure they obtained powerful positions, albeit not necessarily in the same see. Archbishop Anno of Cologne, regent for King Henry IV of Germany, appointed his nephew Cuno, first as archdeacon of Cologne, and then to the archiepiscopal see of Trier. Unfortunately the lay protector of the see objected to Cuno's appointment and fatally attacked him; he put Cuno in chains, threw him down a rock and stabbed him to death. This story is a testament to the opposition such attempts at clerical autonomy might meet when put into action.[114] The role of nepotism in twelfth-century England is made particularly clear by the career of Gilbert Foliot, who both benefited from it, and practised it in turn. He began his career as abbot of Gloucester (1139–48), a position he seems to have owed to two uncles: one, Reginald, abbot of Evesham had been a monk there, the other, Milo, earl of Hereford, was castellan of Gloucester. He subsequently became bishop of Hereford (1148–63) and then bishop of London (1163–87). His relations stretched throughout the English church: one of his maternal uncles was Robert, bishop of Lincoln, another relative, Richard of Ilchester, a royal clerk who became archdeacon of Poitiers and then bishop of Winchester (1174–88). When he had reached a position of authority, Gilbert seems to have used his influence in turn: Robert Foliot, whose relation to him is unclear but probable, became bishop of Hereford. He made at least three, and probably four, appointments of family members to the chapter of Hereford during his episcopate and eight appointments of family members whilst bishop of London, including two of his nephews. Some benefited twice over: Ralph Foliot became archdeacon of Hereford, royal justice and canon of London. It has thus been estimated that of the thirteen of Gilbert Foliot's relations known to have held ecclesiastical office, at least ten owed their promotion to him.[115] The existence of clerical dynasties like this throughout the period indicates that the Church was often regarded as a resource to be exploited for family benefit.

That the eleventh-century reforms made relatively little difference to the importance of family to individual careers becomes clear when one considers two cases where a nephew did not succeed his uncle as bishop. In the tenth century, Bishop Ulrich of Augsburg (d. 973) requested that the German emperor appoint his nephew, Abbot Adalbert of Ottobeuren as his successor, but according to Gerhard, his biographer, the people of Augsburg objected and Ulrich's request was not heeded.[116] The story hints, as does that of Burchard of Worm's initially unsuccessful attempt to succeed his brother, at political negotiations in which the current bishop might not always be able to succeed in appointing his successor, precisely because he was not alive at the time of the election: to be successful the candidate required powerful living backers. Family control of sees was thus by no means always assured in the tenth century. Two centuries later, Gerald of Wales failed in his attempt to succeed his uncle as bishop of St David's in southern Wales in 1176. According to Gerard's own account, the archbishop of Canterbury suggested his name to King Henry II but the king refused to consider it on the grounds that he was too closely related to the southern Welsh nobility, and he did not want to give power to them.[117] Gerald's account may not be accurate but it points to the political norms of the period: powerful clans could and did still expect to control bishoprics, but kings could and did have the right of veto in elections in the later twelfth century. Gerald, like Adalbert almost two centuries earlier, failed in his attempt to succeed his uncle not because a new Puritanism had rendered such nepotism obsolete, but because of the particular political circumstances of his case.

Episcopal elections might often be contested with force as well as words. In the end what seems to have been important in deciding who should become bishop was who had the more powerful connections, both secular and ecclesiastical. The following case illustrates their significance in which the control of the see was contested between two families. In 1008 Theodoric was elected to the see of Orléans. At his consecration a rival claimant, Odolric, in an attempt to prevent Theodoric's election entered the church with an armed retinue and tried to disrupt the ceremony. Theodoric's own retinue responded in kind. Despite this armed intervention, and also a legal challenge mounted on the grounds that Theodoric should be deposed from office as he had committed and confessed to homicide, Theodoric retained his office. He was only deposed some fourteen years later, sometime after reaching a settlement with Odolric that he should succeed him.[118] Theodoric came from a noble family with important ties to the neighbouring archdiocese of Sens; his relations included two powerful clerics, the archbishop of Sens and the abbot of Saint-Pierre-le-Vif in Sens. King Robert the Pious also supported his election. Odolric came from a similar background, but his family had more local ties: his father was the castellan of Pithiviers, north-east of the city, and his maternal uncles included the bishop of Beauvais and Count Odo II of Blois. Robert-Henri Bautier has suggested in a political reading of the rivalry between Theodoric and Odolric that their conflict represents an extension of that between King Robert the Pious and Count Odo II of Blois for control of the city of Orléans.[119] As this case demonstrates, bishoprics could act as focuses for political power and competition amongst noble elites. Neither man was an unreformed secular aristocrat just fighting for control of ecclesiastical revenue; rather they acted at the head of groupings of nobles who used episcopal office not only to display but to perpetuate their hereditary authority and wealth.

Many bishops acted like Theodoric and Odolric in their own family's interest, but the surviving letters of other bishops suggest that several felt themselves to be members of a separate, clerical caste with its own interests, detached from that of their lay relations and counterparts. Most of Bishop Rather of Verona's surviving correspondence is addressed to his fellow bishops, with only five out of sixty-six extant works and letters directed to lay people, including those to the Emperor Otto I and his wife. Rather himself had an eventful career; he was three-times bishop of Verona (931–34,

946–48, 961–68) being deposed in the face of royal and local opposition to his actions, and one-time bishop of Liège (953–55).[120] Rather's letters testify to his continuous plotting to be restored to office, and the support of royal bishops, in particular that of Archbishop Bruno of Cologne and Archbishop William of Mainz, was crucial to his career. The survival of his letter collection, as a personal compilation sent by him to the bishop of Freising, also testifies to this episcopal self-consciousness on the part of the author and his correspondents. The letter collection of the early eleventh-century north French bishop, Fulbert of Chartres, reveals a similar degree of awareness of how clerical identity should be set apart from the secular world.[121] He was at the centre of several clerical networks; over three quarters of his correspondents are abbots, archbishops, bishops, and clerics. Those of his letters which his students thought worth preserving show a conscientious bishop trying to maintain his church's position and income in the world, and to protect his clergy, as becomes clear in the series of letters he sent following the murder of his subdean Evrardus by the servants of the neighbouring bishop, Ralph of Senlis.[122] The attack took place because Bishop Ralph and his relatives thought that a member of their family should hold the office of subdean of Chartres. Fulbert's failed attempts to bring the conspirators to trial demonstrate both his respect for canon law and sense of responsibility for his own clergy. The case shows the problems caused when a family which thought it had a right to a particular office came up against a reforming bishop with a very different conception of how clergy should be appointed, and thus how they were defined. Finally, the letters of a mid-twelfth-century bishop, Arnulf of Lisieux (1141–81) are mainly addressed to bishops and abbots, revealing similar patterns and connections.[123] Collections such as these three indicate a strong sense of clerical community amongst author and recipient. At least two of these collections, those by Fulbert and Arnulf, were compiled for use in the schoolroom as examples of both the learning of individual bishops and of the sort of letters a bishop and his secretariat might be expected to write. Lay correspondents may therefore have been edited out at this stage; even if they were, the surviving letters testify to the vibrant culture of education which existed in certain sees throughout this period, and that such a culture helped to perpetuate a sense of the clergy as an elite, set apart from the laity.

And yet in many ways these bishops seem very similar to their secular counterparts. As we have already seen to be the case in early eleventh-century Orléans, they had their own substantial retinues, usually armed, and would even on occasion lead them into battle. The Bayeux Tapestry depicts Bishop Odo of Bayeux riding into battle wielding something described in the rubric as a 'baculum' (a staff – although it looks more like a club), not a sword, in obedience to church law which forbade clerics from carrying any sort of weapon. Bishop Ulrich of Augsburg, portrayed by his biographer as a conscientious and attentive bishop, led his militia into battle against the Magyars at the Lechfeld in defence of the Reich in 955, although he later, we are told, obtained permission from Otto I to confer on his nephew Adalbero his secular responsibilities for military service and attendance at court, leaving him free to serve God and to attend to his diocese, which he did, touring it four times a year.[124] Although bishops rarely fought themselves, their men made an important contribution to the armies of the Ottonian rulers: in 981, for example, Otto II asked Bishop Reginald of Eichstätt to send fifty armed warriors, the bishops of Regensburg and Salzburg to send seventy, the bishop of Würzburg sixty, that of Augsburg one hundred, and those of Freising and Constance forty, to reinforce those already in his Italian army.[125] Nor was such behaviour confined to the east Frankish Reich. In west Frankia Archbishop Aimo of Bourges led seven hundred men to their death in 1038 at the battle of Cher.[126] In England in 1056, according to the Anglo-Saxon Chronicle, Bishop Leofgar of the frontier see of Hereford 'abandoned his chrism and cross, his spiritual weapons after his ordination as bishop, and seized his spear and sword and went thus to the campaign against Gruffydd, the Welsh king, and they killed him there, and his priests with him'.[127] Such behaviour must have been common amongst the English clergy living on the Celtic frontiers, for the early eleventh-century Northumbrian Priests' Law, in acceptance of reality rather than the aspirations of canon law, fined priests for bringing weapons into church rather than demoting them.[128] Actual participation in battle is rather different to sending troops to battle, and these two English examples, which are not especially typical, may reflect the particular demands made on clergymen in frontier areas where there were few local secular lords to lead defence against external attacks.

Bishops also played significant roles in royal government, and rulers often rewarded clerks in their household with appointment to such sees. Indeed clerks were crucial to the running of the royal household. Those who served in the royal chapel often went on to become bishops in east

Frankia, but even once they did so, their royal service did not cease.[129] Bishop Burchard of Worms' biographer reports how he was so heavily involved in secular business – royal councils, conversations with the king, synodal cares and the 'diverse rumblings of the world' – that he sought refuge from 'the tumults of the world' in a cell he had built specially on top of a hill outside the city.[130] The links between office and bishopric could be formalised: archbishops of Mainz generally served as chancellor of the east Frankish kingdom, and those of Cologne as archchancellor of Italy, for example.[131] Bishops and clerics often served as diplomats. For example, Bishop Oda of Ramsbury negotiated the safe return of Louis d'Outremer to west Frankia on behalf of King Athelstan in 936; Bishop Cenwald of Worcester escorted Edith, sister of Athelstan to the court of King Henry the Fowler where she married his son, Otto I; Bishop Brihteah of Worcester similarly accompanied Cnut's daughter Gunnhild to Germany for her wedding in 1035.[132]

Equally significant is the episcopal contribution to government at a more local level. In northern Italy many bishops gradually acquired comital authority, and thus public authority, in the course of the tenth and eleventh centuries.[133] Whilst this did not happen overtly in England in the eleventh century, bishops were expected to act as presidents of the shire court, and thus to be involved in royal grants of rights and dues, as well as the trial and punishment of criminals. In Osbert's *Life* of Dunstan we are told that the bishop 'refused to celebrate Whitsun Mass until three false moneyers had received due punishment'.[134] In towns throughout Europe, not just in Italy, bishops often acted as lords, assuming public responsibilities. Burchard of Worms, for example, rebuilt a ditch and built a wall around the city in order to restore its security and encourage people to live there;[135] elsewhere bishops acted as masters of water, and building, attempting to imitate Rome and acting as leaders for their own communities.[136]

In doing so, they consciously followed earlier precedents as to how bishops should behave. The biographer of Bishop Otto of Bamberg (d. 1139) explicitly compared his subject's charity, when he fed the starving and visited the sick during a famine in 1125, with the work of Pope Gregory the Great, under whom the Church of Rome assumed responsibility for feeding the poor of Rome.[137] Such precedents derived ultimately from Christ's precepts in the Gospels: the authors of the *Lives* of bishops often depicted their subject as imitating Christ, in particular his concern for the poor, the sick, and weak, and also for peace. Burchard, bishop of Worms (d. 1025), according to his biographer Ebbo, would tour the city in the early hours of the morning looking for people sleeping rough, to whom he would give alms; indeed, he gave away so much of his personal wealth that he died with only three *denarii* in his purse.[138] Episcopal biographers also often portrayed their subjects as peacemakers. The tensions often generated between the bishop and local lords necessitated such skills. Ebbo, for example, describes the rivalry which existed between Bishop Burchard and Duke Otto of Suabia for authority within the city. Criminals escaping from episcopal justice would take refuge in the duke's household, leading to ongoing warfare between the ducal and episcopal households: 'as a consequence many limbs were hacked off and many murders occurred on both sides'.[139] Duke Otto's death led to the situation being resolved; Bishop Burchard not only made peace with the ducal household, but also brought up Otto's son, the future king Conrad II, within his own household. Similar struggles between the local lord and bishop are recorded in other towns as well, including the Flemish Bishop Lietbert's clashes with the local castellan in eleventh-century Cambrai.[140] A century later in Umbria his biographer described how the Italian Bishop Ubald of Gubbio (d. 1160) acted as peacemaker both within the city – he was struck with a stone when trying to break up a fight between its citizens, an action which led both sides to accept his injunction to 'separate and keep the peace' – and between the city and the emperor Frederick Barbarossa.[141] Such tales about bishops as peacemakers show that their role as local lords thus inevitably led them into conflict with other authorities. Such portraits are very one-sided, as suggested by the records of the struggles between rapacious bishops and urban communes in late twelfth-century France. Their biographers chose to remember their subjects as imitating Christ through their rule in part, perhaps, because their reputations were contested. They made a deliberate decision to depict episcopal culture and rule as distinct from that of the secular lay world in such situations, and in order to do so drew upon well-established norms as to how bishops were expected to behave.

Such portraits, bound as they are by earlier precedent, make it difficult to investigate the extent to which episcopal culture differed in practice from that of secular lords. The bishop's palace represents one way of doing so. An important marker of episcopal authority in the urban landscape of most cities, architecturally such buildings were often indistinguishable from those of secular magnates, being centred around a hall where the bishop conducted his court. But Maureen Miller has shown how, in the course of the twelfth century, episcopal palaces in northern Italy developed their own distinctive architectural style and decoration: episcopal halls became much longer than secular ones and decorated with scenes from the life of the founding father of the see.[142] She suggests that this change occurred at the time when bishops were being eased out of local government as communes took charge of Italian cities. Changes in political circumstances rather than a reforming programme *per se* ensured the separation of clerical from lay culture.

Nevertheless, when viewed across three centuries, what is remarkable about the lives of individual bishops is how little they changed. The roles they played in the wider world remained remarkably static, and whilst changes occurred in the emphasis given to age-old ideals of clerical behaviour, it is less clear how far these led to any great changes on the ground for how conscientious bishops lived at any point in the period. Let us turn now to see how far similar patterns can be identified in the evidence for the lives of local priests.

Priests

Their superiors expected priests serving local churches to play a central role in the lives of all Christians. As ministers of the rites for pastoral care – baptism, penance, communion, and those for the sick and the dying – they should oversee every Christian's entry into the world, and the community, and exit from it. They should act as moral arbiters, and live pure lives, set apart from those of their flock. It is, however, very difficult to recover specific information about the lives of actual local priests in this period and therefore the extent of the impact which the episcopal reformers' agendas had upon them. It is nevertheless worth asking to what extent the aspirations, which go back to at least the ninth century, for priests to emerge as a separate caste, living an exemplary life, and acting as moral leaders of their flocks, were realised in this period. In order to answer this question we will consider it in four parts: firstly how were local priests appointed and by whom? Secondly, from which ranks of society were they drawn and therefore to what extent were they distinct from their lay flock? Thirdly, what was the status of local priests within local communities; what roles did they play, and how were they regarded by those they served? Finally, how far was it their education and lifestyle which distinguished local priests from their congregations?

Appointment of local priests

Local churches comprised a valuable element of local lordships.[143] Local lords and local communities usually built such churches, as we saw in the previous chapter; the appointment of clergy to them consequently remained in the hands of the lords who owned them, both lay and ecclesiastical. In 947, for example, the bishop of Gerona consecrated the church of Sainte-Marie de Fenestre, founded by a group of laymen, and granted the church the tithes, first fruits and offerings of two villages 'so that the priest serving the altars may hold and possess it validly'; the principal lay founder, Gothmar, then conveyed the church and its possessions to Rodegar the priest 'so that as long as he lives he shall hold and possess it . . . and serve the altars without disturbance or molestation from me or anyone'.[144] The bishop became involved because of the need to consecrate the new church: it was the lay founder who appointed the priest and granted him the revenues for his lifetime. It was also common for such grants to be made to the priest and to his heir in the next generation. In the late tenth century, for example, the bishop of the west Frankish see of Chartres granted a church to Canon Gerald and a single heir 'to possess, rule and manage according to canonical authority', as long as they were ordained priests.[145] The reference to the need to be canonical priests was relatively unusual; more often such grants were conducted in similar terms, and seemingly for similar motives, to other land transactions with no such requirement.[146] Yet the charter evidence contain hints that the appointment of a priest to a particular church often involved more than the control of revenue. Glismont, a Lotharingian noblewoman, for example established an oratory in 1052 with the stipulation that the priest appointed should celebrate three masses a week for the dead, and keep the church in good repair.[147] Local priests continued to be appointed to churches in similar fashion throughout the period, but from the twelfth century onwards the grant of local churches to monasteries meant that increasing numbers of these appointments were made by abbots rather than lay lords.[148]

The social origins of the parish clergy provide clues both to how they were appointed, and who by, and thus to their status within the local community. Yet the evidence is complex, defies systematisation and is less plentiful than in the later Middle Ages. In a world in which lay and ecclesiastical lords appointed men to serve local churches one might expect local priests to be of relatively low status. That this was often the case in early tenth-century east Frankia is clear from a canon issued by the Council held at Hohenaltheim in 916 which built on ninth-century precedents to specify that freed serfs who were subsequently ordained priests must stay with the lord who had had them ordained:

> *If anyone for love of God chooses one of his serfs, teaches him letters, grants him liberty, makes him a priest (by request to the bishop) and . . . gives him food and clothes, but afterwards, flown with pride, he refuses to celebrate mass and the canonical hours and to sing psalms for his lords and will not obey them properly, saying that he is a free man and can become the man of anyone he choose [he should be excommunicated, and if obdurate, degraded from the priesthood and lose his free status.]*[149]

The life of the early eleventh-century Suabian hermit, Heimerad, confirms the reality behind such injunctions: born a serf on the estate of a noblewoman, when he grew up he was ordained and remained in her service, until she gave her permission for him to leave, which she did as she found him too eccentric.[150] This pattern – freed serf becomes a priest and enters his lord's service – probably also lies behind the provision made in the will of the Anglo-Saxon noblewoman Siflæd that Wulfmær and his children should sing the office in the church at Marlingford, Norfolk, so long as they were in holy orders.[151]

As this example suggests, the office of local priest was often hereditary. In England the late eleventh-century Domesday Book records examples of sons inheriting their office as priest from their father in Bedfordshire, Wiltshire and Somerset.[152] This practice continued in England into the late twelfth and thirteenth centuries as claims about hereditary succession to benefices were brought before the royal courts. For example, in a dispute over who had the right of advowson to the church of Dunston in the diocese of Norwich, the jurors testified 'they had never seen any parson presented to the church, but always the parsons held it, one parson after another, from father to son, down to the last parson lately deceased'. This man's sole heir was his daughter, who was consequently awarded the advowson.[153]

The presence of such sacerdotal dynasties can be read in two ways: either as the perpetuation of unreformed patterns of behaviour, in which priestly families treated the local church like any other form of landholding, as a resource to be exploited for the family's benefit, or as evidence for the development of the clergy as a separate, hereditary, caste. The Cistercian monk, Ailred of Rievaulx (*c*.1110–67) was descended from a dynasty of priests in northern England: his great grandfather was the priest in charge of Hexham and its estates in the mid-eleventh century; his grandfather was treasurer of the community at Durham, and passed the church of Hexham on to Ailred's father, Eilaf. In 1113 Eilaf gave up his hereditary tenure and allowed Archbishop Thomas of York to set up a community of canons, but retained his life interest in certain lands; in 1138 Eilaf restored all the lands he held to Hexham and entered the community of St Cuthbert at Durham on his deathbed.[154] Ailred followed his father into the church as a career cleric before entering the newly established Cistercian house at Rievaulx in North Yorkshire. Whilst reformers like Archbishop Thomas of York undoubtedly looked down upon such families, the family's close connection with the religious life thus continued into the next generation.[155] Here family and clerical identities became transformed to fit with the new behavioural norms.

Hereditary priests seem to have been in decline across these centuries. There is a good deal of charter evidence for priests donating churches to monasteries throughout this period suggesting that the priesthood was no longer regarded as a status to be inherited but rather one defined as much by education and behaviour as birth, thus conforming to the long-established ideals of church reformers. In a changing world, families found new ways alongside existing ones to retain control of the resources represented by their local church. Local studies of the twelfth century suggest that throughout Europe many families of the lesser nobility appointed members of their own family to the ministry. In the twelfth-century Limousin, in south-western France, the brothers of local knights or the nephews of existing incumbents often became local priests.[156] Similarly in the twelfth-century Tirol, the priests of local churches often came from local noble families.[157] In England the monastic founder and reformer, Gilbert of Sempringham (d. 1189), was born the son of a Norman knight in Lincolnshire. According to his *Life*, his father approved of his son's decision to enter the religious life and 'provided him with a competency from his own wealth. Finally he presented him, following the custom of the county, to the lord bishop as rector of the vacant parish churches of

Sempringham and Torrington, which were built upon his demesne'.[158] Gilbert went on to serve two successive bishops of Lincoln as a clerk before returning to the parish to found the religious houses for which he is better known. By 1215 local priests were by no means always freed serfs, subservient to their lay lord, but rather often themselves members of the local elite, either as the owners themselves of the churches they served, or as close relations of the owners.

Roles of local priests

Priests, and the holding of local churches, remained embedded in structures of local lordship in the twelfth century, as earlier. For priests often played important roles within the households of magnates, both ecclesiastical and lay. They acted as tutors: both abbots Odo of Cluny (d. 942) and, two centuries later, Guibert of Nogent (d. 1124) began their studies under priests in their parents' households.[159] Principally they acted as administrators: lords often used their control of local churches to reward the clerks serving in their own households. The right to nominate members of their household to parish churches was one which they sought to retain, even when, under pressure from critics of simony and lay investiture, they had formally handed ownership of a church to a monastic community. Thus in the late twelfth century Earl William de Mandeville agreed with the monks of the East Anglian monastery of Walden that he could retain, in his lifetime, the right to present his own clerks to the seven churches which he had given to the community, on payment of a pension to the community by both himself and the incumbent.[160] Here the parish church is treated as a source of income, and thus as a reward for service. But such cases suggest local lords regarded local priests as being of relatively high status. But many of these priests were absentees, serving the lord rather than the local community.[161]

How were those who actually ministered in local communities regarded by those they served? Narratives such as the miracle recorded in the late twelfth-century collection from the shrine of Our Lady of Rocamadour in south-western France credited a local priest with high esteem from his parishioners: it tells of how, when the priest fell ill, members of his flock visited and nursed him, and that when he died, they petitioned the Virgin to restore him to life: 'Deprived of the good shepherd the priest's flock were afraid they would be devoured by greedy wolves. And so with a combination of speaking, sobbing, and weeping they begged the Virgin to bring the father back to live and to restore him to them', which she did; he woke up and got off his bier as it was being carried to his grave.[162] This account set out to realise the reformers' prescriptive ideals of the priest acting as an *exemplum* to his parishioners considered above; it belongs to the world of aspiration. Yet the archbishop of York took this picture of the priest as defender of his flock literally when he promised in his campaign against the Scots in 1138 to call out each priest to his diocese to go into battle with crosses and relics at the head of their parishioners.[163] And the high esteem accorded to priests in such narratives is borne out in the documentary evidence. The commissioners of the Domesday Book recognised the priests' importance within their local communities in 1086, choosing the local priest, together with the reeve and six men, from each vill to testify to the inquiry.[164] Alongside the reeve, that is the official of the lord, the priest is recognised as holding the highest office within the vill. Priests, especially when they were members of hereditary dynasties, might be relatively wealthy members of the local community. Charter evidence from early ninth-century Brittany confirms the view that priests might often be amongst the wealthier members of their community, controlling relatively significant proportions of land, acting as moneylenders, as surety for transactions, as scribes for the recording of local transactions; judicial proceedings were sometimes held in the church or even in the priest's house.[165] A similar picture exists for northern Spain in the tenth century.[166] High status at a local level is not, however, inevitable; in Bury St Edmunds there were thirty priests, deacons and clerks recorded for 342 new houses, suggesting that for these men at least the ministry could not be a full-time job, and that it was by no means inevitable that the holders of such positions would always act as leaders within their own communities.[167]

Reforming the lives of local priests

The office itself might often be hereditary, deeply embedded both in the lives of the local communities it served, and in the structures of local lordship, with consequent expectations of reciprocal service. Yet as the Bury St Edmunds example cited above suggests, many of those who held priestly office may have been absent, serving as clerics at court, leaving their work to lowly paid vicars. Throughout this period the prescriptive evidence reveals, as we have already seen, reformers anxious to separate the lives of the higher clergy from those of the laity, focusing in particular on the sins of simony and nicolaitism, and on the need to educate priests in both the knowledge required for the delivery of pastoral care and as to how they should behave. At first sight it looks as if the reformers' aspirations failed – but did they? Further investigation of both documentary and narrative evidence suggests that a more complex picture underlies the apparent gulf between reality and aspiration.

Perhaps the most obvious way in which reformers sought to distinguish local priests from their lay flock was through their injunctions about the need for the higher clergy to be chaste and celibate. Hereditary dynasties of priests, such as Ailred of Rievaulx's ancestors, show such injunctions were not always honoured. Whilst Ailred's family's possession of the church of Hexham ended with his father's giving up their possession of the lands in 1138, they are not particularly typical. The twelfth-century cathedral chapters at both Hereford and Lisieux included canons who had inherited their office from their fathers.[168] At a lower level the practice of clerical marriage continued in many areas of Europe: sons of priests continued to attest charters throughout the twelfth and into the thirteenth century in both England and Normandy. In twelfth- and thirteenth-century Castile clergymen's concubines felt sufficiently secure of their status to claim clerical privilege in legal disputes.[169] Yet local studies in Italy suggest that the reformers may have had a greater impact there. In the tenth and eleventh centuries married priests commonly feature in documents, but in the diocese of Verona from the early twelfth century onwards references cease to be made in leases and other notarial documents to the wives, concubines and children of priests.[170] A similar pattern occurs further south in the Lazio where references to priests' wives, concubines and children disappeared in the early eleventh century.[171] The decline in the public recognition of such relationships suggests, at the very least, the effectiveness of reformist propaganda even if such relationships did not always disappear in practice. Yet the difference is particularly striking when compared to the English and Spanish evidence. It may be that in Italy the reforms took hold, at least amongst record keepers, in a way which failed to occur elsewhere in Europe.

The attitude displayed by contemporary writers to priests' wives is similarly varied, and suggests that the demonization of priests' wives and concubines which characterised the work of the reformist polemicists of the eleventh century was tempered by that of less extreme north European reformers. The Italian author Peter Damian (*c.*1007–72), a member of the reforming circles which surrounded the papal reformers of the 1050s and 1060s, characterised priests' wives as sexually rapacious agents of the devil:

> *Through [these women] therefore the devil devours his elect food, while he tears the very holy members of the church with his teeth just as with two millstones of suggestion and delectation, and when he joins [the priests] to [their sexual partners] he transposes [the priests] into his own guts.*[172]

Both he and Pope Gregory VII also described in gleeful terms how such women died in fires, and were thus destroyed.[173] The demonization of such women is usually ascribed to changes in theology which increasingly emphasised Christ's real presence in the Eucharist, and thus the need for those who administered the Eucharist to be pure.[174] Yet it is possible to find much more positive depictions of priests' wives in the work of north European reformist writers. Writing in southern England over a century later (*c.*1184), John of Ford countenanced an example of hereditary priesthood, and wrote in approving terms of Godrida, who was the wife of the priest, Brichtric, of the village of Haselbury in Somerset and the mother of Osbern, who succeeded him. Part of a circle interested in promoting pastoral care and the reform of the clergy and laity in the late twelfth century, John dedicated his work, a life of the village hermit Wulfric of Haselbury, to the pastorally minded reformer Bishop Bartholomew of Exeter (1161–84) and Archbishop Baldwin of Canterbury. In it he tells how when Godrida was making an alb for the priest to wear in his service at the altar she received a miraculous message via the priest from Wulfric, enclosed in his cell attached to the church, that she had made a mistake in her work.[175] Godrida seems to be portrayed as the Good Wife from the Book of Proverbs who manages her husband's home, spins flax and wool, and makes clothing for all her household.[176] Her role as helpmate to the priest is lauded rather than criticised. But Godrida is described here as Osbern the priest's mother, not as Brichtric the priest's wife, perhaps because by then she had been widowed, or perhaps because by the time John wrote it had become no longer acceptable for a man depicted as a model priest, as we shall see Brichtric was, to have a wife. Indeed, elsewhere in the work John reports the story of a priest's former concubine who had converted from her sinful former life to live a religious life in the 'friendship of Christ'.[177] Yet, whilst John chooses not to depict Godrida as the wife of priest, but rather as the mother of one, he nevertheless allows a much more positive view for women than that put forward a century earlier by the papal reformers.

Tales such as this point to the positive role which women might be allowed to play in the service of the altar. As we have seen, canon law, originating in the Merovingian period, treated women as polluting and prohibited them from living in the priest's house or entering the chancel. In the early ninth century Bishop Haito of Basle prohibited women from approaching the altar, even with washed linens.[178] Yet Godrida is not unique; the making of sacerdotal vestments is a role assigned to women in other accounts of the lives of reformers. John of Görze's tenth-century biographer records how John's widowed mother served the brothers of the reformed Lotharingia monastery by making vestments for the community.[179] According to the life of the early eleventh-century bishop, Burchard of Worms, after he became bishop Burchard summoned his sister, Mathilda, and ordered her to get her women to make vestments for him and his clergy, and subsequently appointed her an abbess, despite her protestations that she was a worldly woman who knew only her psalter.[180] Such atelier households are not uncommon. William of Malmesbury, in his early twelfth-century account of the life of the tenth-century English reformer, Dunstan, described how he was invited by a married woman to visit her house in order to draw a pattern for the embroidery for a priest's stole for her girls to use in their work. Dunstan took his harp with him and played a well-known antiphon to which the women 'chattered a cheerful response', but despite this devotional atmosphere, after the visit became known at the royal court Dunstan was accused of practising the 'evil arts' and lost the king's favour.[181] This monastic author used proximity to women to explain Dunstan's loss of royal support; although the real cause probably lay in the complicated court politics of the tenth century, none of William's twelfth-century audience found his account improbable or unreasonable. Nor is such needlework confined to the written page: there still survives the belt of red silk Emma, the wife of the ninth-century ruler Louis the German, gave Bishop Witgar, embroidered with the words 'The shining and most holy Queen Emma gave this belt to Witgar, a man filled with sacred breath'.[182] Here a queen made one of the most intimate of the sacerdotal garments, one which, according to the ninth-century author Hrabanus Maurus, signfied for both priests and monks their chastity and continence.[183] Women, that is queens, noblewomen, and even priests' wives, were allowed to serve the church by making priestly vestments at the same time as reformist writers presented them as a threat to sacerdotal purity. Indeed their textile work put them at the heart of the church's activities, worn as it was in the service of the altar, at the same time as ecclesiastical legislation excluded them from approaching the altar and touching the Lord's chalice. The eleventh-century reformers' rhetoric against women as polluters of a pure clergy is thus only one strand of thought in the Church at the time; clerical writers throughout this period also found other more positive roles for women, including clerical wives.

But how did priests learn to serve the altar? Many hereditary priests must have learnt on the job. Even future bishops were often trained in the households of other bishops: Bruno, son of Otto I of Germany, and future archbishop of Cologne and duke of Lotharingia, was brought up in the household of Bishop Balderich of Utrecht from the age of four.[184] Such practice was even more common at parish level. John of Ford describes how one father trained his son to succeed him.[185] Osbern, we are told, served at his father Brichtric's mass during his lifetime; one Sunday when Brichtric was blessing the water in the church Osbern found that the aspersorium was missing because he had taken it home, and therefore had to borrow that from the adjoining cell of the hermit, Wulfric. Osbern, we are told, also served at Wulfric's own masses as a young man (*adolescens*). Brichtric is depicted in glowing terms as a man well versed in his ministry: 'serving devotedly day and night in prayers and psalms, and in as much as his ministry allowed, he celebrated perpetually keeping watch in his church', riding home for dinner and returning as soon as he had eaten. When he succeeded his father, Osbern is described in similarly laudatory tones as often coming to the church at dusk to sleep in it rather than go home.[186] Such on-the-job training may have been quite effective, but it risked men falling into the faults which the prescriptive legislation we examined earlier suggested to have been all too common: not looking after church vessels properly (what was the aspersorium doing in the priest's house?), or mumbling the words without proper understanding.

The opportunities cathedral schools and monasteries offered for educating the clergy are discussed elsewhere, as is the fact that the higher clergy embraced and supported such initiatives. But the training of the pastoral clergy became an issue not only for their episcopal supervisors, but also for their lay patrons. Sometimes therefore we find laymen seeking a monastic education for their priests. In 904, for example, Rathod gave the monastery at Beaulieu the villa of Chauviac, on condition that his relative Guinebert hold the villa until such time as the abbot and monks granted him a church or other honour suitable for his life as a clerk, following which the abbot would gain ownership of the villa and be free to dispose of the land.[187] The grant in other words seems to be a sort of bursary, consequent upon Guinebert's education at Beaulieu. Rathod not only sought to provide a living for his relative, but viewed the monastery as providing training for the pastoral life.

Communities of canons, living a common life of prayer and celibacy, also became important providers of education for local priests. Such communities became popular throughout Europe in the course of the tenth and eleventh centuries. In the diocese of Verona, for example, from the late tenth century onwards communities of clerics known as *scolae* (schools) were established in both urban and rural churches; although their initial support came from the clergy, over the course of the eleventh century they received increasing numbers of benefactions from lay patrons in return for prayers for their own and their family's souls.[188] In eleventh-century England earls and their families favoured establishing communities of canons over donating to established monasteries.[189] These Italian and English communities were not intended explicitly for educating the clergy; what little we know of their internal life emphasises the importance of communal living, eating, sleeping and praying together. But such communities are part of a more general move to promote the purity of the higher clergy; their lay patrons supported them because they valued the purity of their clergy and the efficacy of their prayers for both the living and the dead. Their emphasis is on praxis. As we saw earlier in this chapter, the synodal evidence suggests that bishops emphasised the importance of praxis and that priests must know certain rites and prayers. Living in community offered an opportunity for educating clerics in these forms of knowledge – learning on the job, as it were. We shall examine these communities in more detail in the next chapter. For now it is enough to acknowledge that they also offered opportunities for a more systematic education than the father–son on-the-job training they often replaced.[190]

Such canonical communities offered one way in which the pastoral clergy differentiated themselves from the lives of their lay congregation. Another way emerges towards the end of our period. From the second half of the twelfth century onwards, associations of parish priests emerge in the towns of northern Europe: in Cologne (1172), Liège (1185), Amiens (1205), and Lyons (1151).[191] Quite what the motives behind such associations were is unclear: a clue might be found in that founded in the Italian diocese of Orvieto by the urban clergy to defend their interests against those of the cathedral clergy in the 1140s and 1150s.[192] To this extent, at least, priests emerged as a separate caste at the end of our period. That they did so owes as much to their own efforts, and those of their lay patrons and congregations as that of their bishops.

Conclusions

Did a great change take place in the way the pastoral clergy were expected to behave, and increasingly did behave, in the course of the eleventh century? Was there, in Maureen Miller's words, 'a profound reorientation of loyalties' on the part of the pastoral clergy away from the lay world, to a separate clerical one?[193] Can we ascribe to the papally led reforms, as R. I. Moore has done, the beginnings of 'a project to divide the world, both people and property, into two distinct and autonomous realms, not geographically but socially'?[194] We have seen that there is little new about the ideals taken up by the eleventh-century reformers; they had been voiced by earlier reformers and previous attempts had been made to enact them. Rather the project had begun with the Carolingians, and their texts and laws provided the foundation for the reforming aspirations of their tenth-, eleventh- and twelfth-century successors.

But these three centuries are characterised as much by continuity as by change. Throughout this period bishops' and local priests' lives remained closely tied to the world: noble families controlled appointments to bishoprics and local churches, to the general benefit of the family's wealth and authority. Their lives remained enmeshed with those of their lay counterparts: bishops continued to reside at court, priests to live in a local lord's household, and eat at his table, as Wulfric is described as doing whilst still a priest before he became a hermit.[195]

And yet important changes did occur. The enormous increase in higher education establishments in the eleventh and twelfth centuries allowed men to pursue a career as secular clerics within the Church. Whilst local priests continued to marry, concubinage became more discreet and less socially acceptable amongst the higher clergy. Increased lay support for canonical communities points to an increase in demand for the delivery of services by priests more remote from the problems of the world; to that extent the pastoral clergy increasingly began to live up to the expectations laid down by the Carolingian reformers.

Notes and references

1 *Grégoire le Grand, Règle pastorale*, ed. B. Judic, F. Rommel and C. Morel, Sources chrétiennes 381, 382 (Paris, 1992), II. 1.

2 'Ut non malum exemplum sint populo episcopi. Bonum exemplum populis se ipsos episcopi et sacerdotes debent praebere et ostendere, non solum dictis, verum et factis.', *MGH Concilia VI: Concilia aevi Saxonici I: 916–60*, ed. E.-D. Hehl and H. Fuhrmann (Hannover, 1987), 22.

3 One twelfth-century Irish bishop set out the episcopate's formal responsibility for the 'two churches', of monks and pastoral clerics in his diocese: *Gille of Limerick (c.1070–1145): Architect of a Medieval Church*, ed. J. Fleming (Dublin, 2001), 150–151.

4 Mansi, *Concilia* XVIII, 263–307.

5 *Sermo lupi ad anglos*, ed. D. Whitelock, 3rd edn (London, 1963).

6 Matthew 5.13, 5.14.

7 M. Andrieu, 'Le sacre épiscopal d'après Hincmar de Reims', *Revue d'histoire écclesiastique* 48 (1953), 22–73.

8 C. van Rhijn, *Shepherds of the Lord: Priests and Episcopal Statutes in the Carolingian Period* (Turnhout, 2007).

9 *Règle pastorale*, ed. Judic; for an English translation, see Gregory the Great, *Pastoral Care*, trans. H. Davis (London, 1950).

10 Theodulf, *Capitula I*, c. 1, *MGH Capitula Episcoporum I*, ed. P. Brommer (Hannover, 1984), 104–05.

11 Ibid., 76–100.

12 M. Miller 'Religion Makes a Difference: Clerical and Lay Cultures in the Courts of Northern Italy, 1000–130', *American Historical Review* 105 (2000), 1095–1300 at p. 1098. See also R. I. Moore, 'Family, Community and Cult on the Eve of the Gregorian Reform', *Transactions of the Royal Historical Society*, 5th series 30 (1980), 49–69; J. Laudage, *Priesterbild und Reformpapsttum im 11. Jahrhundert* (Cologne, 1984).

13 C. Leyser, 'Episcopal Office in the Italy of Liudprand of Cremona *c.*890–*c.*970', *English Historical Review* 125 (2010), 795–817.

14 A. Murray, *Reason and Society in the Middle Ages* (Oxford, 1978); R. I. Moore, 'Family, Community and Cult'.

15 Hrabanus Maurus, *De institutione clericerum*, *PL* 107, 299.

16 *The Decrees of the Ecumenical Councils*, ed. N. P. Tanner, 2 vols (London, 1990), I, 242.

17 See n. 10 above.

18 C. 6, *MGH Concilia VI*, 81; see also the council of Trosly (909), c. 9, Mansi, *Concilia* XVIII, 288–94.

19 Cc. 1, 4, ibid. 191, 192.

20 Mansi, *Concilia*, XIX, 503, 749–50; C. J. Héfèle, *Histoire des conciles d'apres les documents originaux* IV.2 (Paris, 1911), 830, 891, 919.

21 C. 3, *MGH Constitutiones et acta publica imperatorum et regum 911–1197*, I, ed. L. Weiland (Hannover, 1893), 547.

22 For example, see the Councils of Westminster of 1102, 1108 and 1125; *C&S*, II, 675, 694–704, 733–74.

23 Regino, I, q. 18, I. clxxxiv–xcv, 26, 76–80.

24 Burchard, *Decretum*, II. 107–118, *PL* 140, 644–46.

25 The *Scriftboc*: Oxford, Bodleian Library, Ms Junius 121, ff. 88r–v, ed. and trans. by A. J. Frantzen at http://www.anglo–saxon.net/penance/index.html (accessed 19th August 2012). Interest in the issue in eleventh-century and twelfth-century England is demonstrated by the addition of texts on the punishment of sins and the treatment of priests' children to Cambridge, Corpus Christi College, Ms 190 at these times: M. Budny, *Insular, Anglo-Saxon and Early Anglo-Norman Manuscript Art at Corpus Christi College, Cambridge: An Illustrated Catalogue*, 2 vols (Kalamazoo, MI, 1997), I, 543.

26 R. Amiet, 'Une "Admonitio synodalis" de l'époque carolingienne. Étude critique et édition', *Mediaeval Studies* 26 (1964), 12–82, c. 8 at p. 43; J. Avril, 'Les Precepta synodalia de Roger de Cambrai', *Bulletin of Medieval Canon Law*, New series 2 (1972), 7–15.

27 E.g. *The Register of Eudes of Rouen*, ed. and trans. Brown and O'Sullivan.

28 *XL Homiliarum in Evangelia Libri duo*, I.4, *PL* 76, 1091–92.

29 E.g. Regino, I.ccxli, 132; Atto of Vercelli, *De pressuris ecclesiasticis*, II, *PL* 134, 74; Burchard, I.113, 583.

30 Hohenaltheim, c. 7, Trier, cc. 8, 9, *MGH Concilia VI*, 22, 81–2; Atto, *Capitulare*, *MGH Capitula episcoporum III*, ed. R. Pokorny (Hannover,

1995), c. 24, 273–4; Amiet, 'Une "Admonito Synodalis"', cc. 33–34, pp. 49–50.

31 C. 2, Mansi, *Concilia* XIX, 265–68. English translation: Philippe Buc, 'Document 4', in *The Peace of God: Social Violence and Religious Response in France around the Year 1000*, ed. T. Head and R. Landes (Ithaca, NY, 1992), 331.

32 Theodulf of Orléans, *Capitula II*, c. 4; Radulf of Bourges, *Capitula*, c. 18, *MGH Capitula Episcoporum I*, 150, 246–47; Amiet, 'Une Admonitio Synodalis', c. 34, p. 50. It continued into the eleventh century: see Bourges (1031), c. 12, Mansi, *Concilia*, XIX, 504–05.

33 Cushing, *Reform and the Papacy*; Little, *Religious Poverty*; Moore, *First European Revolution*; Murray, *Reason and Society*.

34 S. Wemple, *Atto of Vercelli: Church, State and Christian Society in Tenth-century Italy* (Rome, 1979), 128–33.

35 Rather of Verona, *Die Briefe des Bischofs Rather von Verona*, ed. F. Weigle, MGH Die Briefe der deutschen Kaiserzeit I (Weimar, 1949), 71–106; trans. *On Contempt of the Canons*, in *The Complete Works of Rather of Verona*, trans. P. L. D. Reid (Binghamton, NY, 1991), no. 28, 372–73.

36 Numbers 19.22.

37 Mansi, *Concilia*, XIX. 741–42; Cf. Council of Limoges (1031), c. 3, Mansi, *Concilia*, XIX, 503.

38 T. Reuter, 'Pastorale Pedum Ante Pedes Apostolici Posuit: Dis- And Re-investiture in the Era of the Investiture Contest', in R. Gameson and H. Leyser, eds, *Belief and Culture in the Middle Ages* (Oxford, 2001), 197–210.

39 E.g. Council of London (1075), c. 7, *C&S* II, 614; H. Clover and M. Gibson (eds), *The Letters of Lanfranc, Archbishop of Canterbury* (Oxford, 1979), 72–79; Lateran II (1139), cc. 1 and 2, *Decrees*, ed. Tanner, I, 197; Lateran IV (1215), c. 63, ibid. I, 264. Tours (1163) Toulouse (1119) Rheims (1148), Mansi, *Concilia*, 00; Westminster (1175), *C&S* II, 965–92.

40 Wemple, *Atto of Vercelli*, 133–5.

41 C. 22, Mansi, *Concilia*, XIX, 505.

42 Humbert, *Libri III Adversus Simoniacos*; Reg. VI.5b (c. 8), *Das Register Gregors VII*, ed. E. Caspar, MGH Epistolae selectae II (Hannover, 1920–23), II, 401; translated in H. E. J. Cowdrey, *The Register of Pope Gregory VII, 1073–1085. An English Translation* (Oxford, 2002), 282.

43 Reg. VI.5b, ibid. II, 400; H. E. J. Cowdrey, *Pope Gregory VII, 1073–1085* (Oxford, 1998), 507–14 at p. 508.

44 cc. 1–2, Reg. VII.14a, ibid., II, 480–81; the translation by Cowdrey is at p. 340 of his edition (cited in n. 42).

45 Amiet, 'Une "Admonitio Synodalis"', cc. 37–39, 50–51; Rather, *Synodica*, trans. Reid, *The Complete Works*, 449; cf. Regino, I, q. 23–26, 28.

46 Visiting taverns: Council of Africa (419), c. 7; litigiousness: Isidore of Seville, *Regula monachorum*, c. 17, Council of Westminster (1175) c. 10, *C&S* II, 979, Lateran IV (1215), c. 16, *Decrees*, ed. Tanner, 243; drunkenness: *RC*, c. 23; hunting: Council of Agde (506), c. 55; arms: Council of Meaux (845/6), c. 37; see also F. Prinz, *Klerus und Krieg im früheren Mittelalter* (Stuttgart, 1971).

47 Avril, 'Les 'Precepta synodalia', 11; Lateran II, c. 20, Tanner, ed., *Decrees* I, 221.

48 John of Ford, *Wulfric of Haselbury*, ed. M. Bell, Somerset Record Society 47 (1933), c. 1, 13.

49 Giles Constable, 'Introduction: Beards in History', in *Apologiae duae. Gozechini epistola ad Walcherum. Burchardi ut videtur abbatis Bellevallis, Apologia de barbis*, ed. R. B. C. Huygens, CCCM LXII (Turnhout, 1985), esp. 103–14. Examples of episcopal legislation include: 'Canons of Edgar' (1005x8), c. 47, *C&S*, I, 330; Council of Bourges (1031), c. 7, Mansi, *Concilia* XIX, 504.

50 Cited by R. Mills, 'The Signification of the Tonsure', in P. H. Cullum and K. J. Lewis, eds, *Holiness and Masculinity in the Middle Ages* (Cardiff, 2004), 109–26 at p. 111.

51 'Nullus presbiter in itinere sine orario, id est stola, incedat. Nullus uestrum uestimentis laicabibus et diuersis coloribus induatur', Amiet 'Une *Admonitio Synodalis*', c. 66–67, 60.

52 Tribur (895), Extravagantes, c. 8, *MGH Capitularia Regum Francorum*, ed. A. Boretius and V. Krause, 2 vols (Hannover, 1883–97), II, 248.

53 Regino I. 343–45, 347 at pp. 182–84; Burchard, II. 208–09, 661.

54 *RC*, 114 (Latin), 143 (English translation).

55 Rather of Verona, *Praeloquiorum libri VI and Other Works*, ed. P. L. Reid, F. Dolbeau, B. Bischoff and C. Leonardi, CCCM 46A (Turnhout, 1984); *Praeloquia* 1.5.6, trans. Reid, 160–61. Cf. Ephesians 4.21–4: 'If so be that ye have heard him, and have been taught by him, as the truth is in Jesus. That ye put off concerning the former conversation the old man which is corrupt according to the deceitful lusts, and be renewed in the spirit of your mind, and that ye put on the new man which after God is created in righteousness and true holiness.'

56 Atto, *Capitulare*, c. 15, 270.

57 G. Constable, 'Introduction', Burchard, *Apologia de Barbis*, in *Apologiae Duae*, ed. R. B. C. Huygens, CCCM 62 (Turnhout, 1985), 47–149 at p. 54, n. 27.

58 C. 13, R. Somerville with S. Kuttner, *Pope Urban II, the Collectio Britannica and the Council of Melfi (1089)* (Oxford, 1996), 256–57, 262.

59 C. 13, ibid., 256–57, 262. For discussion of *scissis vestibus* see p. 290.

60 Mansi, *Concilia*, XXI, 438, 458; Lateran II, c. 4, *Decrees*, ed. Tanner, p. 197.

61 Avril, ed. 'Les Precepta synodalia' de Roger de Cambrai', c. 6, 10.

62 D. M. Wilson, *The Bayeux Tapestry* (London, 1985), Plate 17. The identification of the cleric as Anglo-Saxon is not wholly clear, but is likely as he is depicted standing next to a woman with an Anglo-Saxon name, Ælfigyva.

63 *'A' Life of Norbert, Archbishop of Magdeburg*, in *Norbert and Early Norbertine Spirituality*, trans. T. J. Antry, O. Praem, C. Neel (New York, 2007), cc. 1, 2, 126–28.

64 Amiet, 'Une "Admonitio synodalis", cc. 87–97, 66–68. This translation draws on that in Rather, trans Reid, *The Complete Works*, 450.

65 Amiet, 'Une "Admonitio synodalis"'.

66 As suggested by *ordo* 5D, *Die Konzilsordines der Früh-und Hochmittelalters*, ed. H. Schneider, MGH (Hannover, 1996), 278–84.

67 E.g. W. Hartmann, ed., 'Neue Text zur bischöflichen Reformgestzgebung aus den Jahren 829/31. Vier Diözesansynoden Halitgars von Cambrai', *Deutsches Archiv für Erforschung des Mittelalters* 35 (1979), 368–94; *C&S*, I, 422–27; Carine van Rhijn of the University of Utrecht is currently working on these texts.

68 Hartmann, ed., 'Neue Text'.

69 M. G. Cheney, *Roger, Bishop of Worcester 1164–1179* (Oxford, 1980).

70 *Complete Works*, trans Reid, 450.

71 Based on that in R. Somerville and B. Brasington, trans, *Prefaces to Canon Law Books in Latin Christianity. Selected Translations 500–1245* (New Haven, CT and London, 1998), 99–104.

72 S. Hamilton, *The Practice of Penance, 900–1050* (Woodbridge, 2001), 43–44; L. Körntgen, 'Canon Law and the Practice of Penance: Burchard of Worms's Penitential', *Early Medieval Europe* 14 (2006), 103–17.

73 S. Hamilton, 'The Rituale: The Evolution of a New Liturgical Book', in R. N. Swanson, ed., *The Church and the Book*, Studies in Church History 38 (Woodbridge, 2004), 74–86; A. Gaastra, 'Between Liturgy and Canon Law: A Study of Books of Confession and Penance in Eleventh-and Twelfth-century Italy' (University of Utrecht Ph.D. thesis, 2007), ch. 2.

74 S. Hamilton, 'Pastoral Care in Early Eleventh-century Rome', *Dutch Review of Church History* 84 (2004), 37–56.

75 H. Gittos, 'Is there any Evidence for the Liturgy of Parish Churches in Late Anglo-Saxon England? The Red Book of Darley and the Status of Old English', in F. Tinti, ed., *Pastoral Care in Late Anglo-Saxon England* (Woodbridge, 2005), 63–82.

76 C. Cubitt, 'Images of St Peter: the Clergy and the Religious Life in Anglo-Saxon England', in P. Cavill, ed., *The Christian Tradition in Anglo-Saxon England: Approaches to Current Scholarship and Teaching* (Cambridge, 2004), 41–54 at p. 49.

77 For the idea that the Gregorian reformers sought to make the clergy a 'third gender' see: R. N. Swanson, 'Angels Incarnate: Clergy and Masculinity from Gregorian Reform to Reformation', in D. M. Hadley, ed., *Masculinity in Medieval Europe* (Harlow, 1999), 160–77. J. D. Thibodeaux argues instead that reformist prohibitions sought to create an ideal of clerical masculinity which deliberately rejected various indications of secular manhood: 'Man of the Church or Man of the Village? Gender and the Parish Clergy in Medieval Normandy', *Gender and History* 18 (2006), 380–99.

78 L. Trichet, *La Tonsure. Vie et mort d'une pratique ecclésiastique* (Paris, 1990). Constable, 'Introduction', 73–75, esp. p. 74, n. 136.

79 Rather of Verona, *On Contempt of the Canons*, ed. in *Die Briefe*, ed. Weigle, 96–97; trans in *Complete Works of Rather*, no. 28, 372–73.

80 *PL* 131, 23–24; H. C. Lea, *History of Sacerdotal Celibacy in the Christian Church*, 4th edn (London, 1932), 112–13.

81 H. E. J. Cowdrey, 'The Papacy, the Patarenes and the Church of Milan', *TRHS* 5th ser. 18 (1968), 25–48; K. G. Cushing, 'Events That Led to Sainthood: Sanctity and the Reformers in the Eleventh Century', in R. Gameson and H. Leyser, eds, *Belief and Culture in the Middle Ages: Studies Presented to Henry Mayr-Harting* (Oxford, 2001), 187–96.

82 Andreas of Strumi, *Vita sancti Arialdi*, ed. F. Baethgen, *MGH SS* 30.2 (Leipzig, 1934), c. 4, 1051.

83 Cushing, 'Events that Led to Sainthood'.

84 Andreas, *Vita sancti Arialdi*, c. 4, 1052. English translation: M. C. Miller, *Power and the Holy in the Age of the Investiture Conflict. A Brief History with Documents* (Boston, 2005), 51.

85 Cushing, 'Events that Led to Sainthood'.

86 Andreas, *Vita Sancti Arialdi*, cc. 11–12, 1057–58. The exact nature of the common life is unspecified but perhaps it was similar to that recommended by the Lateran Council in 1059.

87 Cushing, 'Events that Led to Sainthood'; Cowdrey, 'The Papacy'.

88 Arnulf of Milan, *Liber Gestorum Recentium*, ed. C. Zey, MGH SRG 67 (Hannover, 1994) III. 15, 189–90: trans. W. L. North.

89 Moore, 'Family, Community and Cult'.

90 C. Violante, *La Pataria Milanese e la riforma ecclesiastica, i, Le premesse* (Rome, 1955); *idem*, 'Les prêts sur gage foncier dans la vie économique et sociale de Milan au xie siècle', *Cahiers de civilisation médiéval* 5 (1962), 147–68, 437–59; Cowdrey, 'The Papacy, The Patarenese and the Church of Milan'.

91 Cc. 19, 20, Mansi, *Concilia* XIX, 505.

92 Reg. II. 45, *Das Register Gregors VII*, 182–85; Cowdrey, *The Register of Pope Gregory VII*, 135–36. See also the letter sent to the count of Flanders two years later: Reg. IV. 11, ibid., 310–11 trans 220–221.

93 P. Vallicellianum E. 62 and P. Vallicellianum C.6 (c. 89), cited in A. Gaastra, 'Between Liturgy and Canon Law: A Study of Books of Confession and Penance in Eleventh-and Twelfth-century Italy' (University of Utrecht Ph.D. thesis, 2007). The Moslem and Norman invasions of southern Italy in the tenth and eleventh centuries explain why the clergy there felt the need to compile new penitentials; such evidence is lacking for northern Italy at the same time.

94 But lay testimony as to where the bishop had exercised his episcopal duties – consecrating churches, ordaining clergy, calling councils, offering penance to public criminals – was crucial to settling a dispute about the boundaries of the diocese of Orvieto: D. Foote, *Lordship, Reform, and the Development of Civil Society in Medieval Italy: the Bishopric of Orvieto, 1100–1250* (Notre Dame, IN, 2004), 125–44.

95 T. Reuter, 'Ein Europa der Bischöfe. Das Zeitalter Burchards von Worms', and other essays in W. Hartmann, ed., *Bischof Burchard von Worms 1000–1025* (Mainz, 2000), 1–28; S. Gilsdorf, ed., *The Bishop: Power and Piety at the First Millennium* (Münster, 2004); J. S. Ott and A. Trumbore Jones, eds, *The Bishop Reformed: Studies of Episcopal Power and Culture in the Central Middle Ages* (Aldershot, 2007).

96 V. King, 'St Oswald's Tenants', in N. Brooks and C. Cubitt, eds, *St Oswald of Worcester. Life and Influence* (London, 1996), 100–16 at pp. 103, 107–11. See also A. Wareham, 'St Oswald's Family and Kin', ibid., 46–63.

97 M. Parisse, 'Princes laïques et/ou moines, les évêques du Xe siècle', *Il Secolo di ferro: mito e realtà del secolo X*, Settimane 38, 2 vols (Spoleto, 1991) I. 449–513, at p. 463.

98 M. G. Cheney, *Roger, Bishop of Worcester, 1164–79* (Oxford, 1980), 6; Otto of Freising, *The Two Cities. A Chronicle of Universal History to the Year 1146*, trans. C. C. Mierow (New York, 1928), 5.

99 Carlrichard Brühl, 'Die Sozialstruktur des deutschen episkopats im 11. und 12 Jahrhundert', *Le Istituzioni ecclesiastiche della 'Societas Christiana' dei secoli XI–XII. Diocesi, pievi e parrocchie. Atti della sesta Settimana internazionale di studio Milano*, 1–7 settembre 1974, Miscellanea del centro di studi medioevali 8 (Milan, 1978), 42–56 at p. 58.

100 J. Boussard, 'Les évêques en Neustrie avant la réforme Grégorienne (950–1050 environ)', *Journal des Savants*, 1970, 161–96.

101 Adhemar of Chabannes, *Chronicon*, ed. P. Bourgain, R. Landes and G. Pon, CCCM 129 (Turnhout, 1999), 146–47.

102 Boussard, 'Les évêques'.

103 C. B. Bouchard, 'The Geographical, Social and Ecclesiastical Origins of the Bishops of Auxerre and Sens in the Central Middle Ages', *Church History* 46 (1977), 277–95.

104 T. Reuter, 'The "Imperial Church System" of the Ottonian and Salian Rulers: A Reconsideration', *Journal of Ecclesiastical History* 33 (1982), 347–74.

105 Parisse, 'Les évêques du Xe siècle', 462.

106 Cited in Bouchard, 'Geographic, Social and Ecclesiastical Origins'. On criticism see H. Fichtenau, *Living in the Tenth Century: Mentalities and Social Orders*, trans. P. J. Geary (Chicago, 1991), 182–83.

107 Bouchard, 'Geographic, Social and Ecclesiastical Origins'.

108 E. Mason, *St Wulfstan of Worcester, c.1008–1095* (Oxford, 1990), 29–33.

109 *Vita Burchardi Episcopi Wormatiensis*, ed. G. H. Waitz, MGH SS IV, 829–46; *The Life of Burchard Bishop of Worms, 1025*, trans. by W. North available at http://www.fordham.edu/halsall/source/1025burchard-vita.asp (accessed 19th August 2012).

110 Reuter, 'The "Imperial Church System"'. 354.

111 M. Lapidge, 'Dunstan [St Dunstan], d. 988, archbishop of Canterbury', *ODNB*.

112 Raoul of Saint-Sépulchre, *Vita Lietberti episcopi Cameracensis*, ed. A. Hofmeister, *MGH SS* 30.2 (Leipzig, 1934), 838–66; J. S. Ott, '"Both Mary and Martha": Bishop Lietbert of Cambrai and the Construction of Episcopal Sanctity in a Border Diocese around 1100', in Ott and Trumbore Jones, *The Bishop Reformed*, 137–60.

113 *Vita S. Ubaldi*, *AASS Maii III*, 628–39 at pp. 630–31.

114 *Vita S. Conrado seu Cunone*, *AASS Junii* I, 126–34.

115 *Gilbert Foliot and His Letters*, ed. A. Morey and C. N. L. Brooke, eds, (Cambridge, 1965), 34–51.

116 Gerhard, *Vita Oudalrici*, c. 23, *MGH SS IV*, 408.

117 H. E. Butler, ed. and trans. *The Autobiography of Giraldus Cambrensis*, London 1937: *De Rebus a Gestis*, c. 9, in *Giraldus Cambriensis Opera*, ed. J. S. Brewer, J. F. Dimock and G. F. Warner, 8 vols, Rolls Series 21 (London, 1861–91), 59–62.

118 *Vita S. Theodorici II*, *AASS Januarii III*, 403–05; *The Letters and Poems of Fulbert of Chartres*, ed. F. Behrends (Oxford, 1976), 38–44, 72, 74–76; T. Head, *Hagiography and the Cult of the Saints: the Diocese of Orléans 800–1200* (Cambridge, 1990), 257–70.

119 R.-H. Bautier, 'L'Hérésie d'Orléans et le muvement intellectue au début du XIe siècle. Documents et hypothèses', *Enseignement et vie intellectuelle* (Paris, 1975), 63–88.

120 P. L. D. Reid, 'Introduction', *The Complete Works of Rather*, 4–11.

121 *Letters of Fulbert of Chartres*, ed. Behrends.

122 Ibid. 52–65; E. Peters, 'The Death of the Subdean: Ecclesiastical Order and Disorder in Eleventh-century Francia', in B. S. Bachrach and D. Nicholas, eds, *Law, Custom and the Social Fabric in Medieval Europe: Essays in Honour of Bryce Lyon* (Kalamazoo, MI, 1990), 51–71.

123 *The Letters of Arnulf of Lisieux*, ed. F. Barlow (London, 1939); trans. C. Poling Schriber, *The Letter Collections of Arnulf of Lisieux* (Lampeter, 1997).

124 Gerhard, *Vita Oudalrici*, ed. G. Waitz, *MGH SS* IV, 377–428 at p. 394.

125 B. Arnold, *Count and Bishop in Medieval Germany: A Study of Regional Power 1100–1350* (Philadelphia, 1991), 47.

126 T. Head, 'The Judgement of God: Andrew of Fleury's Account of the Peace League of Bourges', in Head and Landes, *The Peace of God*, 219–38 at pp. 225–28.

127 *The Anglo-Saxon Chronicle: A Collaborative Edition V: Ms C*, ed. K. O'Brien O'Keeffe (Cambridge, 2001), a. 1056, pp. 116–17; *The Anglo-Saxon Chronicles*, trans. M. Swanton (London, 1996), 186.

128 C. 37, *C&S*, I, 459. For the suggestion that thirteenth-century bishops on the Scottish border tolerated priests bearing arms, see H. Birkett, 'The Pastoral Application of the Lateran IV Reforms in the Northern Province, 1215–1348', *Northern History* 43 (2006), 199–219.

129 Reuter, 'Imperial Church System'.

130 *Vita Burchardi*, c. 10, 837; trans. W. North.

131 Parisse, 'Les évêques du Xe siècle'.

132 M. F. Giandrea, *Episcopal Culture in Late Anglo-Saxon England* (Woodbridge, 2007), 62–63.

133 G. Sergi, 'The Kingdom of Italy', in T. Reuter, ed., *New Cambridge Medieval History III: c.900–c.1024* (Cambridge, 1999), 346–71.

134 Giandrea, *Episcopal Culture*, ch. 6.

135 *Vita Burchardi*, c. 6, 835.

136 Stephan Patzold, 'L'épiscopat du haut Moyen Âge du point de vue de la médiévistique allemande', *Cahiers de civilisation médiévale Xe–XIIe siècles* 48 (2005), 341–58.

137 *Vita altera S. Ottonis*, AASS *Julii I*, 431.

138 *Vita Burchardi*, cc. 20, 22, 843–45.

139 Ibid., c. 7, 835.

140 D. J. Reilly, *The Art of Reform in Eleventh-century Flanders: Gerard of Cambrai, Richard of Saint-Vanne and the Saint-Vaast Bible* (Leiden, 2006), 296–98. See now Riches, T., 'Bishop Gerard I of Cambrai (1012–51) and the Representation of Authority in the *Gesta episcoporum cameracensium*' (Ph.D. thesis, King's College, London, University of London, 2006).

141 Tebaldus, *Vita S. Ubaldi*, c. 2, *AASS Maii III*, 633–34.

142 M. C. Miller, *The Bishop's Palace: Architecture and Authority in Medieval Italy* (Ithaca, NY, 2000); eadem, 'Religion Makes a Difference', 1095–1130.

143 S. Wood, *The Proprietary Church in the Medieval West* (Oxford, 2006). See also W. Davies, 'Local priests in Northern Spain in the Tenth Century', paper delivered to the International Medieval Congress, Leeds, 2009.

144 Ibid., 536.

145 Ibid.

146 Ibid.

147 Wood, *Proprietary Church*, 443, 555. See also charters from the tenth-century Italian diocese of Lucca which specify that the priest was expected to celebrate the mass, the divine office, maintain the lights in the church, render obedience to the bishop each year, and not alienate any of the church's endowment without the bishop's permission: Addleshaw, *Development of the Parochial System*, 8.

148 U. Rasche, 'The Early Phase of Appropriation of Parish Churches in Medieval England', *Journal of Medieval History* 26 (2000), 213–27.

149 C. 38, *MGH Concilia* VI. 1, 39.

150 Egbert of Hersfeld, *Vita Heimeradi* (c. 1070), *AASS Junii V*, 385–95.

151 J. Barrow, 'The Clergy in English Dioceses, *c.*900–*c.*1050', in Tinti, ed., *Pastoral Care*, 19–20, citing D. Whitelock, ed., *Anglo-Saxon Wills*, 92–93.

152 Ibid., 20, n. 22.

153 C. Harper-Bill, 'The Struggle for Benefices in Twelfth-century East Anglia', in R. Allen Brown, ed., *Anglo-Norman Studies XI; Proceedings of the Battle Conference 1988* (Woodbridge, 1989), 113–32.

154 W. Aird, *St Cuthbert and the Normans* (Woodbridge, 1998), 118; *The Life of Ailred of Rievaulx by Walter Daniel*, ed. and trans. M. Powicke (London, 1950; repr. Oxford, 1978), xxxiv–xxxv.

155 D. N. Bell, 'Ailred of Rievaulx', *ODNB.*

156 J. Becquet, 'Le clergé Limousin au XII siècle', in *L'Encadrement religieux*, 311–15.

157 H.-J. Mierau, *Vita communis und Pfarrseelsorge. Studien zu den Diözesen Salzburg und Passau im Hoch–und Spätmittelalter*, Forschungen zur kirklichen Rechtsgeschichte und zum Kirchenrecht 21 (Köln, Weimar, Wien, 1997), 145.

158 *Liber sancti Gileberti*, ed. R. Foreville and G. Keir, OMT (Oxford, 1987), I. 3, 16–17.

159 John of Salerno, *Vita S. Odonis*, I. 7, *PL* 133, 46–47; trans. G. Sitwell, *St Odo of Cluny* (London, 1958), 9; Guibert de Nogent, *Monodiae*, *PL* 156, I. 4, 843–45; trans. P. J. Archambault, *A Monk's Confession: The Memoirs of Guibert of Nogent* (University Park, PA, 1995), 13–16.

160 Harper-Bill, 'The Struggle for Benefices', 124.

161 For northern Spain see W. Davies, *Acts of Giving: Individual, Community and Church in Tenth-century Christian Spain* (Oxford, 2007), 44–50.

162 M. Bull, *The Miracles of Our Lady of Rocamadour: Analysis and Translation* (Woodbridge, 1999), I. 2, 101–02.

163 Richard of Hexham, *De gestis regis Stephani*, ed. R. Howlett, *Chronicles of the Reigns of Stephen, Henry II and Richard I*, Roll Series 82.3 (London, 1886), p. 161; Ælred of Rievaulx, *Relatio de standardo*, ibid, 182.

164 Blair, *Church*, 493.

165 W. Davies, 'Priests and Rural Communities in East Brittany in the Ninth Century', *Études celtiques* 20 (1983), 177–97.

166 Eadem, *Acts of Giving*, 44–50.

167 J. Campbell, 'The Church in Anglo-Saxon Towns', in D. Baker, ed., *The Church in Town and Countryside*, Studies in Church History 16 (1979), 130.

168 J. Barrow, 'The Clergy in the Diocese of Hereford in the Eleventh and Twelfth Centuries', *Anglo-Norman Studies XXVI: Proceedings of the Battle Conference 2003* (Woodbridge, 2004), 37–53; *The Letters of Arnulf of Lisieux*, ed. F. Barlow (London, 1939), nos 115 and 132. In one, Arnulf condemned one priest who had had an overt relationship with his concubine

for thirty years, and the woman and her daughters assaulted the two priests whom he sent to serve the papal injunction removing him from office; in another letter he recalls how he removed eighteen concubines from his cathedral canons.

169 H. Dillard, *Daughters of the Reconquest: Women in Castilian Town Society 1100–1300* (Cambridge, 1984), 127–32.

170 M. Miller, 'Clerical Identity and Reform: Notarial Descriptions of the Secular Clergy in the Po Valley, 750–1200', in M. Frassetto, ed., *Medieval Purity and Piety: Essays on Medieval Clerical Celibacy and Religious Reform* (New York, 1998), 305–35.

171 Toubert, *Structures*, I, 779–83.

172 Ep. 112, *Die Briefe des Petrus Damiani*, ed. K. Reindel, 4 vols, MGH (Munich, 1983–1993), III, 258–88; the translation is that in D. Elliott, 'The Priest's Wife: Female Erasure and the Gregorian Reform', in C. Hoffmann Berman, ed., *Medieval Religion: New Approaches* (London, 2004), 127 which is closer to the Latin than that in *Peter Damian, Letters*, trans. O. J. Blum, 6 vols (Washington, DC, 1990–2004), IV, 278.

173 Ep. 70, *Briefe des Petrus Damiani*, II, 320–21; *Peter Damian Letters*, trans. Blum, III, 110; Paul Bernried, The *Life of Gregory VII*, in *The Papal Reform of the Eleventh Century: The Lives of Pope Leo IX and Pope Gregory VII*, trans. I. S. Robinson (Manchester, 2004), c. 116, 359.

174 Elliott, 'The Priest's Wife'; H. E. J. Cowdrey, 'Pope Gregory VII and the Chastity of the Clergy', in Frassetto, ed., *Medieval Purity and Piety*, 269–302; E. Frauenknecht, *Die Verteidigung der Priesterehe in der Reformzeit* (Hannover, 1997); Moore, 'Family, Community and Cult'.

175 John of Ford, *Wulfric of Haselbury*, c. 82, 109.

176 Proverbs 31: 10–31, especially verses 19, 22, 24.

177 John of Ford, *Wulfric*, c. 75, 103.

178 Haito of Basle, *Capitula*, c. 16, *MGH Capitula Episcoporum I*, 215.

179 *La Vie de Jean, abbé de Gorze*, ed. M. Parisse (Paris, 1999), c. 45, p. 80.

180 *Vita Burchardi*, c. 12, 837–38.

181 *Vita Dunstani*, I. 6 in *William of Malmesbury, Saints'Lives*, ed. M. Winterbottom and R. M. Thomson (Oxford, 2002), 183.

182 'Hanc zonam reginam nitens sanctissima Hemma Witgario tribuit sacro spiramine plenum', cited by Eric J. Goldberg, 'Regina nitens sanctissima Hemma: Queen Emma (872–76), Bishop Witgar of Augsburg and the Witgar-Belt', in B. Weiler and S. MacLean, eds, *Representations of Power in Medieval Germany 800–1500* (Turnhout, 2006), 57–95 at p. 75.

183 Ibid.

184 Ruotger, *Vita Brunonis Archiepiscopi Coloniensis*, c. 4, *MGH SS* IV, 255–56.

185 Cc. 35, 74, John of Ford, *Wulfric*, 52–53, 102.

186 Cc. 16, 36, ibid., 30–31, 53–54.

187 Aubrun, *Limoges*, 349.

188 M. C. Miller, *The Formation of a Medieval Church: Ecclesiastical Change in Verona, 950–1150* (Ithaca, NY, 1993), 48–54, 111–12.

189 M. F. Smith, R. Fleming and P. Halpin, 'Court and Piety in Late Anglo-Saxon England', *Catholic Historical Review* 87 (2001), 569–602 at pp. 580–82.

190 See above: discussion of manuscript from SS XII Apostoli.

191 P. Desportes, 'Les sociétés confraternelles de curés en France du Nord au Bas Moyen Âge', in *L'Encardrement religieus*, 295–309.

192 Foote, *Lordship*, 67.

193 Miller, 'Clerical Identity', pp. 305–06.

194 Moore, *The First European Revolution*, 11.

195 John of Ford, *Wulfric*, c. 1.

chapter 4

Monks, nuns, canons and the wider world

From the beginning of the holy church two ways of life were instituted for its sons: one to strengthen the debility of the weak, the other to perfect the blessed life of the strong . . . Those who hold to the lower make use of earthly goods; those who hold to the higher despise and abandon earthly goods. The path which by divine favour is turned from earthly things is divided into two parts with almost the same purpose, that of the canons and that of the monks.

Urban II, Privilege for the canons of St Mary's, Rottenbuch, 1092[1]

Once Adelheid had settled all interior matters satisfactorily with God's help, she was impelled to turn her attention to the outside world for she also desired to serve the kingdom of God there, filled thus with faith and hope for the greater reward which the Lord promised when he said 'Seek ye first the kingdom and all else will be granted unto you'.[2]

Bertha, *Life of Adelheid, Abbess of Vilich* (composed *c.*1057)

Medieval churchmen continually contrasted the sinfulness of their world with the purity of the kingdom of heaven and valued those men and women who tried to remove themselves from earthly temptations by leading a religious life. This message provoked fear about personal salvation, leading men and women, in Urban II's words, 'to perfect the blessed life of the strong' by adopting a religious life of prayer cut off from the demands of the world, as monks or canons, nuns or canonesses, hermits or recluses. The popularity of this solution to the anxieties provoked by this teaching is indicated by the increasing numbers of men and women in this period who aspired to a life as far removed as possible from the demands of the earthly world. The central Middle Ages are key to accounts of medieval monastic history, for between 900 and 1200 thousands of new religious houses were established across western Christendom. These years saw the emergence of very different and highly influential monastic orders, including the Cluniacs, the Cistercians, the Premonstratensians and the Austin Canons. Each in their own way wished to renegotiate the relationship between the regular clergy and the world and they are testament to the popularity of this movement.

Only a small proportion of the population ever adopted the religious life: the majority of Christians remained in the world, subject to its temptations, either as secular clergy responsible for ministering to the laity, in Urban II's words strengthening the weak, or as lay men and women. It is the latter, especially the increasingly wealthy nobility, who resourced this great growth in monasticism. It is only towards the end of our period that the lesser nobility and merchants began to patronise these new houses. Lay nobles rather than monastic reformers founded new houses. The reasons for the popularity of the monastic life in this period are thus to be found not in the motives of individual religious, but rather in their relationships with members of the lay majority. Although their way of life focused around escaping from the temptations of earthly life as far as possible, the religious could not afford to reject the earthly world entirely. They depended on property worked by peasants, the gift of lay beneficiaries, to support their lifestyle. But these monastic holdings were situated within wider ecclesiastical and lay power structures which meant that their religious proprietors had to engage with the families of their benefactors, other institutions, and both ecclesiastical and secular officials in order to preserve their rights. Lay gifts of land thus initiated and perpetuated relationships between religious institutions and their patrons across several generations.

This chapter traces the varying nature of these relationships between the religious and the laity across the years 900 to 1200, years central to monastic history which witnessed the flourishing of existing houses and the emergence of new forms of monastic life. It begins by considering how the religious sought to distinguish themselves from the laity before investigating how the religious perceived the lay world, and their role within it. It then turns to explore the roles that members of the laity were allowed, and were expected, to play within religious communities, before finally considering the direct role lay men and women played as benefactors in the founding and supporting of religious houses. Looking through the prism of the religious's relationships with the laity offers an opportunity to re-evaluate developments in monasticism in this period.

The religious life

The histories of monastic communities are characterised in this period by repeated attempts to renew the principles governing the way they lived and prayed. Through their chosen ways of life they sought very consciously to differentiate themselves from, and live apart from, the laity whom they regarded as mired in worldly temptations. The difficulty of reconciling their ambitions to live apart from the world with the practical demands of living within it explains why 'reform' was, as Joachim Wollasch observed, a constant of medieval monasticism.[3] Its main principles had been laid down in Late Antiquity, and its adherents constantly looked back to texts from that time as they sought to restore and renew the principles of the ascetic and coenobitic ways of life laid down then. They modelled themselves on the lives of the earliest Christian ascetics who had gone into the Egyptian desert in the third and fourth centuries in order to devote themselves to a life of prayer, cut off from the demands of the world. The word monk, for example, comes from the Greek word 'monos' meaning alone and was used to designate such men and women.[4] Some of these early ascetics adopted a coenobitic life, living in communities, but others chose to live as hermits. The eremitic strand had been particularly influential in early monasticism, and it also proved to be a powerful strand in the religious life of this period. Hermits and recluses, collectively known as anchorites, wandered through woods preaching and had themselves enclosed in cells attached to parish churches or located within city and monastic gates, from which they delivered advice to both the local community and visiting dignitaries. They also became an important feature of many religious communities in this period, serving as an exemplar of the ascetic life to the other members.[5]

The quest to live successfully apart from but in the world was such an important one that reformers made various attempts to draw up guidance as to how such communities should conduct themselves. Those who adopt a religious life are often described as following a regular life; this means one governed by a rule, *regula* in Latin. It thus refers to any religious community living under a rule. In the central Middle Ages such communities can be divided into two main groups, monks and nuns, on the one hand, and canons and canonesses on the other. The rules followed by both groups are in many ways very similar: in Urban II's words, the higher path which is 'turned from earthly things is divided into two parts with almost the same purpose, that of the canons and that of the monks'. This quote comes from the papal privilege for the male canons of Rottenbuch which explains its gender bias.[6] Leaders of both female and male communities recognised the difficulties and anxieties induced by trying to follow the higher path. The consequent need to reconsider and reframe their relationships with the wider community meant they constantly revisited and amplified the rules which governed the religious lives of both monks and nuns.

The early ninth-century efforts of the Carolingian reformer, Benedict of Aniane, to promote the Rule of Benedict, the sixth-century founder of the south Italian monastery Monte Cassino, meant that by the beginning of our period, the Benedictine Rule had become widely acknowledged throughout Western Europe as the prevailing ideal for monastic communities.[7] The Rule enjoined that monks live in communities, under the authority of an abbot, governed by regular prayer: they should follow the Psalmist's injunction to praise the Lord eight times a day. They thus developed a round of daily services – Matins, Laudes, Prime, Tierce, Sext, None, Vespers, Compline – known collectively as the Office which combined psalms with antiphons, readings and prayers; from the ninth century they also attended one Mass late in the afternoon before Vespers but it also became common to offer a Mass in the morning after Prime, followed by one for the commemoration of the dead.[8] Abdicating individual responsibility in favour of the abbot, they should live together, sleeping, eating, and praying together, holding their property in common. Houses of nuns were similarly influenced by the Rule of Benedict.

Canons also lived in communities governed by a rule. Again the Carolingian reformers had promoted a rule for canons, the 'Institutes of Aachen' at the council of Aachen 816–17; this text was more fluid than that of the Rule of Benedict, from which it quoted extensively. By the tenth century a version now known as the 'Interpolated Rule of Chrodegang' (because it combined the rule composed by Chrodegang, the eighth-century

Bishop of Metz, for his cathedral clergy with the Aachen text and other elements), circulated in continental Europe, although it probably arrived later in England.[9] This rule, like that for monks, demanded that canons say the Office eight times day and night, and live together in community, although the content of the divine office is different from that observed in monastic communities: in particular, the canons observed a rather simpler form for the night office.[10] They differed more significantly from monks in that their lives should be characterised not just by regular prayer but also by pastoral ministry to the lay faithful: the rule emphasised the importance of delivering the main rites of pastoral care and of regular preaching:

> *We must take care lest our people run into any peril through our neglect, lest they become careless without baptism, confirmation, confession or preaching. We have therefore decided that all year round the word of salvation shall be preached to them twice a month, every fortnight, so that with the help of God they may attain to eternal life. It would be better still if there was a regular sermon on every feast day and Sunday; the preaching should be in such a manner that the ordinary people can understand it.*[11]

Unlike monks, the rule allowed canons to hold property individually – members of unreformed houses often chose to live independently in separate houses – and to keep the alms offered to them by the faithful for celebrating Mass, hearing confession or singing prayers for the dead, rather than handing them over to the community.[12] These concessions provided a considerable challenge to the precepts about communal living, and, as we shall see, various attempts were made in this period to reform the canonical life by enforcing the principle of communal living.[13] The history of canonesses differs slightly: the Carolingian reformers codified a separate rule for all female religious, particularly canonesses, which made no equivalent pastoral demands upon them.[14]

Such regulations helped shape the identity of particular communities but the boundaries between monastic and canonical communities were not impermeable. Many reformers in the tenth century, for example, trained in houses of canons but went on to become monks and lead a revival of the monastic way of life.[15] Tenth-century monastic reform movements in Rome, Burgundy, Normandy, Flanders, Lotharingia and England led to new houses being established under the Benedictine rule, but also to many houses of canons being turned into monastic communities.[16] Using the language of purity and renewal, the leaders of these changes set out to rescue canonical communities from the perceived contamination of worldliness and decay by promoting chastity and celibacy and adherence to the Rule of Benedict. Ninth-century canonical reformers demanded that canons fulfil their pastoral ministry in the world; changing expectations as much as falling standards within particular communities may explain tenth-century monastic reformers' anxiety to promote greater separation from the world.

Such rivalries meant it was in the interests of these monastic reformers to play up the differences between the two types of religious, particularly in their attitudes to property, but the similarities between them are equally striking. Both canons and monks lived lives of regular prayer, and both types of religious attached great importance to the separation of their way of life from that of the laity. Particular attitudes to sexual behaviour, dress and physical distance characterised this separation. Both the *Rule of Benedict* and the *Interpolated Rule for Canons*, which drew in part on the text of the Rule of Benedict, emphasised the benefits of enclosure: everything necessary to life – water, mill, garden, workshops – should be on one site so, in the words of the Rule of Benedict, 'there be no necessity for monks to be wandering about outside: that is absolutely no good for their souls'.[17] The Interpolated Rule was equally emphatic about the importance of enclosure: the community's building should be surrounded by strong walls with a single gate, entry through which should be tightly restricted.[18] Whilst both sets of religious took seriously their obligation to care for the poor and travellers, they made it clear they should be accommodated separately from the religious community.[19]

The promoters of monastic change in eleventh-century Italy shared a similar quest for purity to those in the tenth century: St Romuald (d. 1027) 'renewed' the life of those in orders who had taken wives like laymen and practised simony.[20] His critique of the worldliness of contemporary religious life – as practised by both monks and canons – led him to establish houses inspired by eremitic principles. Similar critiques of the sinful lives of contemporary simoniacal churchmen in Florence, both monks and secular clerics, inspired John Gualbert (d. 1073) in *c.*1038 to leave the monastery of San Miniato and establish one at Vallombrosa, which subsequently led to an order; Vallombrosa was also influenced by both monastic and eremitic ideas on the importance of escaping from the values and lifestyle of the earthly life. According to Andreas of Strumi's *Life*, John Gualbert emphasised the importance of a strict adherence to the Rule of Benedict; Andreas may have reported this in defence of his subject against the criticism that he had been too active in the campaign against simoniacal secular clergy in Florence.[21] The late eleventh- and twelfth-century movements which led to new orders being established in France were similarly fundamentalist, notably that which began in the Burgundian house of Cîteaux in 1098 and which led to the widely successful reinterpretation of the Benedictine Rule by what quickly became the pan-European Cistercian order.

At the same time various efforts were made to reform the houses of canons. Rather less is known about canonical communities because many of them lacked the institutional longevity which characterised monastic houses. Nevertheless it is clear that in tenth- and eleventh-century England, Italy and southern France individual reformers promoted the communal life amongst communities of canons, culminating in the Lateran Council of 1059 which promoted the canonical life for secular clergy enjoining that they practise 'the apostolic, that is the common life', eat and sleep together, and hold property in common.[22] Throughout this period those men and women who made a profession (or vow) to live a religious life thus constantly had to negotiate the problems and challenges engendered by living in this world despite their attempts to escape it.

Monastic views of the wider world

Those who promoted the renewal of the monastic or canonical life continuously emphasised its distinction from that enmeshed in the ways of the world. Keen to emphasise their separation from the laity, they often used 'lay' as shorthand for unreformed. Thus Farfa's early twelfth-century chronicle records how in 998 the new abbot decided to reform his house because the monks had abandoned monastic discipline, and instead behaved 'like laymen', as evidenced both by their diet (they were eating meat) and dress. This story is recorded in order to explain how this important Italian monastery just to the north of Rome came to adopt the customs of one of the most influential monasteries in Christendom at the time, those of the Burgundian house of Cluny.[23] Sexual impropriety is not amongst the charges recorded on this occasion but such tales are not uncommon in other accounts of change in individual houses where the lifestyle of the unreformed is often compared to that of the laity.

Instead both monastic reformers and their lay supporters attached considerable spiritual capital to those who had physically withdrawn from the lay world. As the Emperor Henry III of Germany (1039–56) observed in a letter to Hugh, abbot of Cluny (1049–1109): 'the prayers [of monks] become more pure, the more removed they become from secular acts, the more worthy, and thus more nearly their prayers stand out in divine view', and thus they can help those in this world.[24] Such beliefs explain the popularity of allowing children as young as six or seven to enter the order, a practice known as oblation, from the Latin for offering.[25] Parents offered the child, together with a substantial gift to the community, to God in a public rite during the Offertory part of the Mass.[26] The prayers of those who had been enclosed all their lives had especial value for lay patrons because they believed child entrants to have lived a purer life than adult converts.[27] This practice had been especially popular in the early Middle Ages, but the new orders founded in the eleventh and twelfth centuries instead emphasised the importance of adult entry; joining a religious order should be a conscious and personal decision, not one made by parents on behalf of a child. Central medieval reformed houses considered those who had entered the monastic life as oblates to be idle and complacent, lacking the spiritual ambition to strive for perfection. Nor was adult conversion confined to the new orders; established houses such as Cluny also witnessed an increase in late conversions between the mid-eleventh and early thirteenth centuries, which Charles de Miramon has suggested should be interpreted as the outcome of existing relations between monks and their lay benefactors. The monks' renewed interest in the spiritual welfare of their benefactors led them to preach the message that to convert oneself was the ultimate gift of both body and belongings; it met with an enthusiastic response.[28] Child oblation did not disappear, however; whilst the Cistercians rejected the practice, refusing to accept a novice under the age of fifteen, men might be promised to the order as children by their parents but only enter as adults.[29] This change in practice which seemingly reflects a renewed emphasis on individual conscience turns out not to be as clear-cut as it first appears to be.

As well as being a vehicle for effective prayer, their supposedly pure lives allowed monks to serve as exemplars of the life to come to those continuing to live in the world. Monastic writers thus often chose to portray monastic leaders in terms taken from Matthew's account of Christ's Sermon on the Mount (5.14–16):

> *Ye are the light of the world. A city that is set on an hill cannot be hid. Neither do men light a candle and put it under a bushel, but on a candlestick, and it giveth light unto all that are in the house. Let your light so shine before men that they may see your good works and glorify your Father which is in heaven.*

This text could be used to support the role of monks as passive exemplars of the pure life, as writers in both ninth-century Frankish Fulda and tenth- and eleventh-century Burgundian Cluny did. But Gregory the Great (d. 604) had used it earlier in his influential *Pastoral Rule* to argue that monks should not shrink from positions of authority within the Church and, as Phyllis Jestice has suggested, several (but not all) monastic writers from the tenth-century Lotharingian Görze movement cited the text to stress the importance of monks taking action in this world, especially once they became bishops.[30] The Görze reformers thus anticipated the more outward-looking agenda of eleventh-century and twelfth-century monastic reformers such as the Florentine John Gualbert, and Frankish Norbert of Xanten (d. 1134), founder of the Premonstratensian order of regular canons in 1120.[31]

Both Gregory the Great and the Görzian reformers took up a theme also embedded within the sixth-century Rule of Benedict which influenced the lives of canons as well as monks in this period. Chapter IV of the Rule twinned the importance of escape from the demands and temptations of the world, on the one hand, with an emphasis on the importance of active altruism on behalf of the less fortunate within it, on the other:

> *To deny one's very self to oneself in order to follow Christ. To discipline the body. Not to be enamoured of soft living. To love fasting. To give new heart to the poor. To clothe a naked person. To visit a sick person. To bury a dead person. To be a support in time of trouble. To comfort one who is saddened. To make oneself an outsider to the ways of the world. To put nothing above the love for Christ.*[32]

Reformers often debated the balance to be struck in the religious life between the twin ideals of the contemplative life, represented by complete withdrawal from the world, and the active life, represented by the pastoral ministry, on the other. Some communities gave precedence to enclosure and interpreted this passage as an injunction to practise altruism only within the monastery; such was the view of the ninth-century commentary on the Rule of Benedict written by Hildemar of Civitate.[33] Others were much more outward-looking. Such debates lie at the heart of the different interpretations about how to live the regular life which existed in this period. Individual houses of regular clergy seeking to define the lives of their members had to position themselves on the axis between the two, and where they chose to do so had repercussions for their relationship with the laity.

Policing the segregation of the world of the professional religious from that of the laity was a continuous process, and one which had repercussions for their relationship with their lay benefactors. In this period this relationship is seldom a straightforward one. Just as different religious from the same period might take different views of their role within the world, so they perceived the laity in different ways. On the one hand some monks demonised the lay world. The late eleventh-century chronicler, Hugh of Flavigny, for example, described a monk's vision of a journey to hell in which the monk asked his guide, St Michael, what the serpents represented, to which the answer came 'They are lay people'.[34] On the other hand, many contemplatives recognised the great debt they owed to the laity. The eleventh-century Bavarian monk Otloh of St Emmeram (d. post November 1070) wrote that no monk should be ignorant of the fact that he depended on the assistance (*administratio*) of lay people living in the world for his food, clothes and lodging. But just as monks depended on lay people, so lay people required monks; their presence in the sinful world meant they required the prayers of monks both for themselves and their relations. Using a musical analogy, Otloh argued that just as a chord requires both higher and lower notes, so whilst the spiritual life may be superior to that of the secular, their mutual dependence brings them closely together.[35] Moreover, he contended that those lay men and women who lived their life according to the Lord's rule would merit the same celestial joys as monks: if they gave one tenth of their produce as tithe, if they refrained from fraudulent practices, abstained from conjugal relations in Lent and on other holy days, abstained from prostitutes and public displays and struggled to live as far as it is possible for the *illiterati* according to the faith, then their life would be as meritorious in the eyes of the Lord as that of monks.[36] Following the admonitions of the clergy as to how to live a good lay life was as meritorious as living life according to a monastic rule. As we have already seen in Chapter 1, such a positive view of the laity remained current into the twelfth century in the widely circulated *Vision of Tnugdal*.[37] A similar acknowledgement of how crucial lay support might be for new monastic enterprises comes in the comment of the biographer of the early twelfth-century preacher and founder of the double house at Fontevrault, Robert of Arbrissel (d. 1116), who acknowledged that 'nor could this have been done without God who continued to inspire in local people the desire to send food'.[38] In theory it constituted a relationship of mutual benefit, one based on the distinctiveness of the religious from the laity.

How far in fact was the role of the laity as necessary adjuncts to the religious life, as idealised by Otloh of St Emmeram, played out in reality? As we shall see, lay men and women could and did enter the cloister, regular churchmen and women looked out into, and had regular contact with, the lay world. The next section explores the nature of the relationship between regular communities and their lay neighbours in more depth, focusing on the specific roles the laity was allowed to play in the everyday life of religious houses.

The roles of the laity within regular communities

People from all levels of lay society contributed to both the material and religious aspects of life within religious houses, as is clear from the genre of texts known as customaries. These texts first emerged in the tenth century and provide more detailed prescriptions than that offered by any rule for the way in which the regular life should be lived in particular houses, or groups of houses, setting out details as to how the annual liturgy should be conducted, alongside instructions about running the community. Such texts theoretically allowed for the circulation of practice beyond the walls of individual houses, but they were more often aspirational than descriptive. Lanfranc's *Constitutions* for Christ Church, Canterbury for example, drew largely on those of Cluny, a community of which he had no experience, although he had been a member of the Norman communities of Bec and Saint-Etienne, Caen; they then circulated as a text in England beyond Canterbury, reaching as far as Durham.[39] Customaries must be treated as texts; they cannot be taken as evidence for practice within a community which owned a copy, but they can tell us a good deal about attitudes and aspirations within those communities that did.

The authors of monastic customaries sought to preserve the house as far as possible from the contamination inherent in worldly contact. This is clear from the practices they envisioned surrounding the treatment of those entering the community, namely guests, and of the officeholders whose duties brought them into contact with the outside world: the guest master and cellarer. Guests should be housed separately from the community and the office of guest master is regarded as an important one; one-tenth of the income of the monastery was supposed to be reserved for guests at tenth-century Fleury.[40] According to Lanfranc's *Constitutions* the guest master might show lay guests around the monastery, including the cloister, as long as they did not wear riding boots or spurs or go barefoot, but not in the presence of other members of the community. Presumably such forms of worldly attire were perceived as polluting.[41] The office of cellarer posed even more challenges. The perils involved led the Rule of Benedict to direct that the office of cellarer, responsible for organising all the material needs of the community, be entrusted to a 'person of mature character'.[42] It was an office often assigned to adult converts, men with some experience of the world such as the tenth-century monastic reformer, John of Görze. He had experience of administering his own estates and serving at court before his conversion. In his *Life* his assumption of the office of cellarer exemplifies the monastic principle of withdrawal. John, we are told, sought to minimise his contact with the secular world, seldom leaving the confines of the abbey to visit its possessions, and when he did so being careful to eat his meals in accordance with monastic measures. Nevertheless, whilst he showed a cheerful face to those he met, he used to complain to his fellow monks,

> *that such secular conversations could never interest him for even a short time, but rather that through them he would lose something from his own accustomed way of life.*[43]

His resistance to the world signified his devotion to the contemplative life and thus his sanctity. Holding this office allowed him to display these qualities. Lanfranc's *Constitutions* provided a way for the holder of the office and the community to act together to negotiate the challenges raised by such a necessary post for the community's well-being. The *Constitutions* demanded that the community should listen to one of the seventy-three chapters from Benedict's Rule being read aloud every day, and that whenever they came to the chapter concerning the office of cellarer, the office-holder should confess his sins before the whole community; after he is absolved the community should sing Psalm 50 for him. This occasion is not a response to specific sins committed by the cellarer, but rather a ritual acknowledgement by office-holder and community of its inherent sinfulness. It is accompanied by a feast in the refectory.[44] In this combined ritual, performed several times a year, the office-holder humiliated himself before the whole community but at the same time the whole community celebrated his necessary role, rendered thanks for it, and thereby exalted it.

At the same time as customaries emphasise the pollution inherent in worldly contact they testify to the permeability of enclosure. Eleventh-century customaries from Cluny refer to *famuli* – lay servants – some of whom lived in the monastery, others with their families in the town outside its walls. They worked in the fields and woods belonging to the monastery as labourers, and as land agents, and inside it in the guest house, store houses and infirmary.[45] But their role in the monastery's life never became confined to manual and secular tasks. They also took their place in the community's liturgical life: in the *Liber tramitis*, an account of Cluny's customs compiled for Farfa in the first half of the eleventh century, *famuli* are described as decorating the church, holding banners in liturgical processions on Palm Sunday and at Rogation-tide, and carrying relics in processions outside the walls of the monastery.[46] They distributed and collected staffs for the Rogation processions, and prewashed the feet of the poor on Maundy Thursday before the office holders of the community formally washed them in imitation of Christ in the rite for the day.[47] Later customaries suggest the *famuli* even became involved in making the Eucharistic hosts.[48] These roles are ascribed to them in later eleventh-century customaries associated with Cluny and it is probable that they continued to play these roles up until the Abbot Peter the Venerable's reforms in the twelfth century which sought to exclude the *famuli* from the more intimate aspects of monastic life.[49]

Being aspirational texts, customaries, however, do not reflect the tensions which having such laymen within the monastic environs might generate within the community. The abbot of the Bavarian monastery of Tergernsee complained in a letter to the bishop of Freising, written in the late tenth century at a time of famine, about the way in which the house's *famuli* disturbed him with their vehement complaints, demanding food and clothing, and threatening to leave, and went on to list them as the craftsmen working on the church, the two workers in the kitchen – one to gather firewood, the other to look after the kitchen garden, the two bakers, the two ploughmen, the goatherd, the horse groom, the cobblers, the quarrymen and the brewers.[50]

In the eleventh and twelfth centuries, orders such as the Vallombrosans and the Cistercians sought to overcome the tensions generated by the involvement of servants in the life of the community in a new way; they invited the men who served as cobblers, millers, weavers, blacksmiths, shepherds and herdsmen to become full members of the community as lay brothers. They were expected to participate in its religious life, albeit separately, and at a more simplified level, than that of the choir monks. Like them, they made their profession after a novitiate of a year; they were also expected to follow a communal life, living in their own dormitory and refectory. Unlike choir monks, Cistercian lay brothers did not have to attend church eight times a day for the divine office; they were, however, expected to observe the office hours, reciting their prayers wherever they happened to be working.[51] The institution of lay brothers, whilst it preserved social distinctions between noble educated choir monks and illiterate workmen – Cistercian lay brothers were not 'to have a book or learn anything except the [prayers]... it was decreed they should know' – nevertheless offered members of the lower orders the possibility of following a monastic life. It did not, however, solve the intrusion of the world into the life of the cloister. Cistercian granges often required hired hands as well as lay brothers, especially at harvest time, and these labourers might include women: Cistercian statutes from mid-twelfth century Portugal went so far as to prohibit women from setting up huts in front of the grange.[52] The involvement of lay men and women in religious communities throughout this period thus testifies to a more open view of the religious life than that suggested by the emphasis on segregation in many reformist writings.

Lay men and women not only worked in and visited religious houses, they also wished to worship in them. The problem of how to accommodate the laity, especially lay women, who wanted to attend a male community's church preoccupied several religious in this period. Some male houses even built separate churches to accommodate visitors: tenth-century Farfa had two churches outside the monastic enclosure, one in the royal palace for when rulers visited, and one especially for lay women, and in the twelfth century the Cistercians often built separate chapels for the laity.[53] But other religious communities happily served churches with a lay congregation: in tenth-century England the customary known as the *Regularis Concordia*, produced in the context of the monastic reform of both cathedral and monastic communities, testifies to the presence of lay men and women at Mass on feast days, and many monastic communities acted as the custodians of popular saints' cults which attracted large crowds of lay pilgrims.[54]

Within tenth- and eleventh-century traditional monasticism, the liturgical year, far from keeping choir monks inside the monastic church in a perpetual round of daily prayer, afforded them opportunities to join in celebration with the wider lay community. The procession on Palm Sunday in many houses required monks to leave the monastery and process to another church, before returning to the monastery, in imitation of Christ's entry into Jerusalem. In eleventh-century Canterbury the monks processed from Christ Church, through the streets of the city, and out of the gates to the church of St Martin's. Whilst it is not clear how far the townspeople of Canterbury participated in, as opposed to witnessed this procession, other rites for this day, such as one from later eleventh-century Exeter, specified that both the clergy, that is the canons, *and* the people should take part in the procession, going to the 'church where branches of palms and other trees have been collected for consecration' suggesting that there, at least, such processions were regarded as community-wide events in which the clergy and people joined together, carrying palms, in imitation of the original crowd which had welcomed Christ into Jerusalem.[55] Sometimes the world came to them: in the eleventh-century Suabian monastery of St Gallen knights and nobles associated with the monastery joined the monks in their Easter procession through the cloister, before coming together for a feast in the refectory.[56] The early twelfth-century monk William of Malmesbury recorded how women, especially pregnant ones, crowded into the Old Church at Glastonbury at Candlemas in the tenth century.[57] On such occasions – Rogation Days were another – the wider community joined with that of the regular clergy to celebrate significant events in the church's year.

The poor had an especial place in regular communities. The Rules commanded monks to care for the poor and customaries demonstrate how they featured formally in the liturgical life of the monks: several customaries record the washing of the feet of twelve poor men on Maundy Thursday (after they have been prewashed by monastic servants) and their subsequent feeding and payment.[58] The poor allowed monks to fulfil Christ's commandment to care, feed and clothe the needy, and to imitate His humility. Their presence thus helped monks construct a view of themselves as Christ's heirs.

But the emergence of the office of almoner in this period suggests that monastic communities of the tenth and eleventh centuries took a more proactive interest in the care of the poor and the sick. This office is not specified in the Rule of Benedict, but it certainly existed by the second half of the eleventh century when various monastic customaries specify his duties.[59] According to Lanfranc's *Constitutions*, the almoner had to seek out and bring aid to the indigent poor: accompanied by two servants he should leave the monastic precincts each week to visit the houses of poor men and deliver necessities. The almoner must, however, refrain from entering any house in which a woman was present, even if she was sick; in such circumstance he should send help via his servants. The importance of maintaining a monk's purity outweighed his personal duty to visit the sick in such cases. Further evidence for the importance of this active ideal is found in accounts of the *Lives* of regular churchmen and women; acts of charity provide a common trope, as their authors sought to demonstrate how their subjects exemplified the precepts of their Rule, and the ideals of the early Church. In a famine in 976, for example, the English monastic reformer Bishop Æthelwold of Winchester 'snatched a host of poor people from the very jaws of death', spending all the money he had, and breaking down the church's silver vessels and ornaments in order to buy further supplies.[60] His biographer explicitly compared Æthelwold to the early martyr St Lawrence who had similarly used the treasures of his church to feed the poor, but such accounts had their ultimate origins in the Rule's emphasis on Christ's injunctions not to lay up treasure in this life but rather to feed and clothe the needy.[61] The late eleventh-century *Life* of Adelheid, Abbess of the Rhineland community of Vilich, records how in the first decade of the eleventh century she cared for the poor during a famine in Cologne, serving bread and bacon to the healthy, cabbage, beans and meat stew to the ill, and gruel to the dying. She also set aside the revenues from one of the convent's manors to feed and clothe fifteen poor people, and to allow the giving of twelve *solidi* to another fifteen paupers on the feast days of each Apostle and payment in kind on at least three quarter-days.[62] In the words of her biographer: 'Once she had settled all interior matters satisfactorily with God's help, she was impelled to turn her attention to the outside world for she also desired to serve the kingdom of God there.'[63] Such texts represent the significance of this ideal for regular communities, not its practice. Yet there is evidence for the realisation of these responsibilities. Whilst customaries enjoined that one-ninth of the house's income should be set aside for care of the poor, and one-tenth for guests, by the late eleventh century it has been calculated that one-third of Cluny's surplus went on the distribution of alms and the reception of guests.[64] Even if the proportion was weighted towards guests, as seems likely, it suggests that the monks of Cluny took their duties to the indigent seriously. Monks' commitments to charity thus often placed them at odds with their desire to retreat from the world. Giving alms and hospitality inevitably brought them into contact with the world, at the same time as they sought, through the liturgy, to incorporate their *famuli* and the poor into their own world. For both pragmatic and ideological reasons, central medieval monasticism appears to have been more outward-looking than it first seemed.

Canonical communities similarly, and less surprisingly, attached considerable importance to works of charity. Charity's prominence within the outlook of many of these communities comes across, for example, in the prologue to the early twelfth-century institutes of St Maria in Porto composed by St Peter of Onesti which became widely adopted by houses of canons throughout northern Italy. Although Peter cited the Rule of Benedict extensively, unlike his model he clearly prioritised the acts of charity over learning and liturgy:

> *Therefore let them love fasting, let them love the poor, let them gather in guests, let them clothe the naked, let them visit the sick, let them bury the dead, let them serve the oppressed, let them console the sorrowful, let them weep with the weeping, rejoice with the joyful, let them not forsake charity, if possible let them have peace with all, let them fear the day of judgment, let them desire eternal life above all, let them put their hope in God, let them put nothing before the love of Christ, let them obey the*

> *orders of their prelates in all things, let them comply with their own bishop in all things, according to the canonical institutes, and finally let them devote work to spiritual teachings, readings, psalms, hymns, canticles, and let them persevere unfailingly in the exercise of all good works.*[65]

Peter did not introduce a new element into the canonical life, but rather promoted an existing one. Such active altruism, caring for the sick, burying the dead, is a theme found in many other canonical communities of the period. For one of the most obvious changes in this period is the growth in charitable institutions over the course of the eleventh and twelfth centuries; hospitals for the sick and indigent were increasingly being founded on both episcopal and lay initiative, and they were usually administered by canonical communities because their rule not only emphasised such duties but also provided a sufficiently flexible structure to allow for charitable work.[66] Thus charity provided a common bond between monks, canons and laity.

But differences also existed. One of the seemingly more obvious divides between monks and canons concerns the delivery of pastoral care to the laity. In theory monks eschewed pastoral care, whilst canons embraced it.[67] In practice, the exercise of the pastoral ministry by monks seems to have been a recurrent issue throughout this period. Bishops might have a monastic background, a trend which increased in the twelfth century, reflecting the value put on clerical purity by clergy and people alike.[68] But they sought to restrict the monastic delivery of pastoral care at a lower level, as is clear from the canons included by Burchard in his early eleventh-century *Decretum*.[69] Monks made several attempts in both mid-eleventh-century Italy and mid-twelfth-century Germany to defend the pastoral ministry of monks, through the composition of false papal decrees and decretals which circulated in various tracts defending monks' ownership of tithes and right to preach, administer baptism and enjoin penance.[70] As these texts suggest, monastic ownership of parish churches provided the tinder for this debate, leading to discussion about whether monks could serve the churches they owned. Several councils in the late eleventh and twelfth centuries enjoined that monks should only deliver pastoral rites if they had an episcopal license to do so, suggesting it had become a live issue.[71] And yet there is evidence from eleventh-century Flanders and the Rhineland that monks there were occasionally allowed to exercise the pastoral ministry; abbots might also seek exemption from episcopal authority which allowed them to exercise episcopal jurisdiction over the churches owned by the monastery.[72]

Monks also supported pastoral care more indirectly. Charters recording the appointment of priests to serve monastic-owned churches often specify the services the priest should deliver at the same time as they record how the monastery should retain ownership of the tithe income. Clearly what went on in local churches under their control mattered to some monastic communities. Others supported efforts to improve the delivery of pastoral care through the composition and copying of liturgies for pastoral rites. The community at Fulda, for example, copied a sacramentary in a prestigious, lavishly illustrated library copy in *c.*980 which included a supplement of the fundamental pastoral rites: those for the administration of baptism, penance, and the visitation of the sick, and rites for the dying. The monks did not need the rites for baptism, for theirs was a single-sex all male community, and the rites for penance are pitched at a lay rather than monastic audience. Rather this collection of rites, considered together, suggests that the Fulda community thought it important to educate local priests in how to deliver pastoral care properly. The sacramentary is a model, not a book for use in the field, but the rites it contains in this supplement may have been copied out into little portable pamphlets, *libelli*, for use by local priests, probably in churches on Fulda's own lands.[73] Nor is Fulda alone in producing such material: similar, seemingly didactic collections of pastoral rites survive from eleventh- and twelfth-century English monasteries.[74]

The Interpolated Rule of Chrodegang, as we have already seen, charged canons with specific responsibility for pastoral care. In Italy there is evidence that some canonical communities took delivery of pastoral rites very seriously. We discussed the evidence of the small, somewhat tatty, codex now in the Vatican, Ms Archivio S. Pietro H. 58 in more detail in the previous chapter as evidence for widespread concern in clerical education. It is worth revisiting here because it was written in Rome in the first quarter of the eleventh century for the basilica of SS. XII Apostoli, which was probably administered by a house of canons at this time. As outlined above, its contents suggest it was made for a community interested in delivering pastoral care to the laity for it includes all the basic rites a priest would need:

an *ordo* for the Mass, and ones for infant baptism, anointing the sick, administering the last rites and burying the dead, together with a penitential. It also includes a copy of the *vita* of SS Eustratius and His Companions, which is marked up in numbered lections, suggesting it was meant to be read aloud, probably in a communal context.[75] The pastoral ministry remained of interest for many of the canonical communities which were reformed in the eleventh and twelfth centuries, like those following the institutes of St Maria in Porto.

In order to sustain life, however, religious men and women had to interact with the lay world, and at levels beyond material supplies and servants. The property and revenues which communities held in common financed these houses. Sometimes such endowments might be made with very specific expectations. For example, in tenth- and eleventh-century east Frankia, royal monasteries undertook to render the 'servitium regis' to support the itinerant royal court in its travels around the kingdom in return for royal protection and immunity, and rulers endowed them with property for this purpose. Sometimes this service might be to house and feed the royal court, either on monastic estates or in the monastery itself; or to make payment in kind to the nearest royal palace in order to supply provisions for the king's table; or to pray for the king, the royal family and the kingdom; or to advise the court; or to supply men for the king's army.[76] The community should support the work of the king spiritually, intellectually and materially.

Elsewhere expectations are less clear cut, but the extent of houses' property holdings inevitably imposed the demands of their tenants on these communities in their capacity as lords. The property holdings of institutions ranged in size, and the widespread geographical distribution of property owned by some houses brought its own challenges, but the holdings of most institutions lay within a day's ride.[77] Especially important houses held more extensive holdings: Farfa, for example, controlled much of the property in the Lazio, as well as possessing lands in the regions bordering the Lazio to the north and northeast.[78] Although the Burgundian house of Cluny had immense influence in this period, most of its considerable land holdings lay within 15km of Cluny itself, although the fact that it also held lands in Champagne, Savoy, Provence, Lombardy, England and Spain testifies to the widespread regard in which it was held.[79] The role of landlord brought the regular clergy forcibly into contact with their neighbours and tenants. In this role they often acted rapaciously, jealously safeguarding their rights, and expanding their authority at the expense of lesser landowners. Yet, as we saw above in the letters written during a famine by the late tenth-century abbot of Tergernsee, monks also often resented the intrusions of such mundane matters on their time.[80]

Their role as landowners led to the establishment of specific offices for laymen who served as buffers between the community, its tenants and the wider world. Charters and customaries testify to the important role played by lay agents in running extensive monastic estates. The provost, not the abbot, had responsibility for administering the community's properties; in practice this responsibility was often delegated to laymen acting as lay abbots, advocates or land agents on behalf of each house. Tenth-century reformers successfully abolished the practice of appointing laymen as abbots, with responsibility for and use of the monastery's property and income as well as its defence.[81] The office of advocate lasted rather longer. The office of advocate (*advocatus*) or guardian (*custos*) seems to have originated in ninth-century reformers' concern to distance monks from the secular world.[82] The practice persisted into the tenth and eleventh centuries when members of the regional nobility, and local counts and lords assumed the office of advocate for a particular monastery.[83] Advocates acted as a buffer between the community and the wider world, representing it in legal cases, taking action against laymen who attacked its property, and sometimes collecting revenues from property in more distant areas. They might also often be asked to confirm the election of the abbot, and might even, as we shall see below, instigate the reform of a house, by handing it over to a reformer. In practice therefore lay agents usually undertook the day-to-day administration. In the tenth and eleventh centuries, nobles, variously known as the *maior*, *villicus* or *ministerialis*, had responsibility for administering the community's estates in a particular area in return for a proportion of the income. In order to retain control over their agents' activities, monasteries in northern France asked them to swear oaths to renounce all bad practice, and not to buy or sell land without the permission of the provost, and not to take the proportion of profits of justice which belonged to the monks. Such oaths suggest that monks wished to set a good example as landlords, and to curb the excesses of their agents.[84] They also point to the pragmatism which governed monastic relations with the wider community in this area.

Lay relations with religious houses

So far we have been concerned with investigating the ways in which the lay world penetrated that of the regular clergy. In this final section we will consider their relations with their lay benefactors. As members of the regular clergy themselves recognised, the laity's involvement was crucial, founding new houses and sustaining existing ones by giving them lands and other revenues and property. Noble patrons invited clerics in from outside to reform existing institutions, and supported new forms of regular life, including those of regular canons, and towards the end of the twelfth century other pastoral institutions such as hospitals and hospices. These developments in the regular life would simply not have been possible without the active agency of the lay nobility.

Most of the evidence for lay support comes from three types of source: the lives of the founders and reformers of communities; charters; and texts memorialising those associated with the house, both living and dead. The religious composed all these genres and they were generally influenced by pre-existing textual models; for example, the lives of late antique saints inspired the structure and incidents in the *Lives* of central medieval monks and canons. Charters are records of legal agreements between the religious house and another party, and were made for gifts, sales, leases and the settlement of disputes. Written for the house's archives after the act of transfer had taken place, in highly formulaic language heavily influenced by the earlier traditions, they usually survive not in their original form, but rather copied into a codex known as a cartulary, where records were grouped, often by the estate to which they relate. For example, the charter archive of the monastic house of Montier-en-Der, founded on the border between Champagne and Lorraine, purportedly goes back to its original foundation in the seventh century but survives now only in a cartulary copied in *c*.1126–29.[85] Various sorts of texts commemorated communities' benefactors. Monastic houses kept the *libri vitae* containing the names of the house's benefactors and others for whom the members of that community should pray on the high altar. *Libri vitae* are unsystematic accumulations of names of those who wished to be remembered by that community.[86] Necrologies are more organised.[87] Arranged by the days of the liturgical year, the names of those to be remembered are listed on the appropriate day, usually but not always the anniversary of their death.

Twelfth-century customaries provide a clue as to when such books were to be used, specifying that after Prime and the first Mass of the day, a Mass of the dead should be celebrated during which prayers should be said for the dead of the community, those in fraternity with it, the house's benefactors, those buried in the abbey's cemetery, and all the dead, and the names for the following day should be read out in the daily chapter meeting which came immediately after this.[88]

Both *libri vitae* and necrologies acted as records of the communities' counter-gifts to the donations recorded in charters: the giving of a gift represents the desire to record and maintain a relationship between two parties, and social anthropology has long emphasised the importance of reciprocal gift for acknowledging and maintaining that relationship.[89] Lay men and women sought to share in the *opus Dei* of a community of regular churchmen or women, often through gifts of property, revenues or precious objects in return for remembrance by the community. This expected link between the donor's gift and the community's counter-gift of prayer could sometimes be made very explicit: Maurus, a merchant from Amalfi, gave the monks of Farfa a carved ivory casket with the following inscription:

> *Take this modest vessel, appropriate for divine worship, and given to you with devout mind by your people. We ask that our names be known to you everywhere, but a salutary precaution led them to be engraved here. I am rightly called Maurus because I have associated with black people; my children follow me, Johannes with Pantaleon, Sergius and Manso, Maurus and also the brother Pardo. Give absolution for sin, offer a celestial crown.*[90]

Specifying that the casket was a gift and could be used in the liturgy, Maurus requested both that the names of himself and his children be remembered, and absolution for sins. The Farfa community also adapted gifts of precious capes from the mid-eleventh-century Byzantine governor of southern Italy and the German Empress Agnes into liturgical copes, to be worn by members of the community at Mass.[91] In both cases these gifts allowed the donors physically to be part of the monastic liturgy; more usually gifts of land or rights to income supported the religious in their round of prayer. The religious made returns for such generosity in a variety of different ways. Some might be very specific, some much more general. Charters might request burial of the donors or a member of their family in the community's church or cemetery; admittance on the donor's deathbed to membership of the community; specific commemoration by the community of the anniversary of their death through feasts, prayers and, later, Masses; admittance to brotherhood, *fraternitas*, with the community.[92] But many donations, especially in the tenth and eleventh centuries, are recorded as being just 'for the souls' (*pro anima*) of the donor and his or her family, and seem to have had the more general aim of establishing a relationship between the family and the community rather than stipulating a specific return. Maurus's gift to Farfa is slightly unusual in this respect in requesting absolution. In mentioning the names of his children, Maurus is less remarkable, for charters often state that donation is being made on behalf of not only the donor but also their wider family, that is their dead parents, living siblings, children and other family. Both sides sought anxiously to maintain the relationship between benefactor and religious across the generations. As Barbara Rosenwein showed in her study of donations made to Cluny in the century and a half after its foundation in 910, a grant of land seldom represented a one-off grant but rather was used to create a continuous relationship between the community and the benefactor's family. Land would be granted by one generation, but subsequently retained or reclaimed, only for it to be given again by the next generation. Such practices suggest one way in which families sought to perpetuate their relationships with a religious house. The practice by which land granted to a community might be immediately leased back to the donor's family for the current and next generation is another.[93]

These three types of evidence – *Lives*, charters and necrologies – testify to the great growth in the number of religious houses in this period, and in lay support for the different ways in which the religious life could be conducted. Taken together, they provide a complex picture of lay relations from the perspective of churchmen; they suggest, as we shall see, a world in which religious houses acted as the focus for political and social ambitions, family identity and memory, but also personal anxiety and devotion. But the very profusion of this sort of evidence in this period makes synthesis a hazardous, if not impossible, task.

The desire to increase power in particular areas may explain why rulers chose to support the work of particular reformers, as Count Baldwin IV of Flanders did that of Richard of St Vannes, for example, as part of the expansion of comital power within Flanders and into northern Francia and

Lotharingia.[94] Baldwin thus assured himself of support from houses with significant landholdings in areas where his own comital authority was precarious. Monastic patronage not only supported rulers in time of political expansion: families used it as a tool to protect their inheritance in times of instability. Church lands were legally inalienable and, in theory at least, immune from royal confiscation in a way that noble land holdings were not. Thus the protection afforded to church land in law explains why the rate at which families chose to establish or donate to houses increased in times of uncertainty when their right to property might be challenged by a change of regime; such increases have been identified in southern Italy at the time of the Norman Conquest in the 1050s and 1060s, and in England during the unrest of King Stephen's reign in the 1030s and 1040s.[95]

Many modern scholars have been interested in uncovering such patterns, looking for the covert secular motives which underlie the bland statements in charters that the founders made the grant on behalf of the souls of themselves and those of their parents. But can such overt statements be dismissed as formulaic? Is it really possible to divide donors' motives into clear categories, separating the secular from devotional? The history of the foundation of one house, Vilich near Bonn, points to the ways in which they might often overlap.

According to the account given in the *Life* of its first abbess, Count Megengoz and his wife Gerberga decided to establish a convent of canonesses there as a result of a crisis within their family. This was the death of their only son, Godefrid whilst on campaign against the Slavs in 977. According to the *Life*, his parents decided to found a house with his patrimony at Vilich, at the juncture of the Rhine and the Sieg rivers, opposite the modern German city of Bonn, so that although deprived of his earthly inheritance, he would gain a better one in heaven.[96] Godefrid's body was brought back and buried in the church on the site of the monastery, as in due course were those of his parents and three of his sisters.[97] His mother then redeemed her young daughter, Adelheid, from the convent of St Ursula in Cologne, and appointed her abbess of the new community. On Adelheid's death in *c.*1015 her niece succeeded her as abbess. Following their son's death Megengoz and Gerberga themselves decided to separate from each other, and to live a continent life of study, following St James's teaching 'Be ye doers of the word and not hearers only' (I.22). Megengoz stayed in the world 'because of the demands from his own people' but in quiet moments he asked his chaplains to explain in German the divine books; Gerberga oversaw the building of the community and followed a life of divine service, fasting and praying both night and day.[98] The premature death of a son is thus reported to have instigated one couple to change their own lives, to found a convent governed by their daughter, which in turn became a centre for family memory; at least three generations were buried there, testifying to the family's ongoing relationship with the house. This account is that given in the mid eleventh-century *Life of Adelheid* written in elegant Latin by Bertha, a member of the community. It doubtlessly mythologised the origins of her house; in particular, according to Bertha, Gerberga had wished from the beginning that the community should follow the Benedictine rule but Adelheid had initially expressed a preference for the less strict life of a canoness. Her later conversion to the Benedictine Rule was part of the narrative of Adhelheid's move to sanctity, and at the same time the story legitimised the shift by referring to the founder's original wishes. Yet comparing this account with other evidence for lay benefactions to other houses in both Germany and elsewhere will reveal how typical it is of lay benefactions in this period.

Vilich is not unusual in serving as the founding family's mausoleum.[99] It is common for nobles in the central Middle Ages to be buried in monasteries; they recognised prayer for the souls of the dead as necessary, and usually entrusted it to monastic communities who, in a period of instability, and dynastic frailty, could be relied on to pray regularly and continuously for the dead, and to maintain their graves, even after the demise of the family. It had become so universal a practice that the twelfth-century Cistercian order, which sought to restrict the practice of saying specific prayers for the dead and attempted, rather unsuccessfully, to prohibit the burial of benefactors in monastic churches, made an exception for the burial of founders.[100] Only the more wealthy nobility could afford to found houses: the founder of Vilich, Countess Gerburga, was the great granddaughter of King Henry the Fowler of the East Franks. However, lesser nobles imitated their nobles by seeking burial in the same church as their ancestors, even when it was not a family foundation. For example, in an act which echoes Megingoz and Gerburga's burial of Godefrid, sometime between 1010 and 1035 the mother and brothers of a young knight, Guido, donated a manse of land to the Burgundian monastery of Montier-en-Der so that he might be buried where his father and ancestors had been before him.[101] The desire to be buried alongside one's ancestors could be so strong that noblemen would even settle disputes with the monastery in order to ensure its fulfilment; the cartulary of Montier-en-Der records how sometime between 1050 and 1060 a certain Hugh came to church, confessed his faults, and being led to penance, made emendation for his faults, giving his castles to the monastery, for his evil deeds and for the soul of his mother and other ancestors, who were already buried in the church, so that he might be buried alongside them.[102]

By serving as mausoleums, such houses also often became a physical focus for family identity and memory. Three generations of the same family were buried at Vilich: Megingoz and Geburga, their children Godefrid, Irmintrud, Bertrada and Adelheid, and their granddaughter who succeeded Adelheid as abbess. Donation charters suggest that donors sometimes thought in terms of three generations: the foundation charter recording the establishment of Cluny in 910 by William of Aquitaine and his wife Ingelberga mentions that they made the donation on behalf of the king and three generations of William's family: William's parents, and his aunt (whose legacy William used as the endowment for Cluny), themselves and their brothers and sisters, their nephews and all their relatives of both sexes.[103] At other times and in other places only two generations are mentioned. The initial leaders of a religious community, such as Adelheid and her niece, might often be intimately connected to its founders and benefactors. A charter of Henry II confirming Vilich's privileges from 1003 even specified that the abbess should be a member of the founder's family.[104] This trend is not confined to the earlier part of our period but continued into the twelfth century after reformers had begun to highlight the dangers of secular influence on ecclesiastical property.

But religious houses served a wider constituency. They acted as an important focus for the pious devotions of neighbouring local families who, whilst unable to afford to alienate the lands necessary to establish a religious house, nevertheless wished to be associated with and remembered by it. And even if they were not the founders, local families often supplied members of the community. The reformer Robert of Abrissel instigated the foundation of the double house of Fontevrault in *c.*1100 on lands donated by William IX of Aquitaine and his wife Philippa. Its first abbess, Hersende, was the widowed mother-in-law of one its earliest patrons, Gautier of Montsoreau; her assistant and successor, Petronilla, was related to another important benefactor.[105] The early members of the reformed community at Görze in the tenth century shared the same names as their lay patrons.[106] The Lords of Semur-en-Brionnais in Burgundy supplied three generations of monks at Cluny in the eleventh and twelfth centuries: Abbot Hugh of Cluny (1049–1109), his nephews Hugh and Geoffrey, and great nephew Raynald. This family also had close connections with the house they established for women in 1054 at Marcigny, indicating that such connections were not always exclusive.[107] The *Statutes* of Cluny compiled by Peter the Venerable (d. 1156) instituted a feast which suggests the continuing importance of such connections: members of the community should remember all their relations of both sexes on the 24th of January.

But founders' families did not always remain intimately connected with their foundations, for a variety of reasons. For example, Walter Espec, a prominent courtier of King Henry I, established the North Yorkshire Cistercian abbey of Rievaulx in 1132. He died childless in 1158 and his nephews, whilst they made some benefactions to the new house, did not prove as supportive as their uncle. In the absence of a powerful benefactor, the community instead constructed its own network of support. Its foundation charter had been witnessed by tenants of Walter Espec as well as members of his retinue, and many of his former tenants and their children went on to become donors to the abbey. The community's near neighbours also made up a large proportion of its donors.[108] Similar connections between neighbours and patrons have been established by Rosenwein in her study of Cluny's charters from the tenth and eleventh centuries.[109] In other words the decision to patronise a particular house reflected social and political ties beyond those of the immediate family.

Such studies of lay patronage do not address the big question of why the lay nobility were willing to alienate the title to so much of their property in this period, nor why some families all chose to enter the religious life, such as that of Bernard of Clairvaux and his brothers and sister, thus committing what Alexander Murray called dynastic suicide. Murray suggested that the ascetic lifestyle of the professional religious appealed to nobles because it offered such a complete contrast to the values of their class: their power, their wealth, their arms.[110] Certainly personal crisis is a common trope in the lives of individual monastic leaders who converted from secular to religious life as adults. Examples can be found from across the period. According to his eleventh-century *Life* a Flemish nobleman called Gerard (d. 959) was out hunting one day when he was inspired by a vision of SS. Peter and Paul to turn away from his secular life, and to become a monk. He thus founded a monastery on his own lands at Brogne, with the support of his father, brother and other relatives, whose consent to the grant is recorded in the foundation charter of 919.[111] Having established his own house, Gerard went on to reform several other houses in Flanders and northern France. He is unusual in being an adult convert: many other well-known figures of monastic reform in the tenth century in England, France and Lotharingia had a monastic or clerical background. Yet Gerard is not unique. John of Görze, one of the men behind the reform of that community in *c.*933, entered the religious life as an adult, having had experience of running his family's estates on the death of his father.[112] In the late tenth century, Romuald, a young aristocrat from Ravenna, entered the monastery of Sant'Apollinare in Classe as an adult after witnessing his father kill someone in a duel; by becoming a monk he sought to atone for his own and his father's sins. Romuald became dissatisfied with the regular life, as conducted in that particular house, and left to live as a hermit, before ultimately founding a monastery at Camaldoli in the Tuscan diocese of Arezzo (*c.*1022) which sought to combine the regular life with the eremitical: a community of monks at the foot of the hill supported more experienced members of the community living as hermits higher up the mountain.[113] In the mid-eleventh century, John Gualbert of Florence entered the monastery of San Miniato as an adult as a consequence of a family feud, before, after trying the life at Camaldoli, founding his own community at Vallombrosa which was notable for its emphasis on the importance of enclosure and the use of lay brothers to act as buffers between the choir monks and the lay world, on the one hand, and for taking a direct part in the fight against simony in the diocese of Florence, on the other.[114] Towards the end of the third decade of the twelfth century a Languedocian knight, Pons of Léras, decided to give up his life as a brigand; worried about how he should remove the stains of his sins, he decided that the only way to do so was to make satisfaction for his past acts by renouncing the secular world, including his family: his wife and daughter entered a convent, his son a monastery. Joining with six other friends, who were similarly motivated to enter the religious life, they built a monastery at Silvanès, in the diocese of Lodève in 1132, on land donated by a nobleman.[115] It is perhaps no coincidence that the customs followed in all four houses founded by these men from the tenth, eleventh and twelfth centuries highlighted the value of being remote from the world. The similarities between these accounts of the lives of these four adult converts and monastic founders signal the importance which individual conversion played in monastic thought: monastic writers idealised entry into the religious life as a personal decision, a conscious turning away from the lay life and embracing of the values of monasticism.[116]

John Gualbert led religious change in both the monastic and clerical spheres in Tuscany. He and his monks preached vigorously in favour of the reform of the pastoral clergy, as well as setting up houses of reformed monks. Yet it is clear that throughout this period the initiative for reform of individual houses, like their foundation, generally came from the laity. In the tenth and eleventh centuries, lay advocates often instigated change. In 941, for example, Count Arnulph of Flanders invited Gerard of Brogne to become abbot of his family's monastery, St Peter's Ghent, where his parents were buried. The house had suffered in the wake of the Viking attacks of the late ninth and early tenth century, losing many of its lands to the local nobility (including Arnulph's own family), and the community itself had abandoned the monastic for the canonical life. In the words of the restoration charter, at the exhortation of religious and revered men, Arnulph restored the house to the monastic rule, inviting the canons to embrace the monastic life; the majority, however, chose to leave, and were replaced by monks, and Gerard of Brogne became abbot. The count also restored the monastery's possessions. According to the charter, the monks were to follow the Rule of St Benedict, but the election of the abbot required the assent of the count and his successors. Arnulph intended that his family should retain considerable influence over the house. In 944 the count accompanied the abbot to Boulogne to collect the relics of SS. Wandrille and Ansbert; he clearly became very actively involved in the reform of this house.[117] Gerard is also credited with reforming at least two other houses in northern France and Lotharingia which had suffered similarly in the late ninth and early tenth centuries.

Throughout this period, lay benefactors remained central not only to supporting materially the lives of religious men and women but to driving forward change in the ways their lives were conducted within their communities. Arnulph's actions are far from unique; it was not unusual for lay nobles to invite renowned abbots to reform houses for which they felt some responsibility. In Rome in the 930s Prince Alberic set out to restore the monastic life of the city which had similarly suffered at the hands of the Saracens and the lay nobility; Alberic is later remembered as one who 'restored the goods of monasteries which had been taken a short while before by crooked men'. Alberic's actions were not confined to the temporal sphere: in 936 he invited Abbot Odo of Cluny to reform the rules and liturgy of the monastic houses in the city and the surrounding duchy.[118] A century later in Burgundy, sometime between 1035 and 1049, Manasses, count of Rosnay and his son, in order to wipe away their transgressions, handed over the community of canons regular which they had established in their castle to the monks at Montier-en-Der because they had discovered the leader of the community, Guido, to be a renegade monk and had driven him out.[119] The importance of lay initiative continued in the twelfth century as is clear from the support shown for the new orders and the various new forms of spirituality by men such as Walter Espec and his tenants. The Cistercians owed their expansion to the initiative and piety of lay nobles, just as earlier reformers had in tenth-century Flanders, Normandy and Rome, and eleventh-century Burgundy.

Conclusions

The central Middle Ages witnessed the foundation of thousands of new houses across western Christendom. It is impossible to estimate how many; the relative poverty of many smaller establishments, especially houses of canons and canonesses, means they have left little or no trace in the historical record. A couple of regional examples indicate the scale of the change. Bruce Venarde estimates the number of nunneries in England and Wales increased from seventy in *c.*1000 to more than four hundred by 1170. Mathieu Arnoux records the foundation of thirty-two canonries in the province of Rouen between 1119 and 1200.[120] At the same time the number of recorded donations to houses of religious also substantially increased. Periods of political instability, which led families to seek security for their property and spiritual patronage for their well-being, help explain particular local patterns in the growth of foundations and donations. But, whatever their origins, these local developments also fit into a bigger picture which suggests that throughout Latin Christendom there was a gradual increase in the number of houses in the tenth and early eleventh centuries, followed by a much more rapid increase in the late eleventh and twelfth centuries.

Increased diversification in the forms of religious life accompanied this growth. This chapter has focused in the main on monastic female and male houses, and on the conscious diversification in the types of monasticism which occurred, but this period also witnessed a significant growth in the establishment of houses for canons and canonesses. Canons' supporters belonged to a very similar milieu to those of monks. In eleventh-century England, for example, earls chose to establish and support houses of canons rather than the great monasteries. Earl Leofric and his wife sponsored the house of canons at Stow in Lincolnshire whose great church still stands as a testament to their generosity. Harold Godwineson refounded Waltham Holy Cross in Essex as a canonical community. Robin Fleming suggests that in turning away from monastic patronage, these nobles showed themselves to be at the cutting edge of eleventh-century piety, drawing in particular on developments in northwest and east Frankia. These reformed communities of canons in cathedrals oversaw some of the more exciting developments in eleventh-century intellectual culture, in pastoral care, medicine, theology, and law, and trained successive generations of clerics as administrators. By founding their own houses of canons, members of the English nobility gained at the same time their own religious centre, dedicated to their memory, and more pragmatically a source of trained clerks to serve in their own households.[121] The noble entourage of King Henry I also embraced canons, playing a significant role in the establishment of houses of Augustinian canons in both England and Normandy. In doing so they deliberately set out to emulate Henry's royal patronage of these types of house. On top of the pragmatic and pious advantages that such communities offered to their eleventh- and twelfth-century patrons, as we have already seen, the Augustinian canons provided a chance to be seen to emulate the devotional behaviour of their lord and rule: social ambition combined with other factors to explain their decision. From the twelfth century onwards such foundations were not confined to the noble elite: one study of canons in the province of Rouen suggests that members of the urban bourgeoisie and the lesser nobility also began to establish canonries in the course of the twelfth century.[122]

In part this change reflects increasing economic prosperity: it only became possible then for those lower down the social order to afford to sponsor their own foundations. In part it is also a reflection of the increasing significance of charity in the eleventh and twelfth centuries. Whilst, as we have seen, charity remained important within the monastic life throughout this period, it is a virtue which laymen increasingly valued and wished to practise. Thus laymen as well as bishops sponsored the foundation of hospitals for the ill and poor. Often they entrusted such foundations to canonical communities to administer, but not always. In 1065, for example, a man called Joceran gave both a vineyard and his house in the town of Cluny to the monastic community there. The grant specified that his house should become a hospice for the poor, and Joceran appointed one of his servants to run it. The running costs of the hospice should be funded by the vineyard, which would be administered by the monks.[123] In requesting that the monks of Cluny oversee the terms of his grant, he asked them to ensure that this charitable act continued after his death, rather than that he be remembered by them after his death. This act is indicative of a significant development in the nature of devotion in this period, but it was one which grew out of existing trends within monasticism.

Throughout this period religious communities strove to separate themselves from the secular world, an aim in which they were supported by the laity; indeed the laity often led such initiatives. At the same time houses of male religious remained active in the world – as preachers, teachers, and pastors – throughout this period. Such external activities were even expected of female religious. Yet it is clear that female houses, and individual female religious, often played important roles within the lay world and in the ministry to the laity. Mathilda, abbess of Quedlinburg (d. 999) served as regent of Germany during Emperor Otto III's absence in Italy in the 990s. Adhelheid of Vilich ministered to the poor during a famine in Cologne in the early eleventh century. In the early twelfth century Robert of Arbrissel conceived his female house at Fontevrault as supporting his work as an itinerant preacher by providing him with a resting place.

Both male and female religious remained constantly engaged with the lay world at the same time as the laity played a crucial part in their religious life. The ways in which the laity aspired to become part of the life of a particular religious community – by entering into confraternity with the community, by entering the community on their deathbed, by choosing to be buried within the precincts of the community – left their mark on the lives of religious institutions, but they also, as we shall see in Chapter 6, influenced the ways in which lay men and women sought to conduct their own devotions.

Notes and references

1 *PL* 151, 338.

2 *Vita Adelheidis Abbatissae Vilicensis auctore Bertha*, ed. O. Holder-Egger, *MGH SS* 15.2, 754–63 at p. 760; English translation: M. Bergen Dick, *Mater Spiritualis. The Life of Adelheid of Vilich* (Toronto, 1994), 27.

3 J. Wollasch, 'Monasticism: The First Wave of Reform', *NCMH* III, 163–85 at p. 163.

4 C. H. Lawrence, *Medieval Monasticism: Forms of Religious Life in Western Europe in the Middle Ages*, 2nd edn (London, 1989), 1.

5 T. Licence, *The Rise of Hermits and Recluses: England and Western Europe 970–1200* (Oxford, 2011).

6 *PL* 151, 338.

7 M. de Jong, 'Carolingian Monasticism: The Power of Prayer', *NCMH II*, 622–53.

8 *Expositio regulae ab Hildemaro tradita*, ed. Mittermüller, 399–400, 481; M. McLaughlin, *Consorting with Saints. Prayer for the Dead in Early Medieval France* (Ithaca, NY, 1994), 71–72.

9 For the text, see J. Bertram, *The Chrodegang Rules: The Rules for the Common Life of the Secular Clergy from the Eighth and Ninth Centuries: Critical Texts with Translations and Commentary* (Aldershot, 2005). The commentary should be treated with caution: see the reviews by M. Claussen, *The Medieval Review*, 6 August 2006, https://scholarworks.iu.edu/dspace/handle/2022/6209 (accessed 13 August 2010) and J. Barrow, 'Review Article: Chrodegang, His rule and Its successors', *Early Medieval Europe* 14 (2006), 201–12.

10 Interpolated Rule, cc. 15–18, 20–22, 24 (Nocturn, Matins, Prime, Tierce, Sext, None, Vespers, Compline); D. Hiley, *Gregorian Chant* (Cambridge, 2009), 25–29. On the Office, see R. E. Reynolds, 'Divine Office', *Dictionary of the Middle Ages*, ed. J. R. Strayer, 13 vols (New York, 1989), IV, 221–231, and A. Häussling, 'Stundengebet', *Lexikon des Mittelalters* VIII, 260–65.

11 Interpolated Rule, c. 44, *RC*, 206, 257.

12 Ibid., c. 42, *RC*, 206, 256.

13 See n. 22 below.

14 *Institutio sanctimonialium*, *MGH Leges III. Concilia II: Concilia Aevi Karolini*, ed. A. Werminghoff (Hannover, 1906), no. 39: *Concilium Aquisgranense B*, 421–56.

15 J. Siegwart, *Die Chorherren-und Chorfrauengemeinschaften in der deutschsprachigen Schweiz vm 6. Jahrhundert bis 1160 mit einem Überblick über die deutsche Kanonikerreform des 10. und 11. Jahrhunderts* (Freiburg, 1962), ch. 4, esp. pp. 156–62.

16 For an overview, see Wollasch, 'Monasticism'.

17 *RB*, c. 66, 304. See also ibid., c. 4: 'The monastery enclosure and stability in the community constitute, however, the workshop where we labour diligently at all these things', 65.

18 Interpolated Rule, c. 13, *RC*, 194, 241.

19 *RB*, c. 53, 248; Interpolated Rule, c. 45, *RC*, 206, 257–58.

20 This is the view of the author of the Prologue of the *Liber Tramitis Aevi Odilonis Abbatis*, ed. P. Dinter, CCM X (Siegburg, 1980), 3.

21 Andreas of Strumi, *Vita Iohannis Gualberti*, ed. F. Baethgen, *MGH SS* XXX.2, 1080–104; S. B. Gajano, 'Storia e tradizione vallombrosane', *Bullettino dell'istituto storico italiano per il medio evo e Archivio Muratoriano* 76 (1964), 99–215, esp. pp. 163–65.

22 C. 4, *MGH Leges IV: Constitutiones et acta publica imperatorum et regum I*: 911–1197, ed. L. Weiland (Hannover, 1893), no. 384, p. 547. *Laws of Æthelred V* (1008), c. 7: canons to live chastely in communities, eat in refectories and sleep in dormitories; *C&S I*, 365.

23 Gregory of Catino, *Il Chronicon Farfense*, Fonti per la Storia d'Italia 33, 34 (1903), I, 55, 2, 75.

24 'quorum oratio tanto purior, quanto ab actibus saeculi remotior, tanto dignior, quanto divinis conspectibus exstat propinquior', *Epistolae diversorum ad S. Hugonem Cluniacensis*, Ep. 6, *PL* 159, 931–32.

25 For further discussion of Romuald's and John Gualbert's conversions, see below.

26 Whilst the Cistercians rejected the practice, refusing to accept a novice under the age of 15, men might be promised to the order as children by their parents: C. B Bouchard, *Sword, Miter, and Cloister: Nobility and the Church in Burgundy, 980–1198* (Ithaca, NY, 1987), p. 49, n. 8.

27 On the early medieval practice, see M. de Jong, *In Samuel's Image: Child Oblation in the Early Medieval West* (Leiden, 1996); eadem, 'Growing Up in a Carolingian Monastery: Magister Hildemar and his Oblates', *Journal of Medieval History* 9 (1983), 99–128. See also J. H. Lynch, *Simoniacal Entry into Religious Life from 1000 to 1260* (Columbus, OH, 1976), 36–50.

28 C. de Miramon, 'Embrasser l'état monastique à l'âge adulte (1050–1200): étude sur la conversion tardive', *Annales. Histoire, Sciences Sociales* 54 (1999), 825–49.

29 Bouchard, *Sword, Miter, and Cloister* 49, n. 8.

30 P. G. Jestice, 'The Görzian Reform and the Light under the Bushel', *Viator* 24 (1993), 51–78.

31 P. G. Jestice, *Wayward Monks and the Religious Revolution of the Eleventh Century* (Leiden, 1997); T. J. Antry, O. Praem and C. Neel, eds, *Norbert and Early Norbertine Spirituality* (New York, 2007).

32 C. 4, *RB*, 2.

33 *Expositio regulae ab Hildemero tradita, et nunc primum typis mandata*, ed. R. Mittermüller (Regensburg, 1880), 146–52.

34 Hugh of Flavigny, *Chronicon*, Bk II, *MGH SS* VIII, 386.

35 *Dialogus de tribus quaestionibus*, c. 44, *PL* 146, 121; I. M. Resnick, 'Litterati, Spirituales, and Lay Christians according to Otloh of Saint Emmeram', *Church History* 55 (1986), 165–78.

36 *Liber de cursu spirituali*, c. 2, *PL* 146, 144.

37 See Chapter 1.

38 *Les deux vies de Robert D'Arbrissel fondateur de Fontevraud: légendes, écrits et témoignages*, ed. J. Dalarun *et al.* (Turnhout, 2006), 168–69; *Robert of Abrissel: A Medieval Religious Life*, ed. B. Venarde (Washington, DC, 2003), 17.

39 H. E. J. Cowdrey, *Lanfranc: Scholar, Monk and Archbishop* (Oxford, 2003), 154–60; *The Monastic Constitutions of Lanfranc*, ed. D. Knowles and C. N. L. Brooke (Oxford, 2002), xxxix–xlii, xliv.

40 *Consuetudines Floriacenses Antiquiores*, ed. A. Davril and L. Donnat, CCM 7.3 (Siegburg, 1984), c. 13, 24.

41 *The Monastic Constitutions of Lanfranc*, c. 90, 128–32.

42 *RB*, c. 31,176; the *RB* is cited in the Interpolated Rule, c. 11, *RC*, 193, 240.

43 Jean de Saint-Arnoul, *La vie de Jean, abbé de Gorze*, ed. M. Parisse (Paris, 1999), cc. 9–12, 75, 85–6, pp. 48–50, 104, 114–116. English translation from Jestice, *Wayward Monks*, p. 34. On John's modest background, see J. Nightingale, *Monasteries and their Patrons in the Gorze Reform: Lotharingia c. 850–1000* (Oxford, 2001), 94–95.

44 C. 89, *The Monastic Constitutions of Lanfranc*, 126–28.

45 G. Constable, '*Famuli* and *Conversi* at Cluny: A Note on Statute 24 of Peter the Venerable', *Revue Bénédictine* 83 (1973), 326–50.

46 Cc. 12, 54, 70, 168, *Liber Tramitis*, 16, 68, 103, 241.

47 Cc. 103, 183, *Liber Tramitis*, 102–6, 253–55. Cf. C. 32, *The Monastic Constitutions of Lanfranc*, 48–52.

48 Udalrich of Cluny, *Antiquiores Consuetudines Cluniacensis*, III. 13, *PL* 149, 757; Constable, '*Famuli*', 329.

49 Constable, '*Famuli*'.

50 *Die Tegernseer Briefsammlung*, ed. K. Strecker, MGH Epistolae selectae III (Berlin, 1925), no. 34, 38–39; translated by C. I. Hammer, *A Large-scale Slave Society of the Early Middle Ages: Slaves and their Families in Early Medieval Bavaria* (Aldershot, 2002), 136.

51 *Instituta Generalis Capituli*, c. 8; C. Waddell, *Cistercian Lay Brothers: Twelfth-century Usages with Related Texts*, Commentarii Cistercienses Studia et Documenta X (Cîteaux, 2000).

52 *Instituta Generalis Capituli*, c. 7.

53 Hugh of Farfa, *Destructio monasterii Farfensi 890–997, MGH SS* 11.2, 533; Jestice, *Wayward Monks*, 196–97. J. Hubert, 'La place faite aux laïcs dans les églises monastiques et dans les cathedrales aux XIe et XIIe siècles', *I laici nella 'Societas Christiana' dei secoli XI e XII*, Settimana Mendola 3 (Milan, 1968), 473.

54 *Regularis Concordia Anglicae nationis monachorum sanctimonialiumque*, ed. T. Symons (London, 1953), 19. On saints' cults, see Chapter 8.

55 M. B. Bedingfield, *The Dramatic Liturgy of Ango-Saxon England* (Woodbridge, 2002), pp. 98–100, citing *The Canterbury Benedictional*, ed. R. M. Woolley, HBS (1917) and London, British Library, Ms Additional 28188 (Exeter, s. xi $^{3}/_{4}$).

56 Ekkehard IV, *Casus S. Galli*, *MGH SS* II, 142.

57 William of Malmesbury, *Vita Dunstani*, I.2–3, in *William of Malmesbury's Saints' Lives*, ed. and trans. M. Winterbottom and R. M. Thomson (Oxford, 2002), 172.

58 C. 55.5, *Liber Tramitis*, 75–77; c. 32, *Monastic Constitutions of Lanfranc*, 48–52.

59 C. 91, *Monastic Constitutions of Lanfranc*, 132; Bernard of Cluny, *Ordo Cluniacensis par Bernardum saeculi XI. Scriptorem*, ed. M. Herrgott, *Vetus Disciplina Monastica* (Paris, 1726), I. 13, 157–61; Udalrich of Cluny, *Antiquiores Consuetudines*, III. 24, 766–67. D. Méhu, *Paix et communautés autour de l'abbaye de Cluny Xe–XVe siècle* (Lyons, 2001), 198.

60 *The Life of St Æthelwold*, ed. and trans. M. Lapidge and M. Winterbottom (Oxford, 1991), c. 29, 44–6.

61 Mt 6.9–21, 25.35–46.

62 *Vita Adelheidis*, 760 (cc. 5–6).

63 Ibid. c. 5; English trans. Bergen Dick, *Mater Spiritualis*, 27.

64 G. Duby, 'Le budget de Cluny entre 1080 et 1155: Économie dominiale et économie monétaire', in *Hommes et structures du Moyen Age* (Paris, 1973), 63–64.

65 L. Holstenius, *Codex regularum monasticarum et canonicarum*, 6 vols (1759), II, 143, cited by M. Miller, 'Towards a New Periodization of Ecclesiastical History', in S. Cohn and S. Epstein, *Portraits of Medieval and Renaissance Living* (Ann Arbor, 1996), 241; *RB*, c. 53, p. 248.

66 E.g. M. Arnoux, *Des clercs au service de la réforme. Études et documents sur les chanoines réguliers de la province de Rouen* (Turnhout, 2000), 119–39.

67 G. Constable, 'Monastic Possession of Churches and "Spiritualia" in the Age of Reform', in *Il Monachesimo e la riforma ecclesiastica (1049–1112): atti della quarta settimana internazionale di studio Mendola, 23–29 agosto 1968*, Miscellanea 6 (1971), 304–31; idem, 'Monasteries, Rural Churches and the Cura Animarum in the Early Middle Ages' in *Cristianizzazione ed organizzazione ecclesiastica delle campagne nell'alto medioevo: espansione e resistenze*, Settimane 28 (1982), 349–89.

68 Bouchard, 'Geographical, Social and Ecclesiastical Origins'.

69 Burchard II. 158 and III.240, *PL* 140, 651, 724–25.

70 G. Constable, 'The Treatise "Hortatur Nos" and Accompanying Canonical Works on the Performance of Pastoral Work by Monks', in his *Religious Life and Thought (11th–12th Centuries)* (London, 1979), no. 9.

71 Council of Poitou (1078), c. 5, Mansi, *Concilia*, XX, 498; Council of Poitou (1100), c. 11, ibid. 1124. The First Lateran Council (1123), c. 16, forbade monks to exercise any ministry: *Decrees*, ed. Tanner, I. 193.

72 Constable, 'Monasteries, rural churches and the *cura animarum*'.

73 Hamilton, *Practice*, 146–49.

74 E.g. Cambridge, Corpus Christi College, Ms 422 (the Red Book of Darley) and Oxford, Magdalen College, Ms 226 (Pontifical); Oxford, Bodleian Library, Ms Laud Miscellaneous 482 (penitential and ordines for the visitation of the sick and for the dying). H. Gittos, 'Is There Any Evidence for the Liturgy of Parish Churches in Late Anglo-Saxon England? The Red

Book of Darley and the Status of Old English', and V. Thompson, 'The Pastoral Contract in Late Anglo-Saxon England: Priest and Parishioner in Oxford, Bodleian Library, Ms Laud Miscellaneous 482', both in F. Tinti, ed., *Pastoral Care in Late Anglo-Saxon England* (Woodbridge, 2005), 63–82, 106–20; S. Hamilton, 'Rites of Passage and Pastoral Care', in J. Crick and E. van Houts, eds, *A Social History of Britain 900–1200* (Cambridge, 2011), 290–308.

75 S. Hamilton, 'Pastoral Care in Early Eleventh-century Rome', *Dutch Review of Church History* 84 (2004), 37–56.

76 J. W. Bernhardt, *Itinerant Kingship and Royal Monasteries in Early Medieval Germany c.936–1075* (Cambridge, 1993).

77 E.g. All the possessions of the Cistercian house of Fontenoy in Burgundy lay within 25–30km of the abbey, that is, within a day's ride: Bouchard, *Sword, Miter and Cloister*, 200.

78 Toubert, *Les structures du Latium.*

79 Bouchard, *Sword, Miter, and Cloister*, 200–02.

80 See n. 50 above.

81 F. J. Felten, *Äbte und Laienäbte im Frankenreich* (Stuttgart, 1980)

82 C. West, 'The Significance of the Carolingian Advocate', *Early Medieval Europe* 17 (2009), 186–206.

83 E.g. Bouchard, *Sword, Miter and Cloister*, 125–28; H. Platelle, *La justice seigneuriale de L'Abbaye de Saint Amand: son organisation judiciare, sa procédure et sa compétence du XIe au XVIe siècle* (Louvain, 1965).

84 R. F. Berkhofer, 'Abbatial Authority Over Lay Agents', in idem, A. Cooper and A. J. Kosto, eds, *The Experience of Power in Medieval Europe, 950–1350* (Aldershot, 2005), 43–57.

85 *The Cartulary of Montier-en-Der 666–1129*, ed. C. B. Bouchard (Toronto, 2004).

86 E.g. The Durham *Liber Vitae*, on which see D. Rollason, A. J. Piper, M. Harvey, L. Rollason, eds, *The Durham Liber Vitae and Its Context* (Woodbridge, 2004), especially D. Geuenich, 'A Survey of the Early Medieval Confraternity Books from the Continent', ibid., 141–48.

87 Dated but still helpful: N. Huyghebaert, *Les documents necrologiques, Typologie des sources du Moyen Âge 4* (Turnhout, 1972). See now M. Lauwers, *La mémoire des ancêtres, le souci des morts: Morts, rites et société au moyen âge (diocèse de Liège, Xe–XIIIe siècles)* (Paris, 1997).

88 *Consuetudines canonicorum regularium Springirsbacenses-Rodenses*, ed. S. Weinfurter, CCCM 48 (Turnhout, 1978), 22–26.

89 The classic work written in 1925 by M. Mauss, *The Gift: Forms and Functions of Exchange in Archaic Societies*, trans. I. Cunnison (New York, 1967) has been the stimulus for further work, summarised by B. H. Rosenwein, *To Be the Neighbor of Saint Peter: The Social Meaning of Cluny's Property 909–1049* (Ithaca, NY, 1989), 125–43.

90 'Suscipe vas modicum divinis cultibus aptum/Ac tibi directum devote mente tuorum/Nomina nostra tibi quesumus sint cognita passim/Haec tamen hic sgribi voluit cautela salubri. Iure vocor Maurus quoniam sum nigr[os] secutus/Me sequitur proles cum Pantaleone Iohannes/Sergius et Manso Maurus frater quoque Pardo/Da scelerum veniam, caelestem prebe coronam.' R. Bergman, *The Salerno Ivories: Ars Sacra from Medieval Amalfi* (Cambridge, MA, 1980), p. 128 cited by Boynton, *Shaping a Monastic Identity*, p. 171, n. 105.

91 Boynton, *Shaping a Monastic Identity*, p. 167, n. 95.

92 M. Bull, *Knightly Piety and the Lay Response to the First Crusade: The Limousin and Gascony c.970–c.1130* (Oxford, 1993), 115–203; McLaughlin, *Consorting with Saints*; Bouchard, *Sword, Miter, and Cloister*, 171–246.

93 Rosenwein, *To Be the Neighbor of St Peter*, 109–143.

94 D. C. Van Meter, 'Count Baldwin IV, Richard of Saint-Vanne, and the Inception of Monastic Reform in Eleventh-century Flanders', *Revue bénédictine*, 107 (1997), 130–48.

95 V. Ramseyer, *The Transformation of a Religious Landscape: Medieval Southern Italy, 850–1150* (Ithaca, NY, 2006); S. Elkins, *Holy Women of Twelfth-century England* (Chapel Hill, NC, 1988).

96 'Omnium igitur rerum quae huic filio defuncto rectae distributionis sorte ceciderunt Deum heredem fecerunt, ut meliori recompensatione hereditatem meruisset in paradiso deliciarum, qua immatura morte preventus caruit in hac convalle lacrimarum', *Vita Adelheidis*, c. 3, 758; translated Bergen Dick, *Mater Spiritualis*, 15–40. L. Böhringer, 'Der Kaiser und Stiftsdamen. Die Gründung des Frauenstifts Villich im Spannungsfeld von religiösem Leben under adliger Welt', *Bönner Geschichtsblätter: Jahrbuch des Bonner-Heimat und Geschichtsvereins* 53–54 (2004), 57–77.

97 Godefrid's body was brought back by his followers, but the *Vita* does not specify where he was buried; for the evidence that he was buried at Vilich see I. Achter, *Die Stiftskirche in Vilich and Jacob Schlafke, Leben und Verehung der heiligen Adelheid von Vilich* (Düsseldorf, 1968), 140–45, cited by Dick, *Mater Spiritualis*, 76.

98 *Vita Adelheid*, c. 3, 758. Gerberga's behaviour is compared (favourably) with that of a widow who undertakes such acts out of necessity because she did so voluntarily.

99 E.g. Count Ezzo and his wife Mathilda established the monastery at Brauweiler, west of Cologne in 1024, which served as the site for their own graves, those of four of their children, and their grandson: J. Rotondo-McCord, '*Locum Sepulturae Meae . . . Elegi*: Property, Graves and Sacral Power in Eleventh-century Germany', *Viator* 26 (1995), 77–106.

100 *Twelfth-century Statutes from the Cistercian General Chapter*, ed. C. Waddell, (Brecht, 2002), 606.

101 *The Cartulary of Montier-en-Der*, ed. Bouchard, no. 48.

102 Ibid., no. 65.

103 *Recueil des Chartes de L'Abbaye de Cluny*, ed. A. Bernard and A. Bruel, 6 vols (Paris, 1876–1903).

104 *MGH Diplomatum regum et imperatorum Germaniae III: Henrici II et Arduini Diplomata* (Hanover, 1900–1903), no. 40, 47–48.

105 B. Venarde, *Women's Monasticism and Medieval Society: Nunneries in France and England, 890–1215* (Ithaca, NY, 1997).

106 J. Nightingale, *Monasteries and their Patrons in the Görze Reform: Lotharingia c. 850–1000* (Oxford, 2001), ch. 5.

107 Bouchard, *Sword, Miter and Cloister*, 50–51, 357–61.

108 E. Jamroziak, *Rievaulx Abbey and its Social Context, 1132–1300: Memory, Locality and Networks* (Turnhout, 2005).

109 Rosenwein, *To Be the Neighbor of St Peter*.

110 A. Murray, *Reason and Society in the Middle Ages* (Oxford, 1978), 350–82.

111 Gonterus, *Vita Gerardi Abbatis Broniensis*, cc. 3–4, *MGH SS XV.2*, 656–57; D. Misonne, 'Gérard de Brogne: moine et réformateur (d. 959)', *Révue bénédictine* 111 (2001), 25–49.

112 *La vie de Jean, abbé de Gorze*, ed. Parisse, c. 11, p. 50.

113 Peter Damian, *Vita Beati Romualdi*, ed. G. Tabacco, Fonti per la storia d'Italia 94 (Rome, 1957), c. 1.

114 Andreas of Sturmi, *Vita Iohannis Gualberti*, ed. F. Baethgen, *MGH SS* 30.2, 1080–1104; Atto, *Vita s. Joannis Gualberti*, *PL* 146, 667–706.

115 Edited by B. M. Kienzle, 'The Works of Hugo Francigena: Tractatus de Conversione Pontii de Laracio et exordii Salvaniensis monasterii vera narratio, epistolae (Dijon, Bibliothèque municipale, Ms 611', *Sacris Erudiri* 34 (1994), 273–311; translated eadem, 'The Tract on the Conversion of Pons of Léras and the True Account of the Beginning of the Monastery at Silvanès', in T. Head, ed., *Medieval Hagiography: An Anthology* (New York, 2001), 499–512.

116 Bouchard, *Sword, Miter, and Cloister*, 49 citing the *Statutes* of 1134.

117 Misonne, 'Gérard', p. 31.

118 B. Hamilton, 'The Monastic Revival in Tenth-century Rome', *Studia Monastica* 4 (1962), 35–68.

119 *Cartulary of Montier-en-Der*, ed. Bouchard, no. 37.

120 B. Venarde, *Women's Monasticism and Medieval Society: Nunneries in France and England, 890–1215* (Ithaca, NY, 1997), 11–12; Arnoux, *Des clercs*, 20–22.

121 M. F. Smith, R. Fleming and P. Halpin, 'Court and Piety in Late Anglo-Saxon England', *Catholic Historical Review* 87 (2001), 569–602 at pp. 579–84.

122 Arnoux, *Des clercs.*

123 D. Méhu, *Paix et communautés autour de l'abbaye de Cluny Xe–XVe siècle* (Lyons, 2001), 198–99.

part 2

People and churches

chapter 5

Pastoral piety: The religious life of the local church

And it is right that every man learn so he knows the Pater noster *and the Creed according as he wishes to be buried in a consecrated grave or to be entitled to the sacrament; for he who will not learn it is not truly Christian nor ought he by rights to stand sponsor at baptism or at confirmation until he learn it.*

'Canons of Edgar', c. 22 (*c.*1005 × 6)[1]

Here Archbishop Wulfstan (d. 1023) sets out the minimum requirements which should be expected of lay men (and women) if they are to be regarded as full members of the Church. They must know the primary prayer of Christianity, that which taught Christ his disciples, the Our Father (*Pater noster* in Latin) and at least one of the several basic avowals of orthodox belief known as the Creed. Those who failed to do so should be excluded from participation in the fundamental rites of the Christian Church, barred from acting as godparents to the newly baptised, receiving the Eucharist at Mass, and burial in consecrated ground. Ignorance meant they could not take part in the rites which defined entry into, membership of, and exit from the earthly community of Christians. Archbishop Wulfstan's definition is perhaps the closest we have to a statement of what constituted a Christian in the years 900 to 1200. Although he required knowledge of the statement of orthodoxy that is the Creed, his emphasis is on those practices which constitute membership of the Christian Church, on orthopraxy as much as correct belief. At the same time his text records the way in which churchmen presumed Christian belief to be central to the lives of ordinary men and women, marking their entry into, and exit from society, solemnising the coming together of the community at Mass. To these basic services of baptism, the Mass and obsequies for the dying, might be added those for atoning for sin, namely penance and confession, and those which accompanied perhaps the most important rite in lay lives, namely the status-changing event of marriage. Collectively they constitute the liturgy for pastoral care, which bishops deemed to be the responsibility of the local priests based in the local churches being built and rebuilt across Christendom.

We traced the processes by which local churches became parish churches in Chapter 2; as we saw there, the years 900 to 1200 witnessed a substantial growth in the number of local churches throughout Europe. Changing settlement patterns, increased prosperity, lordly ambition, the piety of noble families, and that of groups of freemen acting together all helped generate this increase, and meant that by 1200 the majority of Christians in Latin Europe lived within walking distance of the church which provided pastoral services. By the fifteenth century it is evident that the local parish church had become central to the religious lives of most local communities, at least in northern Europe, but it is no means certain that this had been the case in the central Middle Ages.[2] For local churches served merely as one locus for divine power in the landscape of medieval Europe. Monasteries, or rather the shrines of the saints for which they acted as custodians, offered lay people alternative places of worship which, as we shall see in Chaper 7, proved highly attractive. Similarly people often attached significance to sites in the natural landscape: particular trees, springs and wells were all taken over as sites for Christian shrines and churches in the early Middle Ages but the importance attached to them seems to have its origins in pre-Christian times.[3] The existence of monastic shrines and sites such as holy springs thus must often have constituted powerful rivals to the local church as the focus for the devotions of the lay communities in a particular locality. When therefore did the local church assume the role it played in the late Middle Ages as a centre for community devotion? And how far do the roots of this process lie in the years between 900 and 1200? These are the questions which will preoccupy us in this chapter.

As we shall see, there is a considerable body of written and material evidence from this period which, although at times tendentious, seem to point to the important role which local churches already played in the religious lives of these communities in the central Middle Ages. John van Engen has argued that 'the real measure of Christian religious culture on a broad scale must be the degree to which time, space and ritual observance came to be defined and grasped essentially in terms of the Christian liturgical year'.[4] We thus begin by reviewing the ways in which the major feasts of the Church's year impacted on the lives of the laity; which feasts were they really expected to keep, and how far did they observe them? To what extent did the demands of their daily lives accord with ecclesiastical rhythms? We then move to investigate the ways in which the pastoral rites expected of all Christians developed in these years. What evidence is there for the delivery of baptism in local churches? What evidence is there for regular lay penance and confession and Christian marriage? How were obsequies for the dying to be conducted? By asking what went on inside local churches, we can investigate the various ways in which the services held in them helped to structure the religious lives of their lay congregations and thus how these churches became important to them. In order to do so, however, we need first to consider the considerable challenges facing any scholar wishing to study local piety in this period.

Some problems with the evidence

We know remarkably little about what went on inside local churches at this time except that they became bigger. Archaeological and architectural studies of the church fabric point to the substantial increase in the physical size of local churches in the central Middle Ages. Churches across England, for example, were rebuilt on a grander scale in the century between 1050 and 1150.[5] At Raunds Furnell in Northamptonshire archaeological excavation has demonstrated that the original tenth-century church, which followed a single-cell plan, could only accommodate twenty-nine people; it was enlarged in *c.*1000 to one which could take 104 people and a separate chancel was added at that time, detaching the priest and the high altar from the congregation who were now confined to the nave.[6] In part such enlargement of churches reflects practical need arising from demographic growth, but it may also reflect the desire of lords to assert their authority over the landscape by building new and more impressive structures. Yet such buildings are not just statements of lordly ambition but rather served to draw congregations to them, suggesting that they assumed greater importance for the communities they served. Such rebuilding had social repercussions as well. Writing in *c.*1000 Ælfric of Eynsham reminded bishops about the importance of ensuring that lay congregations behaved with due decorum in church; he criticised the widespread practice of chatting and drinking inside church.[7] John Blair suggests that Ælfric's concern reflects the fact that lay congregations had come to regard their local church as a social centre for the community.[8] It must be remembered, however, that Ælfric's text drew on similar ninth-century prohibitions, but that he thought them worth repeating may reflect particular developments in England at this time.[9] There are also other indications that the local church was assuming importance within the lay community it served. The earliest evidence for the painted decoration of the walls of the naves of local churches in England comes only a century later, *c.*1100.[10] From the thirteenth-century onwards English lay congregations were increasingly being awarded responsibility for maintaining the nave, but embellishments like this hint that they may have assumed these obligations somewhat earlier.[11]

Although excavations like that at Raunds Furnell tell us about the ways in which the space taken up by the local church increased, we know very little about the internal fabric and layout. Were there separate altars in the nave for particular groups in the parish, as there were in the later Middle Ages? Did women stand apart from the men in the nave as they did later? The latter seems likely, for depictions of the rites for baptism and penance show men and women as separate groups, but we do not have specific evidence from this period for this crucial element of the lay experience of worship.[12] Did men of high status stand closer to the high altar? It seems likely that they did, for in the eleventh-century 'Vision of Leofric' the altar of St Clement's, Sandwich is described as screened off by a heavy curtain from the nave with Earl Leofric and King Edward the Confessor standing on either side of the sanctuary during Mass.[13] Here the curtain may anticipate the screens erected between the nave and altar in later medieval churches; it is not very clear either quite when these became introduced. Whilst archaeology is not particularly informative about church interiors, it is rather more helpful, as we shall see, when it comes to tracing the extent to which lay men and women used their local church, and in particular the extent to which they came to be baptised and buried in their local church.

Incidental textual references tell us that bishops expected local church priests to own vessels, vestments, and altar hangings, but these have not survived. Similarly we know almost nothing about the liturgy followed in local church services. Both Ælfric and Archbishop Wulfstan followed their ninth-century sources in setting out lists of books which local priests should own, and surviving booklists suggest that at least one local church, that of Sherburn in Elmet in north Yorkshire, owned books for the Mass and Office, including a sacramentary, a gradual, two gospel books, two epistolaries, a psalter, an antiphonary, and a hymnal.[14] But unlike the service books of cathedrals and monasteries, those from local churches have not survived, probably because unlike monasteries and cathedrals they lacked the institutional structures necessary to preserve out-of-date service books after they had ceased to be used.

Rather what have survived are various types of prescriptive evidence written by the higher clergy for the instruction of local priests. These texts include the sorts of advice and injunctions like those already cited by Ælfric and Archbishop Wulfstan written to support bishops instructing their clergy at diocesan synods. Model sermons testify to the attempts of senior churchmen to educate both local clergy and their lay congregations, handbooks of penitential law to the guidance given to priests in the administration of confession and penance. One particular development we find in this period is the adaptation of elaborate pastoral rites originally composed for large clerical communities for delivery by a single priest. Whilst texts of liturgical rites now only survive in manuscripts from greater churches, there are a few examples which seem to have to been composed in order to educate local priests in the purpose and administration of particular rites. Prescriptive evidence is always difficult to interpret because it is influenced by a very powerful textual legacy, but it is not impossible. Careful investigation of changes and interpolations made to liturgical rites, in particular, can tell us a good deal about how churchmen sought to adapt these rites for local churches, as we shall see. Such analysis also raises the possibility that some of these changes may owe as much to lay needs and demands as clerical aspirations.

In what follows we investigate the changing nature of the higher clergy's aspirations for local churches, and explore the impact local churches had on lay lives. Combining the prescriptive evidence with that of narrative texts and material evidence will enable us to draw up a fresh picture of the degree to which local churches became the focus for the religious lives and identities of the local communities they served. We will thus begin by considering the extent of the impact which ecclesiastical measures of time had on lay lives.

The church year

Church law demanded that everyone should attend church every Sunday and on feast days, not just once but three times a day: for the office at the beginning and end of the day as well as Mass. Regino of Prüm, for example, suggested that the bishop ask the lay jury when visiting a local community:

> *If there is any man who has worked on the Lord's day or special feasts, and if anyone resisted taking part in matins, and mass, and vespers on these days.*[15]

It is not very likely that they did so but, as we shall see in the next chapter, attendance at Mass and the offices is central to contemporary depictions of individual lay piety. Church laws also specified in some detail how Sundays and feast days should be kept: there should be no work, no trade, no public meetings, no courts or judicial hangings, no fasting and no sex. They set out periods of sexual abstinence and dietary fasting which should be followed in the four weeks of Advent which led up to Christmas, the eight days after Epiphany (6 January) and in the forty days of Lent. Some laws also required fasting in the forty days between Easter and Ascension Day.[16] During these times of collective fasting all Christians should abstain from alcohol (except beer), meat, fat, cheese and eggs, except on Sundays.[17] Church law even made provision for lay members of the congregation to monitor each other in keeping all of these obligations. Regino instructed the bishop to ask the lay jury:

> *If any man has not observed the Lenten fast, nor Advent, nor the Major litany [25 April], nor Rogationtide, without permission [for abstention being obtained] from the bishop.*[18]

But the laity were not expected to receive the Eucharist regularly; following ninth-century precedent, most injunctions agreed on a minimum of three times a year, at Easter, Pentecost and Christmas.[19]

The practice expected of the laity was clearly stated and reiterated, but implementing it posed various challenges, as churchmen recognised. The popularity of miracle stories about the dreadful experiences which befell people who dared to work on the Sundays and feast days testify to churchmen's continuing unease about the extent to which their message not to work on the Lord's Day met with widespread resistance. In one mid-eleventh-century miracle collection from Ely the master of a servant girl forced her to gather vegetables on a Sunday, whereupon her fingers became stuck to the stake she had used for cutting the plants until she successfully petitioned St Æthelthryth for help.[20] In a late eleventh-century collection from southern England a man pricked his hand on a thorn whilst clearing a field of brambles 'against the law on the Lord's day', whereupon the wound became infected, and he was only healed through the intervention of St Swithun.[21] In an English twelfth-century collection a woman's arm became withered after milking sheep on Good Friday.[22] A late twelfth-century collection from south-western France records how a woman got a needle stuck in her mouth whilst sewing on a Sunday.[23] The very popularity of this topos in accounts of *miracula* suggests the importance of promoting this pragmatic form of Christianity, one focused on observance as much as belief.

Churchmen recognised it as the local priest's responsibility to remind and chivvy his flock about which feasts and fasts should be kept, when and how.[24] This became particularly the case in deciding which of the many feast days in the crowded ecclesiastical calendar the laity of that area should observe. For there was no universal ecclesiastical calendar at this time and church calendars quickly became cluttered. In general the Church year was divided into two intersecting cycles, the *temporale* and the *sanctorale*. The *temporale*, or Proper of Time, records the mostly movable feasts which are mostly associated with Christ's Life, from His birth at Christmas (fixed on 25 December) through to His Resurrection at Easter, which is celebrated on the first Sunday after the full moon which occurs on or after the spring equinox; His Ascension into heaven forty days afterwards and the Descent of the Holy Spirit at Pentecost ten days after that. The second cycle, the *sanctorale*, or Proper of the Saints, records the fixed dates for the feasts of the saints. The feasts of important early saints, such as the Apostles SS Peter and Paul, were universally observed throughout western Christendom, but many others were more localised to particular dioceses or even particular churches. The compilers of church law thus made various attempts to identify and promote the important feasts which all Christians should observe. One text popular in west and east Frankia in the tenth century directed the bishop to check that all the local priests of his diocese own a martyrology – a list of martyred saints arranged in the calendar order of their feast, perhaps with a short life of the martyr – and that he should also know when Easter falls, and understand how to compute the movable feasts of the church calendar.[25]

As new saints became recognised, and old ones promoted, bishops added their feasts to local diocesan calendars, making additional demands on lay communities, and generating, in some cases, considerable resistance. Tales of how initial lay opposition to keeping the feast of a particular saint could only be overcome through a miracle are a common feature of the large body of miracle stories to survive from this period. One case recorded in a late tenth-century monastic miracle collection from north-eastern France represents this trend very clearly, reflecting both the tensions generated by the clergy's demands that the laity observe new feasts in the appropriate manner by abstaining from work and attending church, and clerical anxiety about getting the laity to observe a new feast. In 964 the relics of Saint Hunegund, the seventh-century founder of the community at Homblières, were translated, and the commemoration of her feast revived; the bishop of Noyon duly instructed all the local priests attending the diocesan synod to promote the new feast. The local priest of Sasnulficurt preached to his congregation that they should observe this new feast on 25 August 964. His initial instructions met with vocal opposition: the villagers decided to ignore the priest's instructions and to focus on harvesting the wheat crop, arguing that the new feast was not being kept by any of their neighbours and in any case they could not afford to not work on that day. The grain harvest is, of course, a crucial time in any subsistence economy and the story captures the reluctance of the villagers to risk the harvest for a new feast. Their resistance is thus attributed to both economic pragmatism and religious conservatism. Yet it was overcome when a girl gleaning on the remains of the harvest left by the reapers discovered an ear of wheat soaked in blood, and, on closer inspection, this proved to be the case for all the grain; on examining the grain, the priest declared it a miracle, and, summoning the community to the church, explained that their sinfulness in working on the saint's day had caused this phenomenon. They then told their neighbours, and the news quickly spread through the region, and everyone gave up work to pray to avert God's wrath.[26] As this tale demonstrates, the local priest played a crucial role in instructing his flock in the demands of the church year. At the same time, the rigorous observance required by the ecclesiastical authorities meant, in a precarious agricultural economy, that lay communities could not afford to observe all the feasts recorded in the diocesan calendar.

This is a fact of which churchmen were well aware, and the prescriptive texts record their efforts to identify and promote the most important feasts in the calendar which all Christians must observe, as opposed to those reserved for clerical communities. That they made various attempts to do so reflects how they endeavoured to ensure a level of conformity across Christendom and across dioceses, whilst at the same time recognising the limits of what could be expected of the laity. Archbishop Wulfstan, for example, enjoined that all the feasts of the Apostles should be celebrated except that of SS Philip and James because it fell too close to Easter that year.[27] One such endeavour is found in Bishop Burchard of Worms's (d. 1025) early eleventh-century collection of church law:

> *That the priests should announce which days are feasts to the people for the year, that is, every Sunday, from vespers [on Saturday] to vespers [on Sunday], and Christmas Day [25 December], [the feasts of] St Stephen [26 December], St John the Evangelist [27 December], the Holy Innocents [28 December], the Octave of Christmas [1 January], Epiphany [6 January], the Purification of Holy Mary [2 February], Easter with Holy Week, the three Rogation Days, the holy days of Pentecost, the feasts of John the Baptist [24 June], of the Twelve Apostles, that of the greatest of all the saints, Peter and Paul who illuminated the world with their preaching [29 June], those of St Lawrence [10 August], the Assumption of Holy Mary [15 August], the Nativity of Holy Mary the Virgin [8 September], the dedication of the Holy basilica of St Michael, the dedication of every oratory, and of all the Saints [1 November], of St Martin [11 November], and those feasts which each bishop in his diocese keeps with the people.*[28]

This seemingly comprehensive list of twenty-six feast days on top of every Sunday cannot be accepted as evidence of the calendar observed by the laity in Burchard's own diocese because it was based on that found in an earlier ninth-century episcopal text.[29] Several different lists of feasts to be kept by the laity circulated in church law in the tenth and eleventh centuries in England and Frankia, and all had their origins in earlier Carolingian legislation.[30] The degree of variation between them, particularly in the choice of feasts, suggests that reformist clergy across these three centuries pondered which feasts above all others should be observed, and adapted their precedents to reflect the current calendar rather than copying them unthinkingly.[31] Pastorally minded churchmen were clearly anxious to impose the liturgical year, with its demands, on the practice of the laity, but how far did they succeed?

Sermons offer a way of answering this question. Many but not all sermon texts were written for clerical audiences, but several envisage the presence of a lay audience. Such references point to those days in the liturgical year when their clerical authors expected the laity to attend church. For example, one episcopal sermon from a collection composed in late ninth- or tenth-century Frankia envisages the presence of a lay audience on Maundy Thursday because married men are warned to abstain from sexual relations with their wives for 'several days' before Sundays and feast days 'so that you can approach the Mass of the Lord with a pure heart and chaste body and receive His body and blood without the judgement of damnation'.[32]

It is therefore worth exploring in more detail one collection of sermons which covers the whole of the liturgical year for such references in order to establish how far the prescriptive lists of feasts and fasts set out in church law were realised in the pastoral literature produced for preachers to the laity. On precisely which days did this compiler expect his sermons to be preached to a lay audience?

The collection chosen for this case study is the two series of Catholic Homilies composed in Old English by the late tenth-century English monk, Ælfric, whilst he was a monk at Cerne Abbas in Dorset, sometime between 987 and 995. They circulated widely in the course of the eleventh century as part of a concerted effort by early eleventh-century English churchmen to educate both the local clergy and laity; they now survive in at least thirty-four manuscripts from the eleventh and twelfth centuries and a further fifty manuscripts of the First Series have been postulated to as once existing.[33] Each series comprises forty homilies to be preached right across the liturgical year.[34] In the Preface to the Second Series Ælfric tells us he composed it to supplement the First Series 'because I thought it was less tedious to hear if one book were read in the course of one year and one in the year following'.[35] Both reformist legislation and literature from late tenth-century England emphasised the importance of preaching on Sundays and other feast days, and Jonathan Wilcox has suggested that Ælfric intended his sermons to be delivered by both local priests based in local minsters and by monastic communities to lay congregations.[36] Their contents demonstrate that they were written for a mixed audience of monastic and secular clergy and laity, but their exact purpose is unclear. The texts of some of the homilies suggest they were used for the delivery of sermons within the service, whilst others may have been intended for devotional reading outside formal services. In both series Ælfric consistently used the second person to address the uneducated laity and the third person to address the learned. It is thus possible to identify those sermons he intended especially for the laity.[37] Ælfric clearly did not always expect the laity to be in attendance: in the sermon for Easter Day in the second series he repeated the explanation of the gospel for the Wednesday of Holy Week because:

> *Some of the explanation of this we have told you in another place, some we tell you now, now you are gathered here. We know that you were not all in attendance here on the day when we had to read that gospel.*[38]

Although church law, as articulated by Burchard of Worms for example, presumed that the laity would attend church throughout Holy Week, Ælfric, ever the pragmatist, did not think they would. Table 5.1 correlates the days for which his use of the second person suggests that Ælfric composed sermons pitched specifically at the laity when he clearly expected them to be in attendance, with the list of days identified in the text by Burchard quoted above. He expected the laity to be in church to hear a sermon on only fourteen out of the twenty-six occasions identified by Burchard and his Carolingian predecessors as compulsory. It thus demonstrates Ælfric to be rather more pessimistic than the authors of the prescriptive legislation.

Table 5.1 ◆ Feast days to be observed by the laity: a comparison of the evidence in Burchard of Worms's *Decretum* (*c.*1020), Ælfric's *Catholic Homilies* (987 × 995), and Wulfstan's 'Canons of Edgar' (1005 × 1008)

List in *Decretum*, II. 57	List in *Catholic Homilies* I and II	Feast days specified in 'Canons of Edgar', c. 54
Christmas Day	∅	
Feast of St Stephen		
Feast of St John the Evangelist		
Feast of the Holy Innocents		
Octave of Christmas		
Epiphany	∅	
Octave of Epiphany		
Purification of Mary (Candlemas)	∅	∅
Quinquagesima Sunday	∅	
Holy Week		
Easter Sunday	∅	∅
Rogation Days	∅	∅
Ascension Day	∅	
Pentecost	∅	∅
St John the Baptist	∅	∅
Twelve Apostles		
SS Peter and Paul	∅	∅
St Lawrence		
Assumption		
Nativity of Mary		
Dedication of the basilica of St Michael		
All Saints	∅	∅
St Martin	∅	∅
St Andrew		
Advent Sundays	∅	∅

In setting out the feasts that the laity really must observe, Ælfric tried to give shape to the laity's experience of the church year. He expected them to attend Mass and to hear a sermon on both Christmas Day and Epiphany but not to come to church on the intervening days, *contra* the expectations of Frankish churchmen in the tenth and eleventh centuries.[39] At Epiphany, which commemorated Christ's manifestation to the world, the preacher should remind the laity of the three things provided for man's salvation: baptism, the Eucharist and penance. The next major feast, the Purification of Mary, also known as Candlemas, came almost a month later. Ælfric ended his sermon for that day in his first series with a lengthy description of this strikingly visual ceremony:

> *Be it known also to everyone that is appointed in the ecclesiastical observances that we on this day bear our lights to church and let them*

> *there be blessed: and that we should go afterwards with the light among God's houses and sing the hymn that is thereto appointed. Though some men cannot sing, they can, nevertheless, bear the light in their hands; for this day was Christ, the true Light, borne to the temple who redeemed us from darkness and bringeth us to the Eternal Light, who liveth and ruleth ever without end. Amen.*[40]

Ælfric's reference to the participation by men who 'cannot sing' may refer to uneducated *conversi*, but is usually interpreted as a reference to the ill-educated laity who lack the Latin and musical training to participate in the chant but can take part in the procession. He describes a simple ceremony in which everyone processes with lights to church in order to have them blessed; surviving liturgical rites for grander clerical communities depict a more complex ceremony in which clergy process from one church to another to have their candles blessed and back again.[41] Evidence that Ælfric was not alone in envisioning that such services might take place at a local level comes from the Red Book of Darley, which seems to have been composed to educate a local priest, and includes a text for blessing candles at Candlemas.[42]

The next major event in the Christian year came with beginning of Lent. Ælfric obviously expected the laity to be in attendance on the Sundays at the beginning of Lent, rather than Ash Wednesday, the official start of Lent. He used these occasions to remind them of how they should observe Lent. On Quinquagesima Sunday – just before Ash Wednesday – he reminded his audience they should go to their confessor to confess secret sins and make amends.[43] On the first Sunday of Lent he set out how the Lenten fast should be kept, in terms of abstinence, peace-making, and charity towards the poor.[44] Although Ælfric's sermons for Palm Sunday seem to have been directed at the clergy, elsewhere in his writings he assumed that the laity would take part in the rites for that day, an assumption repeated in at least one later eleventh-century rite from Exeter.[45] Thus in his *Second Letter for Wulfstan* he suggests that monks and laity participate in a joint procession on that day:

> *You must on Palm Sunday bless palm twigs and bear them with praise singing in procession and have them in hand, both monks and laity, and offer them after the gospel to the mass priest with the offering song.*[46]

Ælfric was unusual in arguing that there should be no preaching on the three 'still' days of Holy Week: Maundy Thursday, Good Friday and Holy Saturday. Elsewhere in Christendom bishops clearly expected the laity to attend church, and to be preached to, on these days. One late ninth- or tenth-century Frankish collection included thirteen sermons for Maundy Thursday, the day when public penitents who had been formally cast out of the church on Ash Wednesday were publicly reconciled by the bishop. The text of these sermons is aimed at the lay audience, rather than the public penitents themselves; the laity are encouraged to reflect on their own misdeeds, and encouraged to live a life of sobriety and temperance.[47] Unsurprisingly, Ælfric expected everyone to attend Mass and to take communion on Easter Sunday, explaining 'We will now disclose to you through the grace of God concerning the Holy Eucharist to which you are now to go'.[48]

The next major feasts Ælfric expected the laity to participate in were the three Rogation Days of fasting which preceded the celebrations of Christ's Ascension to heaven forty days after his resurrection. As Easter is a Sunday, Ascension Day is always a Thursday, and thus the Rogation Days fall on Monday, Tuesday and Wednesday. Ælfric explained their importance thus:

> *These days are called litanies (litaniae), that is, prayer days. On these days we should pray for abundance of our earthly fruits and health for ourselves and peace and what is yet more forgiveness for our sins.*[49]

Rogation Days formed a late spring festival to petition God's blessing on the crops and livestock. In both series his sermons for these days are aimed at the laity. In the first series he used them to explain the Lord's Prayer and the Creed, and in the second series to explain the duties of the laity: chastity in marriage, correction of children, truthfulness of merchants, and the importance of intercessory prayer.[50] Evidence from other sermon collections confirms the idea that Rogationtide played an important role in lay instruction but it is hard to know how the services themselves were conducted. A procession went across the countryside between the third and ninth hour of each day; it was accompanied by relics and chanting; the relics were put down at various points and the Gospel read. Church law warned against treating Rogationtide as a festival, suggesting that it often may have been; it should be a time for penance rather than for horseracing and other games.[51] Despite their significance in the Christian calendar, Ælfric's sermons for both Ascension Day and Pentecost, some ten days later, seem to have been pitched at a clerical audience, as were those for the feasts of St John the Baptist and SS Peter and Paul. He expected the laity to attend church on the feast of the Assumption of Mary but the sermons for the remaining feasts of the church year seem to have been pitched at the clergy.

This summary gives the impression that preaching to the laity ceased in the second half of the year, and suggests that the higher clergy did not expect the laity to attend church then as frequently. Such a pattern might fit in with the labour demands of an agrarian calendar which were at their most demanding over the summer and autumn, although the spring season was also rigorous and coincided with the demands of Easter and Rogationtide. Any conclusions about the overall pattern of religious life must, however, also take into account the fact that Ælfric composed his *Catholic Homilies* with an avowedly didactic purpose. He thus privileged the events of the Christian story rather than the lives of the saints, whose feasts predominated in the second half of the year; a self-consciously literary production, the *Homilies* are intended, in Malcolm Godden's words, 'to tell the basic Christian story sequentially from the beginning as far as the constraints of the calendar would allow'.[52] Yet they also show an attempt being made by one popular author to tailor his material to his expected audience: emphasising the tenets of the Christian story were what mattered, because the laity – whilst assumed to be Christian – were also thought to be in need of education.

Senior churchmen thus attached considerable importance to teaching the laity the basics of Christianity, and fretted about the degree to which they were properly Christian. They continued to be anxious throughout this period about the extent of other influences on the cycle of daily life for the laity. As we have already seen, the immediate demands of tasks necessary for the agricultural year such as harvest might prevent lay communities observing feast days. The persistent influence of earlier pagan traditions also remained a concern. The compilers of church law collections continued into the fourteenth century, for example, to include injunctions against the laity keeping the new year according to pagan rites.[53] Whilst scholars have long been interested in the ways in which the early church adapted pagan feasts to the Christian calendar – the feast of St John the Baptist is often linked to the summer solstice, for example, and that of Christmas to the winter one – the repetition of injunctions against paganism in church law suggests unease remained amongst churchmen about the extent to which their flocks had been Christianised. Burchard of Worms copied Regino's prohibitions against celebrating the new year, and at the same time included others inveighing against other superstitions, such as those who regard the new moon as auspicious for the building of a new house.[54] Yet, when one moves outside the closed circle of church law, in which churchmen looked to earlier textual precedents, it is clear that churchmen often presided over more syncretic rites for curing illness, and protecting crops. In one text, recorded in Old English in *c.*1000, for 'how you may better your fields if they will not grow well or if some harmful thing has been done to them by sorcery or poison', earth from the field should be brought into church, and masses said over it, before being replaced, accompanied by the Lord's Prayer and petitions to the Holy Cross. This text also includes a verse to be said by the ploughman when cutting the first furrow.[55] Such a rite complements the Latin blessings found in service books which accompanied the Rogationtide processions from the church and around the land in order to bless the cattle, earth and woods in late spring.[56] In an agrarian economy such syntheses must have been common, but they also point to the presence of other concerns and other influences on the annual lives of the laity than those of the liturgical year.

The cycle of the agricultural year was also refracted back into the laity's relationship with their local church through the payment of tithe and other church dues. The idea that the faithful should pay a proportion, usually a tenth, of their produce for the support of the poor and the maintenance of the church had a long history, but it is only in the ninth century that the actual relationship between payments and tithes is first set out. In some areas the tithes were subdivided into four parts, for the priest, the maintenance of the church building, the poor and the bishop; in other places there was a threefold division for the priest, the building and the poor. They were only one of several types of church due, the nature of which varied between different localities. In England, at least, the payment of tithes in return for pastoral care only became formalised in the late ninth and tenth centuries.[57] By the early eleventh century, Archbishop Wulfstan of Worcester and York anxiously told his clergy to remind people about the payment of tithes and set out the following timetable:

> *And it is right that priests remind the people about what they must render to God as dues in tithes and in other things. And it is right that they be reminded of this at Easter, a second time at Rogation days, a third time at midsummer [St John the Baptist's Day], when most of the people is assembled. First plough alms fifteen days after Easter, tithe of young animals by Pentecost, 'Rome-money' by St Peter's day, [tithe of] the fruits of the earth by All Saints' day, church-scot at Martinmas, and light dues three times a year: first on Easter Eve, and a second time on Candlemas Eve, the third time on the eve of All Saints' day.*[58]

The timetable used eight of the universal feasts included in Burchard's calendar of those the laity should observe (as demonstrated in Table 5.1 above) and clearly linked them to the agricultural cycle: ploughing, animal husbandry, and crop harvesting. Payment schedules such as Wulfstan's gave the laity an additional reason to take notice of, and observe, the annual liturgical cycle of the Church, especially as the payment of secular dues seems usually to have been measured by the liturgical calendar. Plough alms are seemingly an innovation of Archbishop Wulfstan; Rome money is unique to England and represented a yearly payment made to the papacy by the English.[59] Whilst the specific details of the payment schedule are far from universal, churchmen throughout the medieval west expected members of the laity to pay regular tribute to the Church across the liturgical year.

Several Old English sermons link the payment of tithes explicitly to the agricultural year. Ælfric divided the payment of tithes into three parts, and in one of his homilies for the Twelfth Sunday after Pentecost (harvest time in late summer) emphasised the biblical precedents for tithe payments and how, whilst the first two parts finance the minster, the third part goes to the poor, widows, orphans and foreigners.[60] One sermon attributed to Archbishop Wulfstan linked tithes to the harvest even more explicitly:

> *Through Christ's goodness, most beloved brothers, the days are near when we must gather the harvest, and so giving thanks to God, who has given, let us consider our offering or rather our repayment of tithes. For our God, who has deigned to give us everything, thinks it right that he should receive tithes from us that will no doubt benefit us rather than himself.*[61]

He berated those who refuse to pay tithes with the threat of destruction:

> *He [God] asks for first-fruits and tithes, and yet you refuse. Avaricious man, what would you do if he were to take nine-tenths for himself and leave you the tenth? Surely this is what happened when your crops brought meagre yields because his blessing of rain was withdrawn, or when hail battered your vintage or when it failed as a result. Why does this happen? The nine-tenths were taken from you because you refused to pay tithes.*[62]

He emphasised the importance of tithes in support for the poor and outlined how they were divided into four parts. Wulfstan based his text largely on that of the sixth-century homilist, Caesarius of Arles, but it nevertheless clearly links the payment of tithes with the harvest.[63] But that churchmen thought such sermons necessary again hints at a certain level of lay resistance – understandable in a subsistence economy – to these economic demands. Complaints about local churches being used as storehouses, repeated regularly from the ninth century, point to the physical demands which the Church made of the laity in these regions. The copious numbers of surviving charters and leases which record the transfer of rights to tithes between lay noblemen and churches and between different ecclesiastical institutions indicate their importance for the economy of lordship. Tithes represented a significant burden on the peasantry, but in linking payments to the feasts of the church year, churchmen set up another, less benign way, which brought the laity regularly into contact with their local church and the demands of their faith.

Church laws, as we have seen, went into detail about how feasts, including Sundays, and periods of fasting should be observed. Taken together with the homiletic evidence they demonstrate that churchmen sought to promote a very pragmatic form of Christianity. They outlined which feasts should be kept, when, and how, and clearly sought to scale down their requirements to those which might reasonably be expected of the laity. Their expectations may have been limited, but they were firmly stated, and it is clear from sermon evidence that higher churchmen made various efforts to ensure the lay community attended church and kept the feasts of the church year on a regular basis. Christian feasts thus provided a framework for communal activities – ploughing, harvesting – and for collective celebrations such as harvest. But even though we can see churchmen scaling back their demands of ordinary Christians to ones which might more easily be met, we are still a long way from being able to know the extent to which they were realised. The next step to solving this conundrum is to turn to the evidence for the delivery of pastoral care itself: the routine rites which marked the life course of ordinary Christians, those for baptism, penance, marriage, and dying. What can we know of the services for pastoral care provided by the priests of local churches? And how far is what we know confined to the 'ought' world of reformers' prescriptions? Or does any evidence survive which suggest their aspirations were implemented and realised? In asking these questions we are thus able to explore the extent to which the local church in this period became the focus for the lives and religious loyalties of the communities of ordinary lay men and women which they served.

Baptism

Baptism signifies the entry of the individual into the Church, and thus the local community of Christians. Medieval churchmen emphasised its importance in countless sermons and homilies in which they explained baptism's role within the life of both the individual and the community. The audience for such texts is not always obvious; many are too complicated and learned to have been easily understood by anyone except the highly educated clergy, even those written in the vernacular, but others, as we saw above, were seemingly composed for a wider audience of laity and less educated clergy. In a sermon for delivery on Christmas Day, for example, Ælfric (d. *c.*1010) described baptism in simple terms suitable for a lay audience:

> *Each man is filled with sins and is born through Adam's transgression, but he is afterwards born to Christ in the holy community, that is in God's church, through baptism. That water washes the body and the Holy Ghost washes the soul from all sins, and the baptised man is then God's son.*[64]

Ælfric's text is far from unique; the evidence of other vernacular sermons written in England from the late tenth to the twelfth centuries suggests that conscientious churchmen constantly reiterated the message that baptism is necessary for salvation.[65] At the same time they helped promote another view, one of community cohesion in which every individual was 'born to Christ in the holy community'. Depictions of the rite of baptism in manuscripts from east Frankia and southern Italy also stress this view of baptism as a collective act. The miniature illustrating the baptismal rite in the late tenth-century Fulda sacramentary depicts the scrutiny for baptism with women with presumably female children on the right, and the men with male children on the left approaching the clergy in the centre.[66] One late tenth-century Exultet Roll from southern Italy illustrates the baptism of infants by depicting men standing near the font, women behind it, with boys and girls in front of the font.[67] These images represented an idealised picture of baptism, the entry of these children into the wider community as part of a shared and public ceremony.

These portraits of baptism as a collective, formal ceremony in which members of the local community came together to witness groups of children being baptised together, are echoed in the rites found in many liturgical books from the period. The baptismal liturgy had its roots in late antiquity when infant baptism had been unknown; these rites had originally been intended to prepare adult converts, known as catechumens, for entry into the Church over a course of preparatory ritual educative 'scrutinies' during Lent. These 'scrutinies' extended over three, seven or even nine meetings, in which they were instructed in prayers and the Creed, ending with their baptism on Holy Saturday, the day before Easter. But by the ninth century infant baptism had become the norm; this shift led to the clumsy adaptation of this lengthy ritual structure originally intended for adults to one suitable for children. One can trace this process of adaptation in the encyclopaedic collection of liturgical rites now known as the tenth-century Romano-German Pontifical. The modern edition includes two baptismal services: the first sets out a long and elaborate process stretching from the Wednesday of the third week in Lent, when the first of seven scrutinies began, and culminating in the baptism of the infants on Holy Saturday. It envisages a collective, very public rite in which all the male and female children are brought to church by their godparents, their parents and other people who can take charge of the infants when needed. For example, at the first scrutiny meeting, the children are called into church, with boys on the right, and girls on the left: after renouncing Satan on the child's behalf, salt is exorcised and placed in the mouth of each child 'as favour for the afterlife', and then the godparents sign the infants on their foreheads with their thumbs saying 'In the name of the Father and of the Son and of the Holy Ghost', and the sign of the cross is made first by the acolyte, and then by the priest on each child's forehead, and then the catechumens are told to wait outside until the Mass is finished. They are handed over to someone whilst the parents of the children and the godparents make offerings, which are placed on the altar, and the names of those men and women acting as godparents are read out loud, and included in the prayer for the living. The infants to be baptised are supposed to return with their parents and godparents another five times, before returning for the seventh and final scrutiny at the third hour on Holy Saturday when:

> *[They return] with their godfathers and godmothers and are arranged . . . in the order their names are written, with males on the right and females on the left, and they return the Lord's Prayer and Creed, or rather the godfathers and godmothers who are to receive them [from the font] do so for them.*[68]

They are then told to return at the seventh hour to be baptised. First the Easter candle is blessed, then the font, and finally the children, followed by the baptism of the children, and their subsequent confirmation. It is difficult to believe that any priests or lay people were prepared to commit to a ceremony of this length, or to postpone baptism for that long – for as we shall see, church law penalised those parents and priests who allowed children to die unbaptised. The second rite is much more pragmatic; it sets out a one-stop rite.[69] It similarly presumed that this would happen only occasionally, and outlined a collective and public rite. Male children should be on the right, females on the left, and first male, and then female children should be baptised in the font, with the clergy and people standing around. After they had been baptised, the children should attend Mass, communicate, and if the bishop is present they should be confirmed. As this rubric suggests, separate confirmation was rare.

The innate conservatism of ecclesiastical traditions explains why this liturgical and iconographic evidence subscribed to norms laid down in late Antiquity. It presents a picture of the rite which is actually at variance with that in penitential and church law from the central Middle Ages. For legislation suggests that individual infant baptism within a few days of the birth was the norm, rather than a collective Easter baptismal ceremony. Texts advised that children should be baptised within seven or nine days of their birth, and that parents and priests who failed to baptise infants promptly should do penance.[70] In early tenth-century Lotharingia, Regino of Prüm advised the bishop, on his visitation, to enquire of the community whether any children had been smothered by their parents, either before or after baptism, again presuming rapid baptism of babies to be the norm.[71] If a priest is not available to baptise the child, laymen are encouraged to do so if the child's life was in danger; one west Frankish penitential specified that sick children who have been immersed in water in the name of the Trinity by ordinary Christians did not need to be re-baptised.[72] In such circumstances it is unlikely that godparents would be able to take a formal part. But both artistic representations of baptism, and the prescriptions for how the rite should be conducted found in many liturgical books, continued to depict it as a collective, formal, annual ceremony in which the community came together to witness groups of children, presented by their godparents, being baptised together.

It is hard to reconcile these illustrations and rites with the expectations of the prescriptive evidence that children will be baptised on an individual basis. It has been suggested that sometimes the liturgical rite for the baptism of the sick was used for *ad hoc* penance, and in the ninth century Hrabanus Maurus argued that it was absurd to make parents choose between perjuring themselves by swearing their child was mortally ill in order to have a child baptised, or risk the infant dying suddenly unbaptised.[73] But the rite in a sacramentary composed somewhere in southern England in *c.*1061, and now known as the Red Book of Darley, shows specific attempts being made to come up with a suitable rite for individual, *ad hoc* penance. This rite is written for a single child rather than for the several children.[74] Moreover, the rubrics (but not the prayers) are in Old English, rather than Latin, and those for baptism have been adapted to make clear the role of the godparents in giving the responses on behalf of the child, an aspect missing from the Frankish rites discussed above. This rite, Helen Gittos has suggested, is composed for use by a priest to serve his local community; the vernacular rubrics suggest an attempt being made to educate the minister and ensure he understood what he had to do, whilst the rite itself is intended for the circumstances in which he found himself. The contents of the Red Book of Darley are so complex that it is unlikely to have been made for use in a local church, but its concern with specific instructions suggests it was probably written to train those who would serve such communities.[75]

Its authors may have been responding to a new development: the location of baptism in local churches for the first time in England which necessitated detailed training of local clergy. For the material evidence suggests that it is only in the eleventh century that local churches across northern Europe began to acquire stone fonts. Very few stone fonts survive from before the eleventh century but the steep increase in numbers from the mid-twelfth century onwards has been linked to the localisation of baptism.[76] They are to be found in small, local churches all over northern Europe, from Devon in the south west of England to Saxony in the east of Germany and testify to the considerable investment made by local patrons and churchmen in the delivery of baptism within local communities. The work of skilled craftsmen, the fonts were manufactured in quarries before being sent out to churches. A local atelier responsible for a group of eight pedestal fonts in north Devon has been identified, whilst a single workshop at Bard Bentheim in Saxony was responsible for at least 120 fonts which were exported down river valleys and along the coast to southern Germany, Jutland and northern Holland.[77] The acquisition of fonts usually coincided with the building or rebuilding of local churches which is likely to have accompanied a change in status from minster to parish church. Many are elaborately carved structures with a complex iconography, suggesting that they were a valued part of the church fabric. Whether plain or elaborate they are all testimony to the practice of baptism within local churches from the late eleventh century onwards, if not before.

The picture in parts of southern Europe is rather different. In many parts of northern and central Italy, *pievi* succeeded in retaining control over the baptismal rites of subordinate churches within a sizeable area into the later Middle Ages. The reasons for this different pattern of pastoral provision are not very clear. On the one hand, they may reflect the continuation of earlier medieval patterns of authority, and of the powerful interests of the clerical communities which controlled baptismal churches; control of many *pievi* in the eleventh and twelfth century was handed over to monasteries who had a vested interest in preserving the *status quo*. On the other hand, as Maureen Miller has demonstrated, in the diocese of Verona the emergence of new communities in the twelfth century led to the recognition of new churches as having baptismal status.[78] She suggests that uncontrolled growth in the number of churches established in the diocese in the course of the eleventh and early twelfth centuries offered the bishop a chance to assert his leadership over his diocesan clergy by establishing a hierarchy of baptismal churches and dependent chapels.[79] Verona is perhaps exceptional; elsewhere in other Italian dioceses monasteries retained a greater control over baptismal churches, an interest which was probably primarily financial, as it was elsewhere in Europe. Clearly the fusion of pastoral need with ecclesiastical and secular claims to authority was worked out in different ways across the European landscape with a consequent impact on the organisation of pastoral care.

In Italy the retention of baptismal churches also impacted on the experience of ordinary men and women in the distances they were required to travel to get their children baptised. In the cities, at least, baptism may even have remained an annual, collective ceremony which took place at Easter. Erlembald, the leader of the Patarene movement in Milan protesting against corruption in the clergy, we are told by a hostile chronicler, prevented the baptism of many catechumens at Eastertide in 1074 by entering the baptistery of Milan cathedral, and knocking over the chrism in a grand gesture, on the grounds that it was not valid as it had been consecrated by a bishop whom he regarded as guilty of simony.[80] Their experience would have been rather different to that of villagers in England who could expect to take their children to their local church to be baptised as and when they were born. The different histories of England and Italy as regards the location of baptism reflect the impact of authority on local church provision as much as pastoral need.

A similar combination of secular, ecclesiastical and pastoral needs played out in the significance attached to godparents in this period. By the ninth century the widespread adoption of infant baptism meant the onus for instructing uncomprehending infants had passed from the clergy to their godparents, who stood sponsors for them and presented them for baptism. The liturgical rites, as we have seen, emphasised the godparents' responsibility for the child's welfare, symbolised perhaps most compellingly by the instruction that the priest should put the infant in the water, and the godfather should remove him. This is illustrated in one south Italian Exultet roll in which the godfathers present the infants to the priest at the font, whilst the godmothers stand behind it with towels ready to receive those who have just been baptised.[81] Godparents should make the responses to the priest's catechesis on behalf of the child, and to teach their godchildren the Creed and Lord's Prayer when they were old enough. Hence the concern of bishops in Lotharingia, east Frankia and England with ensuring that everyone knew and understood these two texts. Regino of Prüm included in his early tenth-century collection a text instructing each priest to teach all his parishioners the Creed and the Lord's Prayer, and to ask that they recite them to him from memory when they come to confession in Lent, and to deny communion to anyone who was unable to do so; no one should be allowed to act as godparent unless they could recite these two texts before the priest. Regino regarded the failure to teach godchildren these texts as a sin worthy of confession and meriting penance.[82] There is no precedent for Regino's text but it draws on Carolingian material which, as we have already seen, also shaped the concerns of English churchmen in the early eleventh century: hence Wulfstan's prohibition on Christians who do not know these prayers becoming godparents. That vernacular translations of the Lord's Prayer and Creed circulated with manuscripts of Ælfric's sermons suggests that some English churchmen sought to realise Archbishop Wulfstan's injunction that knowledge of these two prayers is fundamental to membership of the Church.[83]

Being a godparent established a relationship of spiritual kinship between the child, the child's family and the godparent. As an institution it served an important social dimension, and the elite used it to make lifelong social and political alliances. Abbot Hugh of Cluny, for example, as godfather to King Henry IV of Germany, was able to act as mediator between the king and Pope Gregory VII in the negotiations leading up to Henry's submission before the pope at Canossa in January 1077.[84] Breaking the bonds created by that relationship was akin to treason: the Emperor Otto III punished his godfather, John Philagathos, the former Archbishop of Ravenna, for usurping the papacy in 997 by having his nose, ears, and tongue cut out, and his eyes put out; John Philagathos had traduced the bonds of what should be a close relationship.[85] The scandal of this case echoed across various writings of the period, testifying to the widespread shock felt at the way this kindred relationship had ended. As with other social relationships at this time, gift giving marked the beginning of the relationship between godparent and child. The gifts made by godparents to their godchildren on this occasion even had a special name – *filiolagium* or *filioladium* – demonstrating the widespread nature of the practice. Documented examples reveal the substantial nature of such gifts which amongst the elite usually comprised lands. The consequent alienation of ecclesiastical property led to criticism of monks and nuns assuming this role. The north French cartulary of Saint Père de Chartres, for example, reveals how the monastery had lost its estate at Gondreville because 'a certain abbot of this place gave [this estate] in gift to a certain boy whom he had received from the holy font; the boy's relatives, in spite of the unwillingness of the monks, possess the property up to the present day'.[86] Our knowledge of such cases is biased towards the high elite, but it seems reasonable to assume that the social advantages of such relationships, albeit on a smaller scale, permeated lower down the social order, and that the institution of spiritual kinship served to strengthen relationships between different groups within more local communities.

The physical evidence of stone fonts and records of gifts by godparents take us beyond the aspirational world of prescriptive clerical texts and testify to the importance of the lived experience of baptism to local communities. Infant baptism served as a naming ceremony for formal entry into secular society, and children who had not been baptised remained officially nameless. An eleventh-century charter of Saint-Victor in Marseilles, for example, records the family of 'Peter and my wife Teuca and my sons William and Jaufred and two others who have not been regenerated by water and the holy spirit [i.e. baptised]' and were thus formally unnamed.[87] Peter of Cornwall, writing in *c.*1200, recorded the story of a child known as 'Paganus' because 'he was a long time a pagan, living twelve years before he was baptised'. As this soubriquet suggests, by this time it had become unusual for children to get to the age of twelve without being baptised.[88] The rite's popularity signifies its importance in signalling the child's entry into the earthly as well as the heavenly community.

Regular baptismal practice need not, however, imply widespread understanding of its significance by the laity. But records of superstitious beliefs amongst the lay population point to the ways in which churchmen believed it to be understood, and misunderstood, by the laity. Burchard of Worms recorded a series of penances for superstitious practices which, as they have no precedents in the surviving penitential tradition, are likely to represent common practice within the early eleventh-century Rhineland.[89] He prescribed a penance for those who regarded the souls of the unbaptised as haunting the living:

> *Have you done what some women do at the instigation of the devil? When any child has died without baptism they take the corpse of the little one and place it in some secret place and transfix its little body with a stake, saying that if they did not do so the little child would arise and*

> *would injure many? If you have done so, or consented to, or believed this, you should do penance for two years on the appointed days.*[90]

He enjoined a similar penalty on those who meted out the same treatment to the corpses of a woman and her child who died together in the course of childbirth. Yet Burchard also included a penance against a superstition which suggests that the laity did not regard infant baptism as fully efficacious:

> *Have you done what some women are accustomed to do? When a child is newly born and immediately baptised and then dies, when they bury him they put in his right hand a paten of wax with the host, and in his left hand put a chalice also of wax, with wine, and so they bury him. If you have, you should do penance for ten days on bread and water.*[91]

These superstitions all point to widespread lay anxiety about the fate of infants who died soon after birth. They also point to a limited, if perverse, understanding of orthodox theology. The fear of those who died unbaptised suggests some understanding of church law's view that the unbaptised were condemned to hell. The desire to give the newly born who died soon after baptism the insignia of the Eucharist indicates, perhaps, a recognition that baptism signified entry into the Church, and a knowledge that partaking of the Eucharist was essential for practising Christians. Alternatively, it may also represent lay knowledge of the last rites for the dying which included the taking of the Eucharist, the *viaticum*. Both scenarios point to a relatively detailed knowledge of ecclesiastical practice, and a desire to ensure that children be saved in the afterlife, whilst the very mild penance given for this practice – only ten days penance – implies that Burchard recognised that such superstition arose from the best of motives. Yet such superstition also implies a lay belief that these infants were not yet full members of the community, combined with a concern to ensure that they become so. Archaeological evidence suggests that this view may have been more widespread. It is rare to come across child graves in pagan burial grounds, but late Anglo-Saxon cemeteries in both Norwich and around the small church at Raunds Furnell in Northamptonshire have been found to include a significant proportion of infant graves.[92] As only the baptised could be buried in consecrated ground, these graves are physical testimony to the widespread acceptance, and understanding, of the Church's message that baptism is necessary to membership of the Christian community.

The revisions made to tailor the collective, annual, adult baptismal liturgy to an *ad hoc* rite for individual infants, when combined with the substantial material evidence for fonts in local churches, the burial of children in Christian cemeteries and the changing nature of church status in many areas to allow for baptism in the locality, point to the fact that across the medieval west local churches had become the focus for the initiation ceremonies of the newest members of the communities they served. Churchmen's ambitions for universal baptism were gradually being realised at all levels of society.

Confession and penance

If eleventh-century parents in England and the Rhineland were so anxious about the fate of their dead children in the afterlife, how did they feel about that of their own souls? And how did they try to allay these concerns? By 900 the Church had a well-established procedure for dealing with the consequences of sinful behaviour: penance. This is a process by which individual Christians seek to atone for their sins through confession, through penitential acts which demonstrate their repentance, and through good works, in order to ensure their salvation at the Last Judgement.[93] The rites and laws governing penitential practice had been laid down by the beginning of the tenth century. Law collections such as that by Regino of Prüm suggest that churchmen expected all Christians to confess their sins – however minor – to their priest at least once a year. They reserved more serious sins to the bishops, and expected these penitents to undergo a rite of public penance. But were their assumptions realised? How far did penance become part of the normative experience of ordinary lay men and women?

It is clear that churchmen envisaged that the local church would act as the focus for a collective annual penitential ceremony in which the entire congregation came together at the beginning of Lent to atone for their sins and make peace with each other. At the beginning of our period, Regino of Prüm included in his collection the following canon 'On confession and penance':

> *Priests ought to admonish the people subject to them so that everyone who knows himself to be wounded with the mortal wound of sin should on the fourth day before Lent [Ash Wednesday] return with all haste to the*

> *life-giving mother church where, confessing with all humility and contrition of heart, the evil which he has committed, he shall receive the remedies of penance according to the scale fixed by canonical authorities . . . But not only he who has committed some mortal sin but also every person who recognises that he has polluted the immaculate robe of Christ which he received in baptism with the stain of sin shall hasten to come to his own priest and with purity of mind most humbly confess all the transgressions and all the sins by which he remembers he has incurred offence against God, and whatever is enjoined on him by the priest he will do, as if it was uttered by the mouth of Almighty God, he shall diligently listen and most cautiously observe.*[94]

This text tells us what Regino thought should happen at local level. It is not a description of actual practice, but rather a reflection of earlier traditions: Bishop Theodulf of Orléans in the early ninth century had enjoined that confession should be made to priests in the week before the beginning of Lent and quarrels settled, so that all entered the Lenten season of feasting and almsgiving with pure minds as preparation for communion on Easter Sunday.[95] Other texts also stressed the importance of annual confession as a time for settling quarrels. Archbishop Ruotger of Trier (915–31) instructed his priests to make sure all the faithful confessed their sins in both word and thought to the priest in the week before Lent began and accepted penance for them. Peace should be restored, all grudges and disputes abandoned, following the words of the Lord's Prayer, 'Forgive us our trespasses as we forgive those who trespass against us'. They should remind their flock how to behave in Lent, hear individual confessions, give a penance commensurate with the guilty deed, remind the penitent of the importance of confessing bad thoughts as well as deeds, and accept his confession.[96] Ruotger's text remained in his diocese, but Regino's circulated more widely, and in the eleventh century it became copied into Burchard of Worms's popular *Decretum*. The popularity of texts such as this suggest other churchmen of the time shared these men's aspirations for annual Lenten confession in local churches.[97]

Narrative texts provide further support for this picture of penance as embedded in the local community. Tales of good penitents situate them confessing their sin, and performing penance, within their local community and its church. Perhaps the best example of such a story is that recorded by

Ekkehard of St Gall, writing in the mid-eleventh century, albeit about events which supposedly took place in the ninth century. He describes how penance was conducted in one local community, recounting the circumstances surrounding the conception of one member of the community of St Gall, Iso. His parents were preparing for the Easter celebrations on Holy Saturday, after the Lenten period of fasting and abstinence, when his father unexpectedly came upon his mother taking a bath, and both became overcome by desire. They realised immediately that they had sinned, and reproached themselves so loudly that soon their entire household knew what they had done. They therefore went immediately to the priest, and confessed their sin before him and the local community; the priest accepted their repentance and granted them forgiveness, but gave them a penance which was to stand by the doors of the church for a day and a night and to be excluded from communion for that time, which included one of the greatest feasts in the Christian year, Easter Sunday. Anxious to participate in the annual Easter communion, Iso's parents visited a neighbouring priest to ask for absolution, but he refused, and they therefore performed their penance, standing at the back of the church, fasting and crying, dressed in penitential sackcloth. At the end of Mass on Easter Sunday, however, someone whom they took to be a priest from a neighbouring village rushed into the church, led them up to the altar and gave them communion, ordering them to change out of their sackcloth, and to celebrate Easter. This priest was subsequently discovered to be an angel, as the neighbouring priest had spent the entire day in his parish in front of witnesses.[98] Tales such as this sought to promote penance as voluntary, performed by penitents because of their own awareness of sinful behaviour, rather than because priests told them to do so. At the same time, this story situates penance within the context of the local community; it was not secret, but nor was it seen as a matter for great scandal. By quietly performing their penance, Iso's parents atoned for their sin and were accepted back into the community. Their story points to an attempt by leading churchmen to promote the practice of regular, voluntary penance. It also underlines the presumption that it would take place in the local church.

The delegation of such an important rite to priests in local churches generated a good deal of anxiety amongst senior churchmen as to whether it was being imposed correctly. Such concerns were not new; the reforming bishops of the ninth century had been similarly worried, and had composed and copied a large number of penitential texts to support local priests in this work. Clergy in the central Middle Ages thus inherited a tremendous body of material which they continued to copy and adapt. The sheer volume of surviving material points to the considerable effort made by senior churchmen to promote the practice of penance amongst the laity: at least 300 manuscripts survive from before 1000, and they continued to be copied and composed afterwards.[99]

Penitentials are usually quite short works. By the tenth century they had come usually to consist of an *ordo* for how to hear confession and enjoin penance, followed by a list of possible offences with the appropriate penance. Sometimes this list took the form of questions about whether the penitent had committed a series of offences, followed by the appropriate penance. These questions might potentially cover a huge range of offences, from what would now be regarded as serious crimes to minor infringements of religious practice and superstitious belief. For example, the questionnaire at the beginning of Book XIX of Burchard of Worms' early eleventh-century *Decretum* began by asking:

> *Have you committed murder voluntarily, not because of necessity or because of war, but because of your passion, so that you may steal the things of him you have killed? If you have done so, you ought to fast, as is customary, on bread and water for 40 days continuously, what is popularly called a carina, and observe this for seven sequential years.*[100]

But it also included questions about superstition like this one:

> *Have you collected medicinal herbs with incantations to others, not with the Creed and the Lord's Prayer, that is, with singing the 'Credo in Deum' and the 'Pater noster'? If you have done otherwise, 10 days penance on bread and water.*[101]

Burchard's text is unusual amongst penitential texts in some ways because it is extremely long, covering some 194 questions. Most penitentials are much shorter – some ten to thirty questions – and often concentrate on more serious offences. Burchard's text is part of his collection of canon law in twenty books, and the length of his penitential probably reflects his wish to be comprehensive. The problem for modern scholars is knowing what to make of all such lists, for they are usually made up of texts copied or adapted from earlier precedents. Both of Burchard's questions cited here, for example, are based on texts found in Regino's *Libri duo*, which in turn have earlier textual precedents.[102] Diligent analysis of the minor editorial decisions made by compilers when selecting this material suggests that the compilers of such texts did not blindly copy them, but rather selected and adapted their sources to fit local circumstances.[103] At the same time, they added new information: Burchard, for example, included a lot of material not found elsewhere on superstitions common amongst women.[104] It seems that whilst they built on earlier precedents, compilers adapted their material for new circumstances and contemporary problems.

But Burchard was a bishop and his *Decretum* survives in the libraries of cathedrals and great monasteries across Europe. Who constituted the audience for his work and that of other penitentials? Some modern scholars think these texts were intended primarily as guidance for bishops and their officers, when exercising jurisdiction over particularly heinous sinners, whilst others have suggested they were composed as guides to educate local priests in their pastoral duty of hearing annual confession.[105] Burchard, for example, stated in the preface to his *Decretum* that he had compiled its twenty books of church law for the instruction of the clergy of his diocese, and one modern scholar, Ludger Körntgen, has suggested that the lengthy questionnaire at the start of book XIX is intended to help priests memorise the contents of this diverse collection.[106] The encyclopaedic range of sins in the *Decretum* make it unwieldy as a practical guide, but a very helpful educational tool for training priests in how to administer penance. The picture is not clear-cut, however, for many of the other penitential texts from this period were copied with other legal texts and survive in manuscripts made for cathedrals and other institutional libraries, suggesting that they were intended for bishops and their officers.[107] It is much more difficult to identify amongst the surviving manuscripts any codices made for local churches, and consequently we lack evidence for the actual practice of penance in a local church context. Nevertheless it is clear that the higher clergy made a concerted effort to educate priests in how to administer penance. Some codices even link penitential texts explicitly with other pastoral rites. Thus the clergy of S. XII Apostoli in early eleventh-century Rome included a penitential in a codex alongside rites for baptism, visitation of the sick, and the obsequies for the dying, amongst other texts aimed at training priests in their pastoral duties; and in mid-eleventh-century Worcester, the monks included two penitentials alongside the rites for sick and the dying in one manuscript.[108] Both manuscripts seem to have been intended to educate the local priests in their duties, and point to a concern amongst senior churchmen in these two regions with the promotion of penance at the local level.

The inclusion of guides on how to hear confession, *ordines*, which generally precede the list of sins, also point to a more pastoral context. These rites are generally written for a single priest to hear the confession of an individual penitent; such occasions were not particularly private and one particular text from Italy records how the priest, sitting before the altar, should hear confession and give penance to individual penitents in turn.[109] Confession in such circumstances might not be private but it would be personal, part of an individual's relationship with his priest. It also had a very public dimension. Iso's parents, we are told, deliberately reported what was a private sin, engaging in sexual intercourse at a time when it was forbidden by the ecclesiastical calendar, to their household and confessed their sin before the local community.

A different, and rather more formal practice, existed for those guilty of truly heinous sins which had offended the public weal, *poenitentia publica* (public penance). Like confession, public penance is also associated with the Lenten period. At the beginning of Lent those judged to merit public penance should present themselves, accompanied by their local priests, at the doors of the cathedral. There they are met by the bishop. After they had been given their penance they are led into the cathedral, where ashes are placed on their heads; dressed in sackcloth they are driven out of the Church building, just as Adam had been expelled from paradise. They are formally reconciled with the Church in a public rite held on Maundy Thursday at the end of Lent. Liturgical public penance, however, was reserved to the bishop, and lay outside the usual experience of most ordinary lay Christians.[110] As a practice, it had its roots in Late Antiquity, but the shape of public penance in this period owed more to the efforts of reformist bishops in the ninth and tenth centuries. The liturgical records testify to continuous revision and diversity in practice, suggesting that bishops made real efforts to implement it. There are also hints in other episcopal sources that episcopal reconciliation of penitents was regularly conducted. Thietmar of Merseburg, writing in the early eleventh century, describes how Otto III's funeral cortege, passing through Cologne on Maundy Thursday in 1002 en route to Aachen, passed the penitents waiting outside the cathedral to be reconciled.[111] He also reports the burial of a man 'in the southern part of the [cathedral] at the place where the penitents appear on Maundy Thursday'.[112] Public penance also had a fearful reality for those penitents whom Archbishop Ruotger of Trier, writing in the 920s, condemned for nervously telling each other jokes, or stories, whilst waiting in the queue to be reconciled by the bishop on Maundy Thursday.[113]

Ruotger's exasperated reference to the noisy unease of penitents nevertheless points to the underlying anxiety which surrounded the practice of penance. It is suggestive of, but not evidence for, its widespread practice. For this we must turn to the widespread copying and composition of penitential texts and rites in this period; the fact that senior churchmen thought it worth investing time and parchment in such activities, combined with the didactic tone of much of this material, suggests a considerable concern with delivering penance at a local level. Penance clearly mattered to senior churchmen, and they made a good deal of effort to educate local priests in it and ensure they had access to penitential guides. Bishops were clearly keen to see penance administered to local congregations. How far they succeeded is unclear, but all this evidence for clerical activity suggests that annual confession, if not yet universal, was becoming much more common in this period.

Dying, death and burial

Death is universal, but can the same be said for Christian obsequies in this period? How far did the lay men and women who made up the congregations of local churches undergo the last rites on their deathbed? Were they buried in accordance with Christian rites in a consecrated ground? It is remarkably difficult to answer these questions.

The Church assumed the Christian way of death to be universal. The compilers of church law around 1000 displayed very little interest in ensuring that the laity die and be buried in accordance with the rites of the Church. They assumed they would be, and chose instead to regulate how these rites should be conducted: thus they instructed priests only to give the *viaticum* to the sick whilst they could still swallow, and to hear the dying person's confession before anointing her or him with holy oil.[114] Churchmen are instead more preoccupied with regulating the income from these rites, veering between enjoining priests not to charge extortionately for their services, to setting out when and how payments should be made, such as that for *soulscot* which was paid in eleventh-century England at the graveside to the representative of the church in whose territory the dead person had lived.[115] In northern Italy at the same time the illustrators of a sacramentary made for Bishop Warmund of Ivrea (966–1002) presumed that lay people would follow the Christian last rites. The miniatures which accompanied the *ordines* for the dying included lay people as well as clergy in their depiction of the various stages of the process. Their iconography is unique: they make clear that such rites should be administered to lay men in a lay setting. They also set out a clear role for lay women and men in the obsequies: mourning, laying out the dead, and carrying the funeral bier to the graveyard. Dying is portrayed as a family affair. In the first scene the sick man is given absolution by the priest whilst his wife and family look on; in another scene the priest, accompanied by other clerics, anoints the dying man with chrism whilst a distraught woman with unkempt hair looks on, held back by a lay man. She is also there in a scene where the body is washed and wrapped in a shroud by laymen. She is again present at the funeral Mass, and together with the clergy and laymen accompanies the bier to the burial in the cemetery. The message is clear: such rites should be administered to the laity, and dying takes place at home amongst the family and household.

Yet it far from clear how churchmen intended that the last rites should be conducted for ordinary lay Christians. As already discussed with regards to baptism, those liturgical books which survive were compiled, on the whole, for large clerical communities. Designed with the life of a large monastery in mind rather than that of a lay household, however grand, they prescribed a sequence of elaborate rites to accompany the dying person from their deathbed to the grave.[116] These rites had already largely reached their late medieval form in Carolingian monasteries in the late ninth century.[117] The process began when the priest visited the dying person's bedside to hear her, or his, confession. He then anointed the dying person with holy oil, extreme unction, and offered communion, the *viaticum*. These preliminary rites served as a preparation for death itself; there might be a significant interval between the conduct of these rites, and death itself. During that time, someone must be appointed to watch the deathbed, and when it seemed that death is imminent, the watcher summons the brethren of the community to gather around the deathbed, singing the seven penitential psalms and the litany until the moment of death, at which point they should sing an antiphon, 'May Christ receive you who has called you, and may the angels lead you into the bosom of Abraham', followed by a psalm. Thus at the moment of the death the dying person should be accompanied by the prayers and chants of the community as she or he crossed over into the afterlife. Prayers are then said to commend the dead person's soul to God, the corpse is washed and laid out, and carried into the church, where it remains overnight until Mass the next morning. After Mass the body is taken to the graveside and buried. Prayers, psalmody and chants accompany each stage.

These rites could not have been easily adapted for lay communities: they presume the priest will be accompanied by clerics on his visit to the sickbed, and that the whole community of brothers will gather around for the commendation of the soul at the point of death. Yet, as we have already seen to be the case for baptism and confession, various attempts were made to educate local priests in the conduct of these rites. The Red Book of Darley, for example, is much more practical and only mentions a single ministering priest as participating in the obsequies rather than a body of clerics.[118] One vernacular manuscript from the mid-eleventh-century bishopric of Worcester included instructions on how the priest should find out whether the dying person knows his Creed and Pater Noster. If he does, he should sing them. If does not,

> *then let the priest find out for himself during the period of that interval, as it seems to him, whether he knows what is true belief, that is, that he must believe that Father and Son and the Holy Ghost is one God and that he must arise on Doomsday with body and soul and stand at God's judgement and there receive reward for all the deeds that he here in the world previously performed.*[119]

The comprehensive nature of such instructions point to their educational purpose; they are too detailed to be used easily for the actual administration of the rite. Rather, the concern here to explain meticulously what should be done suggests that the person behind its composition is anxious to ensure that priests who administered the last rites understood the rite's rationale. Churchmen in eleventh-century England thus clearly aspired to make Christian rites for the dying universal, and take them out of the monastery to the faithful of local churches.

Elsewhere in Europe it seems that such attempts enjoyed less success. There is a growth in references in the eleventh and twelfth centuries, especially in France, to the practice of lay patrons seeking the privilege of dying as a member of a regular community, with all the accompanying liturgical rites, a practice known as becoming a *frater* or *soror ad succerrendum*. Monastic customaries make provision for the practice, monastic charters record the gifts consequent on such occasions, and monastic chronicles describe individual cases. Orderic Vitalis, for example, records how Ansold entered the Norman house of Maule with his wife's permission and died there three days after making his monastic profession.[120] The very popularity of this practice may indicate dissatisfaction with the nature of the obsequies provided by the priest of local churches. People may have had other motives too: becoming a monk or nun, even on one's deathbed, meant that as a member of the community one would be regularly remembered in the community's prayers.

But even if some members of the nobility who could afford it chose the monastic way of death, the majority of lay Christians died at home accompanied by specifically lay rites – wakes – which bothered churchmen. Ecclesiastical reformers worried that the lay way of death was not sufficiently solemn. In particular their concern focused on wakes as evidence that Christian practices were not followed, and Christian beliefs were insufficiently understood. Regino of Prüm warned that:

> *Laymen who keep watch at funerals shall do so with fear and trembling and with reverence. Let no one presume to sing diabolical songs nor make jokes and dance, as pagans have devised through the devil's preaching. For who does not know it to be diabolical, and not only alien from the Christian religion, but also to be contrary to human nature, that there should be singing, rejoicing, drunkenness, and guffawing, and that all piety and feeling of charity disregarded, as if to exult in a brother's death, where mourning and lamenting with tearful voices ought to resound for the loss of a dear brother . . . Such unfitting joy and destructive songs are through God's authority to be wholly forbidden. For if anyone desires to sing, let him sing the Kyrie eleison. But if he does otherwise, let him be entirely silent. If, however, he will not be silent, he shall be at once denounced by all, or charged under oath/adiured that he does not have God's permission to stay there any longer, but should*

> *withdraw and go to his own house. The next day, moreover, he shall be punished in such a way that all the others may be in fear.*[121]

Whilst there is no textual precedent for Regino's text, concern about wakes seems to have been common. In England Ælfric warned priests against 'joining in the heathen songs and loud laughter of the laity' and eating and drinking in the presence of the corpse. He also recounted the story of how St Swithun punished someone who dared to punish him on one such occasion:

> *At one time men were watching a dead body, as is customary, and there was a certain foolish man, making fun in an inappropriate way, and he said to the men, as if in play, that he was Swithin.*[122]

As well as preaching against the playing of such anti-clerical games at the funeral, he also enjoined against beer-drinking around the corpse. The roots of this concern that the laity mourn the dead with due decorum go back to the ninth century. It continued into the twelfth century when miracle collections recorded lay people playing games and singing popular songs instead of praying for the dead.[123]

Stories like that of the man who dared to mock St Swithun whilst keeping vigil over the dead are indicative of the considerable degree of residual lay resistance to the clergy's efforts to promote mourning in a more decorous and doleful manner. Initially they seem to be at odds with the monastic records of men and women joining communities in order to die supported by the monastic liturgy and to be remembered after their death; such examples suggest that those who could afford it (like all those entering the monastery they made a donation) chose to emulate monks, and accepted the monastic vision for death. But dying *ad succerrandam* remained confined to members of the elite; moreover, it is recorded as being most popular in those societies, such as that of the Limousin in south-western France, in which monasteries seem to have been the focus of lay noble piety. But, as we have seen in earlier chapters, monasteries did not constitute the only focus for lay piety in this period. The evidence of gravestones, of bell towers, poetry, and legal and liturgical texts all point to a world in which men and women expected to be buried within their local community, watched over by members of their family and household, who also prayed for them too.

As we have already seen, churchmen at Worcester cathedral in the mid-eleventh century were interested in educating the clergy of local churches in their pastoral duties. One penitential from mid-eleventh-century Worcester sets out a scenario in which the priest arrives only once the dying man is incapable of speech: in such a scenario those who have been 'standing around' the dying man's bedside may attest on his behalf that he wished to make a last confession and take communion.[124] The presumption is that, just as in a monastery, the family will watch at the bedside of the dying person. At the same time the fictional stories which circulated within clerical communities supposed that it to be normative for a priest to be summoned to the deathbed to administer the last rites. In the *Ruodlieb*, an eleventh-century Latin romance from southern Germany, a priest is called to a dying lay man's deathbed – he has just been stabbed by his wife's lover – and conducts the last rites in this manner:

> *He came and wished to preach the holy faith to him. The old man, groaning often, had not strength except to utter, 'I believe'. The priest then asked him whether he was repenting of the evils he had done. With nods and words he showed that he was penitent. Then, through the body of the Lord cleansed of all sin, as he exhaled his soul, he gave it to the Lord and said, 'Have mercy on a sinner, holy Christ! Forgive those two who snatched away my life from me, and move my sons, I pray, to do the same.' He spoke, then fell silent, and soon afterwards he died.*[125]

The *Vision of Tnugdal*, a mid-twelfth-century account of an Irish knight's vision of the afterlife, which circulated widely across the religious houses of Europe, records how when he fell ill the household behaved in a manner similar to the way a monastic community should behave when a member is thought to be dying:

> *The symptoms of death are present . . . the household rushes around, the food is taken away, the squires shout, the host moans, the body is laid down, bells are rung, the priest comes running, the population is astounded, and the whole city is overcome by the sudden death of the good knight.*[126]

As in the monastery, Tnugdal's is a communal death in which bells are rung and priests summoned. Both the *Ruodlieb* and *Vision of Tnugdal* were composed within monastic contexts, but their authors, in projecting the monastic rites into a lay setting, clearly felt they had a universal applicability. Some authors even assumed the knowledge of the correct procedures for the dying to be widespread. Writing in Old French in the 1130s, Geoffrey Gaimar recorded how, after William Rufus had been shot whilst out hunting in the New Forest in 1100, he repeatedly demanded the Lord's Body, whereupon the huntsman who was with him gave him some herbs to eat in place of the viaticum.[127] Both men, and their audience, knew what needed to be done to make a Christian death.

But how far were these rites practised outside the realm of literature and the cloister? Members of at least one lay community in early eleventh-century England sought to make their own provisions for burying and commemorating the dead, rather than delegating such rites to either the local priest or monks; these arrangements focused on their local church. The community is Abbotsbury in Dorset, or rather a confraternity based on its church. The statutes of this confraternity make provision for any member who falls ill within sixty miles of the place to be brought home by fifteen men and,

> *if he dies in the neighbourhood, the steward is then to inform the guild-brothers, as many as he can possibly ride to or send to, that they are to come there and worthily attend the body and bring it to the minster, and pray earnestly for the soul.*[128]

The implication is that there is an additional benefit to bringing home a dying man in order to ensure that he dies at home, rather than bringing home a corpse. No explicit provision is made for rites to accompany the death; the focus is rather on prayers after death. This example will be considered further in the next chapter; for now, it is worth noting that the existence of lay confraternities like that at Abbotsbury give the lie to the view that in this period the only good death was a monastic death. In eleventh- and twelfth-century Limousin and Normandy monasteries acted as the focus for the death of noble families, but in eleventh-century England, where canonical communities were more influential, a different, and seemingly more lay-centred model prevailed.

Architectural history offers further clues as to how these rites came to be adapted and followed outside the monastic cloister. A recent study of late eleventh- and early twelfth-century churches with towers in Lincolnshire suggests that towers were added to these churches in order to accommodate a burial rite similar to that set out by Lanfranc in the customary he had drawn up for Christ Church, Canterbury.[129] Lanfranc's rite, composed for a monastic community, emphasised that the vigil over the corpse should be performed in a separate chapel. It is argued that in Lincolnshire the base of the tower performed a similar function, whilst the ringing of the bells, found in the upper chamber of the tower, are also an important part of the rite. The presence of bell towers in the local churches built and rebuilt by the Anglo-Norman elite of Lincolnshire testifies to the spread of the monastic rite of the vigil for the dead – hinted at also in the eleventh-century Abbotsbury statutes – into the wider community. There are too many uncertainties for this thesis to be regarded as anything other than hypothetical: we lack detailed evidence for the liturgy at the level of local churches, and what we know about the liturgy more generally suggests that the presumption of the successful spread of a uniform rite for the dying, even within one diocese, is unlikely.

Archaeological evidence also points to the desire to identify the dead to both the living on earth and to God at the Last Judgement. The emergence of bounded graveyards in the tenth century, often next to churches, is testament both to increased ecclesiastical authority and increased Christian burial. The plentiful evidence of stone and wooden monuments to mark the graves of members of the elite testifies to the fact that correct burial mattered. Excavations in England at Raunds Furnell (Northamptonshire) and St Mary's le-Wigford, Lincoln suggest the presence of post holes for wooden markers beside graves. Elsewhere in tenth-century northern England stone was more plentiful, and some graves were marked by stones decorated in a distinctive Christian Hiberno-Norse style. Whilst most graveyards contain only one or two such graves – usually presumed to be those of the founders of the church – the presence of up to twenty such monuments in the graveyards of urban churches in Lincoln and York testify to the desire of merchants in these towns to emulate the burial of the lesser nobility in rural churches, and display their social status after death.[130] Burial itself in this period was usually marked by burial in a container, such as a coffin or sarcophagus, or at least in a grave lined with tiles or stones. Victoria Thompson has suggested that this interest in enclosing the corpse reflects a concern in homiletic and poetic texts with having a perfect body at the time of the resurrection at the Last Judgement.[131] A similar anxiety to identify the corpse at the Last Judgement perhaps underlies another odd feature of burials in this period: graves from the eleventh century have been found in both England and Germany where the corpse is buried with a lead plaque identifying the dead person by name. For example Cunigunde, the wife of the Emperor Conrad II, was buried at Speyer in the Rhineland with a plaque detailing the names of the thirteen bishops and archbishops who participated in her funeral.[132] Yet it was buried with her, and was presumably intended to be read by God rather than man. These internal and external markers suggest that the elite internalised the Church's message, and conformed to ecclesiastical authority and orthodox theology when it came to burial. They demonstrate that Christian burial mattered to the laity.

The material evidence of graves and churches suggests that in this period the widespread adoption of Christian obsequies for the dead is not a figment of churchmen's overactive imaginations but rather a reality. Fictional tales point to how their clerical authors could assume that the knowledge and practice of Christian obsequies to be universal. Liturgical and legal evidence points to churchmen's attempts to educate their clergy in the correct administration of the last rites to the laity. Stories about laymen joking about saints whilst at a wake point to the amalgamation of lay and clerical ideas, but show the success of Christianisation. There is, therefore, a body of evidence which suggests that the laity internalised and practised, to a large extent, the Christian way of death prescribed by the clergy. It is as well to remember that local churches lay at the heart of the lay experience of death.

Marriage

Knowledge of Christian prayers, the ability to act as godparents, to take part in communion, and to receive a Christian burial are all the outward signs which in Archbishop Wulfstan's eyes, at least, defined a Christian. Unlike marriage, they are universal. For marriage is not universal but rather reserved only to the laity; it is the ability to marry which distinguished them from the clergy. The English monk Ælfric contrasted the classes of clerics and laymen thus:

> *Chastity is befitting to every man, most of all to those servants of God in holy orders. The chastity of a layman is that he keep the marriage law and in the permitted manner, for the increase of people, beget children. The chastity of a man in holy orders, of those who serve God, is that they*

> *abstain entirely from fleshly desires, and it is fitting to them that they beget to God the children which laymen have begotten to this world.*[133]

Marriage defined the laity, and whilst St Paul famously wrote 'it is better to marry than to burn' (I Corinthians 7.9), many Christian writers held a much more positive view of the institution, as Ælfric demonstrates. A century and a half after he wrote, the author of the earliest life of the reformer Norbert of Xanten (d. 1134) recorded how Norbert had encouraged Count Theobald of Champagne and Blois (d. 1152), whom he described as a generous patron of the Church and protector of the poor, 'to continue the good work and beget an heir through marriage'.[134] Procreation through marriage, as long as husband and wife adhered to the prohibitions on sexual relations outlined in ecclesiastical law, constituted one way in which Christians could demonstrate their adherence to God's law, just as clerics following the rule was another. In Ælfric's words:

> *If the men in holy orders keep God's services at the established times and live purely, and if laymen live according to what is proper, then we may know as a certainty that God will be willing to provide for our prosperity and peace among us, and in addition to that to give us everlasting joy with him.*[135]

Many churchmen clearly shared Ælfric's positive view of marriage.

It is therefore all the more remarkable, especially when compared with the evidence for rites for initiation into and exit from life how little involvement the clergy sought in the life-changing rite of marriage. Although canon lawyers, and their subsequent historians, paid a good deal of attention to the law and rites of marriage, they never came wholly under ecclesiastical jurisdiction in the Middle Ages. Marriage thus represents an interesting case for investigating the influence of the Church on lay life. Interesting, not so much because it remained resistant to ecclesiastical influence, but rather because it is possible to catch glimpses in the evidence which suggest that the drive to involve the clergy in the marriage ceremony and the law of marriage came from the laity themselves as much as the clergy. The increased Christianisation of marriage in this period is, it will be suggested, testament to the Church's pastoral success and confirmation of it.

This argument contradicts that of Georges Duby who famously argued for the existence of two models of marriage at this time: a secular model, which allowed marriage to close relations and easy divorce, and a clerical model which emphasised its indissolubility and prohibited marriage to close relatives.[136] The secular aristocratic model was driven by the need for legitimate heirs, which prioritized monogamy, but which also rendered divorce necessary if the marriage was not successful in this respect. In the clergy's eyes worldly marriage mirrored Christ's union with the Church and was thus indissoluble.[137] Duby's theory oversimplifies a much messier reality. Marriage practice varied considerably between different areas of Europe, and between different classes. Churchmen were sometimes even willing to condone divorce.[138]

Churchmen were not wholly clear as to what constituted a valid marriage, making it a much debated question by canon lawyers. Unlike baptism which, for most Christians, had become a single rite by the tenth century, marriage was regarded as the result of a nuptial process made up of several secular as well as ecclesiastical rites. It never constituted a sacerdotal monopoly. One influential text, included in the late ninth-century Frankish Pseudo-Isodorean Decretals, set out the five stages for making a marriage, which might extend over several years.[139] The prospective bridegroom should seek the hand of his prospective wife from the head of her family or guardian (the first stage, petition). If permission is granted, a formal betrothal follows, which is marked by the legal grant of a dower by the groom to the bride, to provide for her if widowed (the second stage, dotation and betrothal). These initial stages might take place some time, even years, before the actual marriage, and would be invoked in situations where one or both principals was too young to marry, but their families wanted to use their prospective marriage to mark an alliance. When the time came for them to marry the priest would bless the bride, and then the groom would ask for her and she would be given to him by her family in a public ceremony which might be accompanied by prayers (the third and fourth stages, the blessing and the handing over). The couple were, in imitation of the Old Testament couple, Tobias and Sarah, to stay continent for two or three nights, devoting themselves to prayer, before consummating their marriage (the fifth and final stage). In this account the role of the priest is confined only to stages three and four. The initial stages – petition, betrothal and endowment – remained secular, familial and essentially private, as did the fifth; the priest's blessing helped to sanctify the public aspects of the rite, but did not in and of itself make the marriage.

The stages prescribed in Pseudo-Isidore are echoed in eleventh-century legal texts from England and Italy.[140] An Old English treatise on marriage, composed in *c.*1000, set out three steps for making a valid marriage: the marriage having been arranged between a man and the woman and her family, the prospective bridegroom should publicly declare 'according to God and proper secular custom' his desire to marry and support her. This vow is followed by arrangements for gifts to be made to the bride's family to compensate for her upbringing, and endowment to support her when widowed; the couple are then publicly betrothed. The marriage proper followed when 'there should by rights be a priest who shall unite them together with God's blessing in all prosperity'.[141] Private inter-familial negotiations are to be followed by public petition, an exchange of gifts to signify betrothal, and a sacerdotal blessing at the marriage itself. The late eleventh-century Italian supporter of Pope Gregory VII, Bonizo of Sutri, followed Pseudo-Isidore more exactly but specified at the outset that the prospective bride and groom must give consent, followed by the betrothal, endowment, blessing, handing over, and consummation.[142] The family's consent, betrothal and dowry are as important as the priest's blessing. Churchmen never regarded the priest's blessing as essential to a valid marriage: they recognised the validity of second marriages but forbade priests from blessing them because they offended the idea of spiritual indissolubility. In the words of Ælfric's *First Old English Letter for Bishop Wulfstan*:

> *The layman may marry a second time, and a young widow may again take a husband, but yet no one may give them a blessing unless she is a maiden but rather they must do penance for their incontinence.*[143]

Sacerdotal involvement is not, therefore, necessary to make a valid marriage.

The law remained firm on this issue, but nevertheless the years 900 to 1200 witnessed an increasing emphasis on ecclesiastical involvement in the marital process. The betrothal and endowment remained secular occasions which might take place some years before the marriage itself. That families routinely chose the marriage partners for their children is clear from Drogo of Saint Winnoc's late eleventh-century *Life* of St Godelieve of Gistel (d. *c.*1070) which describes how:

> *she was sought by many men, mighty as she in honourable morals, so gentle and humble, sweet in her actions and affable in prudent*

> *conversation. Among others who sought the hand of so outstanding a young woman was one called Bertolf. He was a powerful man, exalted in birth and wealth. The dowry he offered made him much more pleasing to Godelieve's parents than the other noble suitors, and the girl was promised in legal marriage to him.*[144]

In the tenth and eleventh centuries the marriage, although marked by both secular and religious rites, remained a primarily domestic occasion. Some books from the tenth and eleventh centuries included texts for blessing the couple, the bedchamber, the bed, and the ring, suggesting a domestic setting for the ceremony itself.[145] Such rites suggest that noble families invited priests into their homes, requesting blessing on the elements which they regarded as important to the conclusion of the process: the rings, which marked the exchange of gifts, the bed and bedchamber which signified consummation of the marriage. But other liturgical collections made provision for a Mass for the marriage, implying a church setting for the ceremony. During this period it seems that churchmen increasingly sought to make them more religious occasions. The raucous nature of the celebrations bothered them. Church law collections prohibited priests from attending weddings, and enjoined priests to avoid the love songs, jokes and lewd gestures common at such events. They also prohibited the laity from dancing at weddings.[146] At the same time, liturgical books begin to record more elaborate rites for the sacerdotal blessing of marriage ceremonies, combining the domestic blessings with the Mass. It is not until the late eleventh or early twelfth century that the location of the nuptial liturgy definitively shifted to a church setting. The early twelfth-century rite composed at Bury St Edmunds but used at Laon in northern France soon afterwards begins at the church door, the ring is blessed with prayers which refer to both partners and,

> *After this blessing has been said the man is asked by the priest if he wishes to have her as his lawful wife. The same question is asked of the woman.*

The man then gives gifts to the woman, and the priest, receiving the woman from the person who gives her away, hands her over to the man, they join hands, and the ring is given and placed on the thumb, index and middle finger, and the bridegroom says, in a new innovation:

> *With this ring I thee wed, this gold and silver I give thee, with my body I thee honour, with this dowry, I thee endow.*

The bride falls to her knees before her new husband as a sign of obedience. The bride and groom then enter the church, where a mass is held, before returning home for the blessing of the bedchamber and the holy couple.[147] By holding the ceremony in public before the church door the rite turns what had been a largely domestic, family arrangement into a public ecclesiastical one. It also prioritises the importance of both parties publicly expressing their consent. Yet this aspect of the rite is not wholly new. In the early eleventh century Burchard of Worms had insisted on the public nature of marriage and imposed a penance on anyone who took a wife without endowing her, or without receiving the priest's blessing.[148] It is clear that over time the priest came to play a greater role in the marriage ceremony, but their presence in the house itself suggests that this may have come about as much because of the family's wish for a sacerdotal blessing as for the Church's desire to regulate marriage.[149]

Charters offer a fresh perspective on the complex relationship between the clergy and laity. Families often recorded the groom's agreement to give a dowry to his betrothed in a charter. One exemplum preserved in a formulary collection from the southern German monastery of St Gall shows how transactions required the consent of both families:

> *I in God's name N. whose father is by name N. and whose mother is by name N. have, as many persons already know, willed legally to betroth to myself a certain woman by name N., whose father was by name N. and mother by name N. with the consent of our parents and kinsfolk, and I am resolved, God willing, to come to the day of our marriage. And I cede to her on the day of our marriage, once the kiss has taken place, and the ring has been put on, some things from my estate which are as follow . . .*[150]

Such Frankish charters composed between the ninth and twelfth centuries often have lengthy, quasi-liturgical preambles full of biblical language, reminding the audience how marriage is sacred, created by God as a proper means of procreation. In the later Middle Ages, sermons on marriage served to promote the clergy's views about the indissolubility of marriage to the laity.[151] Here the laity's desire to record the transaction offered an opportunity for clerical instruction to the audience of elite families.[152] But practice in this regard varied considerably throughout Europe: similar documents produced in this period in England and southern France are resolutely secular, even when recording the marriage of the sister of a bishop.[153] It is therefore difficult to use such evidence for a resolutely lay-oriented view of marriage; here the lay elite's desire to document dotation became combined with the clerical wish to instruct.

Such cases are confined to the noble elite. It is highly unlikely that the vast majority of lay Christians were formally married along these lines. Evidence from the later Middle Ages suggests that the vast majority of marriages were informal. Nevertheless, there are some hints that churchmen expected marital issues to be a real problem within local communities, as indeed the evidence of church courts suggests they were in the later Middle Ages, and that they were anxious to ensure that such cases were properly regulated. Regino expected formal marriage to be sufficiently widespread that he instructed the bishop and his officers when making a visitation to check that all cases where the marriage had been dissolved had episcopal approval. The bishop should ask a lay jury when conducting a visitation:

> *If any man has abandoned his wife, although (she) is unchaste, without the judgement of the bishop.*[154]

Similar questions were asked three hundred years later in northern Italy of the actual jury of one *pieve* in a case which was really concerned to establish who had authority over a particular church, when they were asked whether it was the bishop or the abbot who had dealt with marital cases.[155] Such cases fit with the more general concern – testified to by the Frankish charters' preambles – with promoting the indissolubility of marriage.

The compilers of penitentials and church law collections seem more concerned to regulate sexual relationships than marriage. They are pre-occupied with outlawing fornication, punishing relationships between unmarried people and adulterers.[156] They similarly prohibited marriage between those related through spiritual affinity: godparents could not marry godchildren, or the parents of their own godchildren. They forbade incest, but the number of degrees of relationship outside which relationships were allowed, which varied from four to seven, and the way in which those degrees were calculated, varied between areas, and across the period.[157] In any case, pious men and women seem to have been happy to ignore the Church's teachings on the subject. The Saxon noblewoman Godila, for example, is portrayed as a pious widow by her nephew. He describes her as someone who 'constantly performed as many good deeds as she could but, how, after four years of widowhood, in 1007,

> *[she] married her relative Herman [Count of Werl] doing this without regard for the ban imposed by Bishop Arnulf and heedless of a promise to three bishops who forbade this in the name of God. Because of this the bishop struck her with the sword of excommunication, and thereafter she was denied any hope of future offspring.*

She did not, however, separate from her husband.[158] Nor is she unusual. Noblemen and women in both England and east Frankia often appealed to Rome against such prohibitions, to the chagrin of local officials to the extent that bishops and church councils are recorded as forbidding such petitions.[159] Archbishop Dunstan of Canterbury, for example, is recorded as excommunicating a noble for an illicit marriage, whereupon the nobleman appealed to Rome successfully, but Dunstan refused to have the anathema lifted.[160] To this extent, despite the lay desires for sacerdotal nuptial blessings, marriage remained a much more secular rite than those for baptism, penance and the dying.

Marriage has some parallels with baptism. Both rites are subject to existing secular ties and ambitions. Elite families recognised and established alliances with other groups both through invitations to become godparents to their children and by arranging marriage alliances. But unlike the rite for baptism, marriage remained throughout this period much more independent of ecclesiastical control, partly at least because of the clergy's own ambivalence about their role rather than because of lay resistance to their authority. That elite families sought priestly blessing on the marriage reflects the internalisation of Christian values: they wished such an important, life-changing event, to be protected and recognised. These changes thus reflect the success of the delivery of pastoral care to the elite in this period. But such success is perverse, for the majority of marriages continued to take place without reference to the Church. To that extent this life-changing ritual remained resolutely secular.

Conclusions

From the cradle to the grave, therefore, churchmen expected the laity to mark the stages of their lives through its pastoral rites. The fact that we lack any very clear articulation of the minimum standard of Christian practice expected of the laity reflects the optimism of churchmen in this period: they simply felt no need to produce such a statement in a world in which everyone was Christian. At the same time, as we have seen, members of the higher clergy across Europe in Lotharingia and the Rhineland, England, and northern and central Italy, made an enormous effort to educate local priests, and through them the laity, in the basic tenets of the faith. To do so they used and built on the helpful and full body of materials which they had inherited from their Carolingian predecessors. These laid out very clearly what they expected of the laity but, far from mindlessly copying them, churchmen in our period adapted them and improved on them in various ways in order to deliver pastoral care to their flocks. Their efforts thus paralleled the erection of local churches throughout the countryside which was going on at the same time. Churchmen demonstrated their interest in using these churches to deliver pastoral care not only through legislation but though education, and liturgical books from eleventh-century Italy and England testify to the attempts made by senior clerics to train local priests in the correct delivery of pastoral rites. The evidence of penitentials and canon law collections suggests that bishops in England, Germany and Italy made a similar effort in this field. Taken together they are testament to a series of interlocking efforts made by bishops across Europe to ensure that the newly erected local churches became centres for pastoral care and piety within their community.

The evidence of the churches themselves, with their stone fonts, bounded cemeteries and graves, all serve as tangible evidence for the success of this endeavour. Christians in small local settlements across Europe were baptised and buried in them. At the same time, we need to acknowledge that the written evidence for pastoral care becoming more widespread in this period is patchy and sporadic. Whilst some texts circulated widely, such as Ælfric's vernacular sermons within England and Burchard's *Decretum* across all of Europe, the distribution of others is much more limited. It is also worth acknowledging the limits of ecclesiastical authority: in the arena of marriage, for example, the nobility of Europe remained resistant to ecclesiastical regulation, yet demanded sacerdotal blessing, whilst lesser orders probably eschewed ecclesiastical marriage altogether. In those for entry and exit from life, and even that for confession, the laity appear to have been much more willing to accept and adapt their own lives to ecclesiastical demands. And although the Christian year came to dominate much of lay life it also had to adjust itself to the demands of the agricultural year.

When he translated Theodulf's *Statutes* for his English clergy, Archbishop Wulfstan wore rose-tinted spectacles. He wrote in an uncertain and unstable world, as England came under repeated attack and then invasion from Scandinavia. His demand that adults know the Our Father and the Creed so that they could be active participants in their own salvation is a product of these times: 'how then can every man pray inwardly to God unless he has true faith in God?' In a world which attributed disasters to divine providence, it behoved all the people to renew their faith. Yet, as we have seen, lay Christians were far from passive recipients of pastoral care. Instead their concerns and interested helped shape the way in which churchmen chose to deliver pastoral rites, and in doing so shaped the way that the delivery of pastoral care, centred on the local church, developed in this period.

Notes and references

1 *C&S* I, 322.

2 E. Duffy, *The Stripping of the Altars: Traditional Religion in England 1400–1580* (New Haven, CT and London, 1992); K. L. French, G. Gibbs and B. Kümin, eds, *The Parish in English Life 1400–1600* (Manchester, 1997); K. L. French, *The People of the Parish: Community Life in a Late Medieval English Diocese* (Philadelphia, 2001); E. FitzPatrick and R. Gillespie, eds, *The Parish in Medieval and Early Modern Ireland: Community, Territory, and Building* (Dublin, 2006).

3 For a summary of this material, see the survey by A. Walsham, *The Reformation of the Landscape: Religion, Identity and Memory in Early Modern Britain and Ireland* (Oxford, 2011), 18–79.

4 'The Christian Middle Ages', *American Historical Review* 91 (1986), 519–52 at p. 543.

5 R. Gem, 'The English Parish Church in the Eleventh and Early Twelfth Centuries: A Great Rebuilding?', in J. Blair, ed., *Minsters and Parish Churches: The Local Church in Transition 950–1200* (Oxford, 1988), 21–30; R. Morris, *Churches in the Landscape* (London, 1989).

6 A. Boddington, *Raunds Furnell: The Anglo-Saxon Church and Churchyard* (London, 1996), 22–25, 66.

7 Ælfric, 'Pastoral Letter for Wulfsige III', *C&S*, I, 217–18.

8 Blair, *Church*, 458–59.

9 E.g. Regino, II, 5, q. 88, 250. Cf. 'Canons of Edgar', c. 26, C&S, I, 323.

10 Blair, *Church*, 457.

11 See also the arguments by C. Davidson Cragoe, 'The Custom of the Church: Parish Church Maintenance in England Before 1300', *Journal of Medieval History* 30 (2010), 20–38.

12 E.g. the Fulda Sacramentary depicts the scrutiny for baptism with women and girls on the right, men and boys on the left: *Sacramentarium Fuldense saeculi X. Cod. Theol. 231 der K. Universitätsbibliothek Zu Göttingen*, ed. G. Richter and A. Schönfelder, repr. Henry Bradshaw Society 101 (London, 1972–1977), pl. 42; e.g. illustrations of infant baptism in south Italian Exultet Rolls show men and boys as separate from women and girls: M. Avery, *The Exultet Rolls of South Italy*, 2 vols (Princeton, NJ, 1936), pl. CXVI, CXVII.

13 M. McC. Gatch, 'Miracles in Architectural Settings: Christ Church, Canterbury and St Clement's, Sandwich in the Old English Vision of Leofric', *Anglo-Saxon England* 22 (1993), 227–52; Blair, *Church*, 457.

14 M. Lapidge, 'Surviving Booklists from Anglo-Saxon England', in idem and H. Gneuss, eds, *Learning and Literature in Anglo-Saxon England: Studies Presented to Peter Clemoes on the Occasion of his Sixty-Fifth Birthday* (Cambridge, 1985), 33–89, no. VI.

15 Regino II.5.57, 246.

16 E.g. I Cnut 14–16, *C&S*, I, 478–79.

17 E.g. dietary specification in Burchard, *Decretum*, XIX.9, *PL* 140, 980–81 but also found in earlier sources.

18 Regino, II.5.49, 246.

19 R. Meens, 'The Frequency and Nature of Early Medieval Penance', in P. Biller and A. J. Minnis, eds, *Handling Sin: Confession in the Middle Ages* (Woodbridge, 1998), 35–61 at p. 38; J. Avril, 'Remarques sur un aspect de la vie paroissale: La pratique de la confession et de la communion du Xe au XIVe siècle', in *L'Encadrement religieux des fidèles au Moyen Age*, 345–63.

20 Goscelin of Saint-Bertin, *The Miracles of St Æthelthryth the Virgin*, c. 7, in Goscelin of Saint-Bertin, *The Hagiography of the Female Saints of Ely*, ed. R. C. Love (Oxford, 2004), 119.

21 *Miracula S. Swithuni*, c. 46, in M. Lapidge *et al.*, *The Cult of St Swithun* (Oxford, 2003), 680–82.

22 S. Yarrow, *Saints and Their Communities: Miracle Stories in Twelfth Century England* (Oxford, 2005), 199.

23 M. Bull, *The Miracles of Our Lady of Rocamadour: Analysis and Translation* (Woodbridge, 1999), III. 19, 194–95.

24 E.g. Northumbrian Priests' Law (c. 1008X23) directs that any priest who misdirected his flock as to when feasts should be held should be fined, c. 11, *C&S*, I, 455.

25 *Admonitio Synodalis*, cc. 96–97, 68.

26 Berner US, *De Translationis Corporis S. Hunegundis Virginis Apud Viromanduos*, c. 14, *PL* 137, 70–71.

27 Æthelred V c. 14.1, *C&S*, I, 353. The feast day of SS Philip and James (1st May) would have fallen within the fifteen days after Easter in 1009, 1014, 1017, and 1020; ibid. n. 2.

28 Burchard, II.77, *PL* 140, 640. This list circulated widely in the later Middle Ages as it entered Gratian's *Decretum*, III *De consecratione,* D. 3. C. 1, http://geschichte.digitale-sammlungen.de/decretum-gratiani/kapitel/dc_chapter_3_3941 (accesssed 29 December 2011).

29 Cf. Haito von Basel, *Capitula*, *MGH Capitula Episcoporum I*, ed. P. Brommer (Hannover, 1984), 212. Haito's text emphasised that a bishop should order the celebration of the saint to whom his own church was dedicated: 'dedicatio cuiuscumque oratorii seu cuiuslibet sancti, in cuius honore eadem ecclesia fundata est, quod vicinis tantum circum commorantibus indicendum est, non generaliter omnibus'. This makes more sense than Burchard's text: 'Dedicatio cuiuscunque oratorii et omnium sanctorum'. Burchard also added the feast of the Nativity of Mary to Haito's list.

30 V Æthelred c. 12.2–18,; I Cnut, 14–17, both *C&S* I, 352–54, 478–79; Gratian, *Decretum*, III D.3, de cons. C.I (http://geschichte.digitale-sammlungen.de/decretum-gratiani/kapitel/dc_chapter_3_3941; accessed 21 January 2011).

31 N. M. Thompson, 'The Carolingian *De Festiuitatibus* and the Blickling Book', in A. J. Kleist, ed., *The Old English Homily: Precedent, Practice and Appropriation* (Turnhout, 2007), 97–119.

32 J. McCune, 'Rethinking the Pseudo-Eligius Sermon Collection', *Early Medieval Europe* 16 (2008), 445–76 at p. 458. That of Bishop Herbert de Losinga of Norwich (d. 1119) was also written for a mixed audience: *The Life, Letters and Sermons of Bishop Herbert de Losinga*, ed. E. M. Goulburn and H. Symonds, 2 vols (Oxford, 1878).

33 J. Wilcox, 'Æfric in Dorset and the Landscape of Pastoral Care', in F. Tinti, ed., *Pastoral Care in Late Anglo-Saxon England* (Woodbridge, 2005), 52–62 at p. 61.

34 *Ælfric's Catholic Homilies: The First Series*, ed. P. Clemoes, EETS SS 17 (Oxford, 1997); *Ælfric's Catholic Homilies: The Second Series*, ed. M. Godden, EETS SS 5 (Oxford, 1979); M. Godden, *Ælfric's Catholic Homilies: Introduction, Commentary and Glossary*, EETS SS 18 (Oxford, 2000). All translations are from *The Homilies of the Anglo-Saxon Church. The First Part, containing the Sermones Catholici or Homilies of Ælfric in the Original Anglo-Saxon with an English Version*, 2 vols, ed. and trans. B. Thorpe (London, 1844; repr. 1971) unless otherwise stated.

35 Preface, *Catholic Homilies II*, trans. Thorpe, 2–3.

36 Wilcox, 'Æfric in Dorset'.

37 Godden, *Ælfric's Catholic Homilies: Introduction.*

38 Cited by Wilcox 'Ælfric in Dorset', 54.

39 McCune, 'Rethinking', 454.

40 *Ælfric's Catholic Homilies I*, ed. Clemoes, 76–77; trans. Thorpe, 150–51.

41 M. B. Bedingfield, *The Dramatic Liturgy of Anglo-Saxon England* (Woodbridge, 2002), 50–72.

42 Cambridge, Corpus Christi College, Ms 422, pp. 285–88.

43 *Ælfric's Catholic Homilies I*, trans. Thorpe, I, 164–65.

44 *Ælfric's Catholic Homilies I*, trans. Thorpe, I, 178–81.

45 London, British Library, Ms Additional 28188, ff. 89v–98v: 'On Palm Sunday when the sacrament of the mass has been completed the clergy and the people should proceed to that church where branches of palms and other trees have been collected for consecration' trans. Bedingfield, *Dramatic Liturgy*, 99 n. 21.

46 Fehr, *Die Hirtenbriefe Ælfrics*, 216, cited by Bedingfield, *Dramatic Liturgy*, 97 n. 14.

47 McCune, 'Rethinking', 465.

48 *Catholic Homilies II*, trans. Thorpe, II, 262–63

49 *Catholic Homilies I*, trans. Thorpe, I, 244–45.

50 Ibid. I, 244–95; *Catholic Homilies II*, trans. Thorpe, 315–49, 261–71.

51 Blair, *Church*, 486.

52 Godden, *Ælfric's Catholic Homilies: Introduction*, xxvii.

53 E.g. Regino, I.304, 164, II.51, 246; D. Harmening, *Superstitio. Überlieferungs-und theoriegeschichtliche Untersuchungen zur kirchlich-theologischen Aberglaubensliteratur des Mittelalters* (Berlin, 1979), 135.

54 Burchard, XIX.5, *PL* 140, 960.

55 J. D. Niles, 'The Æcerbot Ritual in Context', in J. D. Niles, ed., *Old English Literature in Context* (Cambridge, 1980), 44–56; K. Jolly, *Popular Religion in Late Anglo-Saxon England: Elf Charms in Context* (Chapel Hill, NC, 1996), 8–9.

56 Blair, *Church*, 486.

57 F. Tinti, 'The "Costs" of Pastoral Care: Church Dues in Late Anglo-Saxon England', in F. Tinti, ed., *Pastoral Care in Late Anglo-Saxon England* (Woodbridge, 2005), 27–51.

58 'Canons of Edgar', c. 54, *C&S* I, 331–32.

59 Blair, *Church*, 441, 444.

60 Tinti, 'The "Costs" of Pastoral Care', 39–40.

61 Thomas N. Hall, 'Wulfstan's Latin Sermons', in M. Townend, ed., *Wulfstan, Archbishop of York: The Proceedings of the Second Alcuin Conference* (Turnhout, 2004), 94–139, at p. 117.

62 Hall, 'Wulfstan's Latin Sermons', 118.

63 The Blickling Homily for the Third Sunday in Lent also emphasised the importance of the payment of tithes and how they financed both the Church and alms for the poor: *The Blickling Homilies*, ed. and trans. R. J. Kelly (London, 2003), 26–36.

64 *Catholic Homilies II*, ed. Godden, i. 6; translated and cited by Bedingfield, *Dramatic Liturgy*, 189; see also Thorpe, *Catholic Homilies*, II, 13.

65 See also Sermo de Baptismate, VIIIc, in *The Homilies of Wulfstan*, ed. D. Bethurum (Oxford, 1957), 175–84; Hall, 'Wulfstan's Latin Sermons', 96–97; T. A. Cooper, 'The Homilies of a Pragmatic Archbishop's Handbook in Context: Cotton Tiberius A.iii', *Anglo-Norman Studies* 28 (2006), 47–64.

66 *Sacramentarium Fuldense saeculi X. Cod. Theol. 231 der K. Universitätsbibliothek zu Göttingen*, ed. G. Richter and A. Schönfelder, repr. Henry Bradshaw Society 101 (London, 1972–77), pl. 42 (f. 214a).

67 M. Avery, *The Exultet Rolls of South Italy*, 2 vols (Princeton, NJ, 1936), pl. CXVI, 13, pl. CXCVII.

68 XCIX. 337, ibid., II, 93.

69 *Ordo* CVII, *PRG*, 155–72.

70 'The So-called "Canons of Edgar"', c. 15, *C&S*, I, 319 (7 days); 'The Northumbrian Priests' Law', c. 10.1, ibid. 455 (9 days). See also Regino, I. 130, 132, pp. 92–94.

71 Regino, II. 5. 4, II. 60, pp. 238, 280.

72 Paenitential Parisiense compositum (N. France), s. xi, in A. Gaastra, 'Between Liturgy and Canon Law: A Study of Books of Confession and

Penance in Eleventh- and Twelfth-century Italy', (Ph.D. thesis, University of Utrecht, 2007), n. 642. On the details of the practice, see Ælfric's letter to Archbishop Wulfstan, *C&S*, I, 250.

73 Cited by Cramer, *Baptism and Change*, p. 140.

74 Cambridge, Corpus Christi College, Ms 422, pp. 367–94 (digital images are available at the Parker Library on the Web: http://parkerweb.stanford.edu/parker/actions/page.do?forward=home). On the vernacular rubrics, see R. I. Page, 'Old English Liturgical Rubrics in Corpus Christi College, Cambridge MS 422', *Anglia* 96 (1978), 149–58; T. Graham, 'The Old English Liturgical Directions in Corpus Christi College, Cambridge MS 422', *Anglia* 111 (1993), 439–46.

75 H. Gittos, 'Is there any Evidence for the Liturgy of Parish Churches in Late Anglo-Saxon England? The Red Book of Darley and the Status of Old English', in F. Tinti, ed., *Pastoral Care in Late Anglo-Saxon England* (Woodbridge, 2005), 63–82.

76 R. Morris, 'Baptismal Places 600–800', in I. Wood and N. Lund, eds, *People and Places in Northern Europe 500–1600: Essays in Honour of Peter Hayes Sawyer* (Woodbridge, 1991), 16.

77 C. S. Drake, *The Romanesque Fonts of Northern Europe and Scandinavia* (Woodbridge, 2001).

78 Miller, *The Formation of a Medieval Church*, 138.

79 Ibid., 136.

80 Arnulf of Milan, *Liber gestorum recentium*, ed. C. Zey, MGH SRG 67 (Hannover, 1994) IV.5, 6, 209–11.

81 M. Avery, *The Exultet Rolls of South Italy*, 2 vols (Princeton, NJ, 1936), pl. CXCVII.

82 Regino, *Libri duo*, I.275, 144. J. H. Lynch, *Godparents and Kinship in Early Medieval Europe* (Princeton, NJ, 1986), 329–332.

83 *Catholic Homilies*, ed. Thorpe, II, 596–99; 'Canons of Edgar', c. 22, *C&S, I*, 322.

84 I. S. Robinson, *Henry IV of Germany 1056–1106* (Cambridge, 1999), 158–59.

85 S. Hamilton, 'Otto III's Penance: A Case Study of Unity and Diversity in the Eleventh-century Church', in R. N. Swanson, *Unity and Diversity in the Church*, Studies in Church History 32 (Oxford, 1996), 83–94.

86 Cited by J. H. Lynch, 'Baptismal Sponsorship and Monks and Nuns, 500–1000', *American Benedictine Review* 31 (1980), 108–29 at p. 128.

87 C. Blanc, 'Les pratiques de piété des laïcs dans les pays du Bas-Rhône aux XIe et XIIe siècles', *Annales du Midi* 72 (1960), 137–47, at p. 137.

88 P. Hull and R. Sharpe, 'Peter of Cornwall and Launceston', *Cornish Studies* 13 (1986), p. 27.

89 C. Vogel, 'Pratiques superstiteuses au début du XI siècle d'après le *Corrector sive medicus* de Burchard, évêque de Worms (965–1025)', in idem, *En remission des péchés. Recherches sur les systèmes pénitentiels dans l'Eglise latine* (Aldershot, 1994), X.

90 Burchard, XIX.v, *PL* 140, 974–75.

91 Burchard, XIX.v, *PL* 140, 975.

92 S. Crawford, *Childhood in Anglo-Saxon England* (Stroud, 1999), 75–91.

93 S. Hamilton, *The Practice of Penance, 900–1050* (Woodbridge, 2001), 2.

94 Regino, *Libri duo*, I.292, 152.

95 Theodulf, *Capitula I*, cc. 36–41, 133–39.

96 Hamilton, *Practice*, 68–70.

97 *PL* 140, XIX.2, 949.

98 Ekkehard IV, *Casus s. Galli*, c. 30, ed. H. Haefele (Darmstadt, 1980), 70–72; M. de Jong, 'Pollution, Penance and Sanctity: Ekkehard's *Life* of Iso of St Gall', in J. Hill and M. Swan, eds, *The Community, the Family and the Saint: Patterns of Power in Early Medieval Europe* (Turnhout, 1998), 145–58.

99 Hamilton, *Practice*, 44; Meens, 'Frequency'.

100 *PL* 140, XIX. 5, 951.

101 Ibid., 961.

102 Regino I, 304, II.v, q. 52, II, 374, pp. 160, 246, 424.

103 A. H. Gaastra, 'Between Liturgy and Canon Law: A Study of Books of Confession and Penance in Eleventh- and Twelfth-century Italy' (Ph.D. thesis, University of Utrecht, 2007); L. Körntgen, 'Canon Law and the Practice of Penance: Burchard of Worms' Penitential', *Early Medieval Europe* 14 (2006), 103–17.

104 Vogel, 'Pratiques superstitieuses'.

105 F. Kerff, 'Libri paenitentiales und kirchliche Strafgerichtsbarkeit bis zum Decretum Gratiani. Ein Diskussionsvorschlag', *Zeitschrift der Savigny-Stiftung für Rechtsgeschichte. Kanonistische Abteilung* 75 (1989), 23–57; R. Kottje, 'Busse oder Strafe? Zur "Iustitia" in den "Libri Paenitentiales"', in *La Giustizia nell'alto medioevo (secoli V–VIII)*, Settimane 42 (Spoleto,

1995), 443–474; R. Meens, 'Penitentials and the Practice of Penance in the Tenth and Eleventh Centuries', *Early Medieval Europe* 14 (2006), 7–21.

106 Hamilton, *Practice*, 31; Körntgen, 'Canon Law'.

107 Meens, 'Frequency'.

108 S. Hamilton, 'Pastoral Care in Early Eleventh-century Rome', *Dutch Review of Church History* 84 (2004), 37–56; V. Thompson, *Dying and Death in Later Anglo-Saxon England* (Woodbridge, 2004), 57–91; eadem, 'The Pastoral Contract in Late Anglo-Saxon England: Priest and Parishioner in Oxford, Bodleian Library, MS Laud Miscellaneous 482', in F. Tinti, ed., *Pastoral Care in Late Anglo-Saxon England* (Woodbridge, 2005), 106–20.

109 S. Hamilton, 'Doing Penance', in M. Rubin, ed., *Medieval Christianity in Practice* (Princeton, NJ, 2009), 135–43.

110 Hamilton, *Practice*, 7.

111 Thietmar, *Chronicon*, IV.liii, p. 192.

112 Ibid. VI.lxxxvi, p. 294.

113 Hamilton, *Practice*, 204.

114 E.g. *Ælfric's First Old English Letter for Wulfstan*, cc. 178–81, *C&S*, I, 295; 'So-called "Canons of Edgar"', cc. 68–9, ibid., 335, 337–38; Regino, I, Praef. q. 19, I. 117–18, 120, pp. 26–28, 86; Burchard, XVIII, *PL* 140, 933–44.

115 V Æthelred, c. 12, *C&S*, I, 352.

116 E.g. that in *The Pontifical of Magdalen College*, ed. H. A. Wilson, Henry Bradshaw Society 39 (London, 1910), 93–100; on this rite see S. Hamilton, 'Rites of Passage and Pastoral Care', in J. Crick and E. van Houts, *A Social History of England* (Cambridge, 2011), 290–308.

117 F. S. Paxton, *Christianizing Death: The Creation of a Ritual Process in Early Medieval Europe* (Ithaca, NY, 1990).

118 Gittos, 'Is There Any Evidence', 74.

119 Thompson, 'The Pastoral Contract', 118.

120 Orderic Vitalis, *Historia Ecclesiastica*, 5.9, ed. M. Chibnall, 6 vols (Oxford, 1969–80), III, 192–98; L. Gougaud, *Devotional and Ascetic Practices in the Middle Ages*, trans. G. C. Bateman (London, 1927), 131–46; Bull, *Knightly Piety*, 143–46.

121 Regino, I.398, 200 trans. in *Medieval Handbooks of Penance*, trans. J. T. McNeill and H. M. Gamer (New York, 1938), 318–319.

122 Cited by Thompson, *Dying*, 83–84.

123 Bullough, 'Carolingian Liturgical Experience', 56–57 citing *MGH SS* VIII, 231–32.

124 Thompson, *Dying*, 73.

125 *Waltharius and Ruodlieb*, ed. and trans. D. M. Katz (New York, 1984), 147.

126 *The Vision of Tnugdal*, ed. and trans. J. M. Picard (Dublin, 1989), 112.

127 I. Short, ed. and trans., Geffrei Gaimar, *Estoire des Engleis* (Oxford, 2009), 342–343.

128 See discussion of confraternities in Chapter 6 below.

129 D. Stocker and P. Everson, *Summoning St Michael: Early Romanesque Towers in Lincolnshire* (Oxford, 2006), 79–92.

130 D. Stocker, 'Monuments and Merchants: Irregularities in the Distribution of Stone Sculpture in Lincolnshire and Yorkshire in the Tenth Century', in D. M. Hadley and J. D. Richards, eds, *Cultures in Contact: Scandinavian Settlement in England in the Ninth and Tenth Centuries* (Turnhout, 2000), 179–212; Blair, *Church*, 468–71.

131 V. Thompson, 'Constructing Salvation: A Homiletic and Penitential Context for Late Anglo-Saxon Burial Practice', in S. Lucy and A. Reynolds, eds, *Burial in Early Medieval England and Wales* (London, 2002), 229–40.

132 Hamilton, *Practice*, 179–80; see also C. Daniell, 'Conquest, Crime and Theology in the Burial Record, 1066–1200', in Lucy and Reynolds, *Burial*, 241–54 at pp. 241–42; Bartlett, *England*, 597.

133 *Ælfric's Catholic Homilies: The Second Series*, ed. M. Godden, EETS s.s. 5 (Oxford, 1979), II. 6.136–66, cited by R. K. Upchurch, 'For Pastoral Care and Political Gain: Ælfric of Eynsham's Preaching on Marital Celibacy', *Traditio* 59 (2004), 40–78 at p. 74.

134 *Version A: Life of Norbert, Archbishop of Magdeburg*, c. 15, trans. in *Norbert and Early Norbertine Spirituality*, ed. T. J. Antry, O. Praem and C. Neel (Mahwah, NJ, 2007), 158.

135 *Ælfric's Lives of the Saints Being a Set of Sermons of Saints' Days Formerly Observed by the English Church*, ed. and trans. W. Skeat, EETS o.s. 76, 82, 94, 114 (London, 1881–1900), 13.133–38; trans. Upchurch, 'For Pastoral Care', 77.

136 G. Duby, *Medieval Marriage: Two Models from Twelfth-century France*, trans. E. Foster (Baltimore, 1978); idem, *The Knight, The Lady and the Priest: The Making of Modern Marriage in Medieval France*, trans. B. Bray (Harmondsworth, 1985).

137 D. d'Avray, *Medieval Marriage: Symbolism and Society* (Oxford, 2005).

138 M. McLaughlin, *Sex, Gender, and Episcopal Authority in an Age of Reform, 1000–1122* (Oxford, 2010), 16–49; M. Aurell, *Les noces du comte: mariage et*

pouvoir en Catalogne (785–1213) (Paris, 1995); C. Bouchard, '*"Those of My Blood": Constructing Noble Families in Medieval Francia* (Philadelphia, 2001).

139 Ps.-Evaristus, *PL* 130, 81; P. L. Reynolds, *Marriage in the Western Church: The Christianization of Marriage during the Patristic and Early Medieval Periods* (Leiden, 1994; repr. 2001), 391.

140 McLaughlin, *Sex, Gender, and Episcopal Authority*, 19–22.

141 *C&S*, I, 427–31.

142 Bonizo of Sutri, *Liber de Vita Christiana*, ed. E. Perels (Berlin, 1930; repr. Hildesheim, 1998), VIII.11, 256–57.

143 c. 156, *C&S, I*, 291.

144 Drogo of Sint-Winoksbergen, *Life of St Godelieve*, ed. M. Coens, *Analecta Bollandiana* 44 (1926), 103–37; trans. B. L. Venarde, in T. Head, ed., *Medieval Hagiography: An Anthology* (New York, 2001), 359–73 at p. 364. On this life, see Duby, *The Knight*, 130–35; R. Nip, 'Godelieve of Gistel and Ida of Boulogne', in A. Mulder-Bakker, ed., *Sanctity and Motherhood: Essays on Holy Mothers in the Middle Ages* (New York, 1995), 191–223; D. J. Defries, 'Drogo of Saint-Winnoc and the Innocent Martyrdom of Godeliph of Gistel', *Mediaeval Studies* 70 (2008), 29–65.

145 E.g. the Red Book of Darley (Cambridge, Corpus Christi College, Ms 422), pp. 276–84.

146 Burchard, X. 10, *PL* 140, col. 817; J. A. Brundage, *Law, Sex and Christian Society in Medieval Europe* (Chicago, 1987), 191.

147 K. Ritzer, *Le Mariage dans les Églises chrétiennes du Ier au XIe siècle* (Paris, 1970) (French translation of 1962 German original); K. Stevenson, *Nuptial Blessing: A Study of Christian Marriage Rites*, Alcuin Club Collections 64 (London, 1982), 68–70.

148 Burchard, IX.1, XIX.5, *PL* 140, 815, 958.

149 Ritzer, *Le Mariage*; M. M. Sheehan, 'Choice of Marriage Partner in the Middle Ages: Development and Mode of Application of a Theory of Marriage', *Studies in Medieval and Renaissance History* 1 (1978), 1–33; repr. in C. Neel, ed., *Medieval Families: Perspectives on Marriage, Household and Children* (Toronto, 2004), 157–91.

150 P. L. Reynolds, 'Dotal Charters in the Frankish Tradition', in P. L. Reynolds and J. Witte, eds, *To Have and To Hold: Marrying and its Documentation in Western Christendom, 400–1600* (Cambridge, 2007), 114–64 at p. 159 (Document 12).

151 D'Avray, *Medieval Marriage*, 73.

152 Reynolds, 'Dotal Charters'.

153 E.g. *Anglo-Saxon Charters*, ed. and trans. A. J. Robertson (Cambridge, 1939), nos 76 and 77, 149–51; R. H. Helmholz, 'Marriage Contracts in Medieval England, and C. Johnson, 'Marriage Agreements from Twelfth-century Southern France', both in Reynolds and Witte, *To Have and to Hold*, 260–86, 215–59.

154 Regino, II. 5. 21, 240.

155 'Atti della causa tre Giovanni Vescovo Bresciano e Gonterio Abate di Leno', in F. A. Zaccaria, *Dell'antichissima Badia di Leno* (Venice, 1767).

156 Brundage, *Law, Sex*, 206–07.

157 P. Corbet, *Autour de Burchard de Worms: L'Église allemande et les interdits de parenté (IXème–XIIème siècle)* (Frankfurt am Main, 2001).

158 *The Chronicon of Thietmar of Merseburg*, VI.86, 294; Corbet, *Autour de Burchard*, 146.

159 E.g. Council of Seligenstadt (1023), c. 18, *PL* 140, 1062.

160 Adelard, *Epistola Adelardi ad Elfegum Archiepiscopum de Vita Sancti Dunstani*, in *Memorials of Saint Dunstan, Archbishop of Canterbury*, ed. W. Stubbs, Rolls Series 63 (London, 1874), 67.

chapter 6

Ordinary piety: Individual and collective prayer

So when you are occupied with much business, make short prayers. In the morning hear the canonical hours properly: Matins, Prime, Terce, Sext, None, and later Vespers and Compline. Hear the hours of the Blessed Virgin every day. Many clerics are hypocrites. Monks and hermits, in order to please men, pretend to make long prayers that they might be seen by men [Matt. 6, 5]. But you, far removed from all vanity and pretence, should hold to the truth discreetly.

(Robert of Arbrissel, *Letter to Countess Ermengarde of Brittany*, c.1106 × 1109)[1]

This advice is taken from a letter written by the monastic founder and preacher Robert of Arbrissel (d. 1116) to one of the leading noble women of northern France, Countess Ermengarde of Brittany (d. 1147). In his letter Robert constructs a model for the pious life of a noble woman which owes much to the liturgical round of the clerical life but which he depicts as distinct from, and indeed, superior to that of hypocritical clerics; short prayers have as much merit as long prayers, as long as the intent is there; personal prayer is as valuable for a lay noble woman as it is for churchmen. Robert emphasizes the importance of discretion and interior piety, of praying 'from the heart, not the lips', and that giving alms, praying, and fasting should be done not for 'human praise' but rather for God.[2] He regards discretion and mercy as universal values to be practised by members of the laity as well as the religious.

As we shall see presently, there is nothing particularly novel in Robert's model of lay personal piety, but it is a picture of lay piety which is markedly different to that offered in the previous chapter. There the focus was on what Carl Watkins has described as 'the ordinary rhythms of parish religion'. As we saw, these placed the onus on *orthopraxis* rather than orthodoxy, on outward practice rather than inward thought, on ritual rather than belief. In this pastoral model the parish priest delivered pastoral care to his essentially passive flock. In the words of one early twelfth-century bishop of Limerick the laity should do as they are told by churchmen and 'carefully avoid evil, earnestly search for good and obey their pastors in everything'.[3] By participating in the religious script that the clergy devised for them to mark the passing of their lives, lay Christians thus demonstrated their inner conformity with the Church's teachings.

Yet records of expressions of personal piety proliferated in the central Middle Ages. The collective rites demanded by church law and performed in the local churches, were accompanied by individual and collective lay devotions which were independent of the requirements made by the Church of all Christians. How therefore is the parochial model's emphasis on collective, priest-orchestrated rites and actions to be reconciled with that in Robert's advice to Countess Ermengarde on personal devotion and action? Both models clearly existed at the same time, but one recommended acts of individual piety, the other participation in more passive rites of collective piety. Robert could be dismissed as offering an impractical, semi-monastic model to an aristocratic woman; yet it is one which he had clearly worked through and conceived as having a very specific lay application. Nor is it exceptional – as we shall see, Robert's recommendations resonate with other contemporary evidence for personal piety amongst the laity. Rather than view these two models as contradictory, they should be seen as in a continual dialogue with each other. Collective clerical rites – such as those for canonical hours – provided the structure for personal observances, but the impetus for lay piety came as much from the laity as the clergy. And piety, be it collective or individual, reactive or proactive, could only be adjudged by exterior actions, as we shall see.

This chapter starts by investigating churchmen's narrative accounts and the evidence of prayer books for the ways in which their clerical authors expected the laity to use existing frameworks for their own devotion. It then turns to consider the other focuses for lay piety, asking how far individual laymen and women sought responsibility for only their own salvation and how far they also prayed for that of their friends and kin. In other words, to what extent is the evidence for lay devotion assembled in this chapter a reflection of individual or collective devotion?

Devotional frameworks for personal piety

The collective rites of the Mass and the Divine Office provided the scaffolding for the practice of personal acts of devotion by members of the laity. In doing so the laity imitated the clergy, for both liturgies already served as the focus for devotion within regular communities of the time. The Divine Office – a daily cycle of seven daily services and one night office, comprised of psalms, readings, antiphons, responsories, hymns and prayers – had deep roots, originating in the early monasteries of Late Antiquity, but the roots for the custom of saying at least two Masses daily, after Prime and Vespers, go back only to the Carolingian monasteries of the ninth century.[4] Churchmen promoted rites for both the Mass and the Office as focuses for lay piety in the years 900 to 1200.

Church law required that the laity attend Mass regularly on Sundays and keep feast days. How far then was daily attendance at Mass thought desirable? There is good evidence for an appetite for displays of such assiduous piety amongst the laity in early eleventh-century Germany. Indeed this practice aroused suspicion in the minds of the German bishops who met at the council of Seligenstadt in 1023 to condemn 'certain of the laity, especially matrons' who have the custom of hearing the Gospel every day, and of hearing special masses for the Holy Trinity and St Michael for purposes of divination'. The council agreed that the masses for the Holy Trinity and St Michael should be said only at the appointed time in the church calendar, and that the laity should hear the daily masses only for the salvation of the living and the dead.[5] The recitation of daily masses for the living and the dead had become the norm in Carolingian monasticism, and this reference is thus evidence both of clerical attempts to extend this practice to the wider lay community and of concern to correct the erroneous practices which might arise as a result.

One twelfth-century northern French abbot went so far as to imagine the Mass as providing an opportunity for a count's own personal devotions. In Hermann of Tournai's account of the murder of Count Charles the

Good of Flanders on 2 March 1127, the count is reported to have ordered his chaplain to sing Mass, and whilst the Epistle was being read, and 'the count was prostrate in prayer with an open psalter so that he might read the Psalms', and at the same time giving alms to the poor, he was murdered.[6] Far from listening to the words of the Epistle, as conceived by those such as Bishop Gille of Limerick who promoted the passive obedience of the laity in collective rites, the count is portrayed as engrossed in his own recitation of the psalms at the moment of his death. Hermann can be accused of adopting this model of lay devotion for rhetorical effect: he depicts the count as making a good death, just as he shows his murderers as doubly damned by attacking a man absorbed in prayer. But in order to convince his audience Hermann could not afford to distance himself too far from reality: several prayer books and psalters made for the personal use of their lay owners survive from this period, as we shall see. Hermann's account is therefore testimony that by the mid-twelfth century nobles would be expected to read their own psalter during Mass, reciting texts routinely used in the divine office, as well as the Mass, and familiarising themselves with the daily round of liturgical prayer. Here the Mass provides a framework for personal devotion: the count's devotions run parallel to the rite administered by the clergy. As such he takes part in the Mass, but on his own terms, and Hermann approves of him for doing so.

Hermann's account suggests that Robert of Arbrissel's advice to Ermengarde is not outlandish. By the twelfth century it had become conventional for churchmen seeking to cast lay members of the nobility in a good light to portray them as reading the psalms and hearing the office. The problem for historians is that much of our evidence comes from monastic authors anxious to spread their ideals of devotion to the laity by constructing lay piety in accordance with monastic fashion. Churchmen seeking to portray particular laymen and women as devout usually described them as hearing the divine office regularly. Thus Odo of Cluny, writing in *c.*930, told how the lay nobleman Gerald of Aurillac 'whether at home or abroad . . . performed the divine office either in common or privately', and always had a Mass said after the night office when he was about to go on a journey.[7] Odo's Gerald is a layman living a monastic life in the world: he abstains from the norms of his class, refraining from marriage and from fighting, choosing instead to go into battle with his sword held backwards. Writing in the early twelfth century, William of Malmesbury described

William the Conqueror as attending Mass, vespers and matins daily, and a little later Hermann of Tournai recorded how Count Baldwin VII of Flanders (d. 1119) attended vespers so regularly that a woman who wished to bring a complaint before him that her cow had been stolen knew to find him in church then.[8] But such stories tell us that participation in the canonical hours indicates to their clerical audiences a pious lay man rather than that such practices were widespread. Indeed, other evidence suggests that such behaviour might be regarded as exceptional, rather than the norm. Byrhtferth of Ramsey reported how the father of Oda, the tenth-century archbishop of Canterbury, disapproved of his son's frequent churchgoing as a boy, but whilst he threatened him, he failed to deflect him from his chosen path.[9] The canon in one eleventh-century penitential from southern Italy went so far as to assign a penance to clerics who neglect to keep the canonical hours but enjoined that lay people 'who know them' should observe them but they need not do penance if they fail to do so.[10] The defeatist tone of this passage suggests the compiler of this text presumed such practices, however desirable, not actually to be very widespread at the time. This presumption also seems to underlie the case Pope Innocent III made for the canonisation of the former tailor, Homobonus of Cremona (d. 1197) in 1199, in which he cited the fact that Homobonus had always attended matins, and routinely frequented the Mass and the other office hours, as indicators of his sanctity, alongside his charity towards the poor.[11]

Hearing the divine office daily thus became a standard feature of clerical portraits of devout laymen in these three centuries, even if the practice itself was not widely followed. But Robert also enjoined Countess Ermengarde to hear the hours of the Virgin every day. The practice of reciting supplementary prayers to Mary throughout the day seems to have emerged only fairly recently in tenth- and eleventh-century clerical communities. In the mid-eleventh century Peter Damian (d. 1072), for example, encouraged the saying of the daily Office of the Virgin amongst both the Italian secular clergy and laity, praising its protective powers for 'whoever strives to recite these hours daily in her honour will have the mother of the Judge as his helper and advocate in his day of need'.[12] It seems to have become popular amongst the Italian nobility only later in the century: her biographer praised Countess Mathilda of Tuscany (d. 1115) because 'day and night she never stopped listening to this office [of the Virgin]'.[13] Here Robert's advice to Ermengarde can thus be seen to fit with the norms of the day.

Robert only advised Ermengarde to pray seven times daily and to hear the hours of the Virgin, but another standard feature of clerical accounts of lay piety is the all-night vigil in which the lay person prayed alone, usually in church. It is also a feature of the lives of churchmen such as Bishop Udalrich of Augsburg, and its extension by clerical writers to lay men and women tells us much about the application of the norms of clerical communities to accounts of lay piety. The night vigil is, for example, a particular feature of accounts of the piety of members of the Ottonian royal family. Both the biographers of the widowed Queen Mathilda (d. 968) described how, after her retirement to the house of canonesses at Quedlinburg in Saxony, she spent her nights in the church in selfless prayer for the pardon of sinners and eternal rest of souls, before joining the rites of the community at the start of the day.[14] Nor is this practice confined to descriptions of female piety: Bishop Thietmar of Merseburg reports that the inner conscience of Mathilda's great grandson, Otto III (d. 1002) was so burdened 'under the weight of many misdeeds' that he 'continually sought to cleanse himself through vigils, earnest prayers, and rivers of tears'.[15] Nor is it peculiar to German portraits: the pious Anglo-Saxon nobleman Leofric (d. 1057) is also described as praying silently at night in church.[16]

We thus have several accounts which project a model of clerical devotion, derived from the liturgical practices of regular communities on to their accounts of lay piety. In doing so these clerical authors constructed a model which served as a suitable framework for the devotions of the notably pious. Robert's advice to Ermengarde hints at how this model might be translated into actual practice for some, but the manuscript evidence of prayer books and psalters provides more tangible evidence how this clerical model impacted directly on royal and noble devotions.

Prayer books and psalters

Hermann of Tournai's account of the death of Count Charles the Good suggests that twelfth-century lay nobles could be expected to own and read psalters, and there is a good deal of documentary evidence from across the period for ownership of both psalters and books of private prayer by members of the nobility. For example, the fact that the Carolingian magnate, Eberhard, margrave of Friuli and his wife Gisela bequeathed a psalter to each of their children in their will of 867 suggests its importance to lay devotion in the ninth century.[17] In the twelfth century, Earl Robert and Countess Amice of Leicester left their personal psalters to the house of Augustinian canons they founded in Leicester.[18] Furthermore, the physical testimony of the prayer books made for lay magnates which survive confirms that they were intended not for the use of their chaplains but rather to support these particular men and women in their own devotions.

Those which survive have a predominantly royal provenance: they include those made for Charles the Bald (d. 877), Otto III (d. 1002) and Princess Gertrude of Poland (d. 1109). Analysis of the prayer book made for the young ruler Otto III suggests that it was made to support his personal observances, rather than simply for use by his chaplain.[19] Its size also supports this presumption: it is small, measuring some 12cm by 15cm, and is only 44 folios long. It is a personal book, made to be read, rather than serve as a choir book. It is also extremely luxurious, being written in gold on purple parchment with five full-page illuminations. Three of these depict a young man: in one he is standing in lay dress between SS Peter and Paul, in the *orans* position with arms outstretched, in another, again in lay dress, he is prostrate, in *proskynesis*, before Christ, and in the third, dressed in the royal regalia, he is seated on a throne, receiving a copy of the book from a cleric. The young man is clearly Otto III himself: this picture, and the accompanying verse on the opposite page, make clear that the book was made for, and given to the young ruler. Its contents suggest the king should use the book himself. The miniatures helped place the ruler next to Christ, reflecting strands of royal ideology, but also provide an ideological context for his own prayers. It also includes the text of the seven penitential psalms (nos 6, 31, 37, 50, 101, 129, 142) which had, since the late eighth century, been a standard feature of private devotion. They are followed by a litany, including a petition for the protection of the king and his princes written in the first person:

> *That you guard us in your will, me your servant and unworthy king, and all our princes, we pray you hear us.*

This litany is therefore to be recited by the king himself, hence the references to '*me* your servant' and 'all *our* princes'; he is not expected to delegate this task to his chaplains. The litany is then followed by prayers petitioning God to guide the orator's acts and thoughts, followed by a sequence of prayers, one of which has an especial resonance. According to its rubric, 'whoever prays this prayer daily shall not feel the torments of hell in eternity'. In it the orator takes responsibility for his own salvation pleading 'I pray you Saint Peter who holds the keys of the kingdom of heaven to absolve *me* from *my* sins on this earth'. Intercessory prayer is not sufficient; the orator attaches importance to prayers he said himself. Whilst this particular prayer is not unique to the Otto III prayer book, as it is found in various eleventh-century collections with a clerical provenance, it provides a helpful perspective to Bishop Thietmar of Merseburg's account of the young man's lonely vigils in which he wept for his sins.

The prayer book made for Otto III omits the canonical hours, but they are found in several other prayer books made for rulers and magnates, including that made over a century earlier for Charles the Bald, and that made in an English reformed monastic community a few years later, sometime in the early eleventh century, now Cotton MSS Nero A. ii and Galba A. xiv. The Galba prayer book includes a collection of prayers in the vernacular to be recited at the canonical hours, which suggests that the book was made to support personal devotions within the structures of the divine office. The prayer to be said at *None*, like that to be said daily in the Otto III prayer book, emphasised the orator's desire for direct communication with the Lord, rather than through an intercessory:

> *My Lord Jesus Christ, you were suspended on the cross, you received the criminal who believed in you into the joy of paradise and let him accompany you. You were a mighty King, even though you hung on the cross; I humbly confess* my *sins to you and beseech you on account of your great mercy to permit* me *to enter through the gates of paradise after my journey from this life.*[20]

Such prayers differ from the usual run of prayers in which the orator acts as intercessor on behalf of others as much as himself. In this prayer, like that in the Otto III prayer book, the orator pleads for himself; such texts are vivid testimonies to the fact that individuals wished to take responsibility for their own salvation. The Galba prayer book was made in, and perhaps for a member of, a monastic community; its similarities with that made for a king demonstrate how the laity and clergy shared a common culture of personal devotion. Such prayers were, of course, to be recited by the individual within the communal office. This practice helped make individuals, both lay and clerical, aware of their own participation in what Diana Webb has called a 'shared spiritual culture'.[21] They represent what Eamon Duffy has called, in his study of later medieval Books of Hours, 'the personalizing of religion'.[22] They are thus evidence for the importance of viewing such personal devotions as on a continuum with those of collective prayer, and lay observances as imitating and on a par with clerical practices.

Prayer for dead kin

The expense of such codices meant ownership had to be confined to the social elite in the central Middle Ages; yet at the same time both prescriptive and descriptive evidence suggests that churchmen strove to promote the practice of lay prayer more widely. In particular they expected members of the laity to assume responsibility for prayer for dead members of their family and friends in order to alleviate their punishment in the afterlife. The Carolingian churchmen gathered at the council of Mainz in 847 articulated this requirement very clearly:

> *Priests should seek a simple confession of sins from the sick who are in danger of death; not, however, imposing on them a quantity of penance, but making it known, and the weight of penance should be alleviated through the prayers and devotions to almsgiving of friends, so if by chance the sick should die soon, they will not be excluded from the fellowship of pardon through the obligation of excommunication.*[23]

Through vicarious prayer and devotion friends helped the dying person to fulfil their penance so as to ensure their salvation in the next life. The churchmen meeting at Mainz merely articulated a practice which had already become widespread amongst the lay nobility of praying for both the living and the dead. The transfer of wealth to ecclesiastical institutions which we investigated in Chapter 4 is evidence that the regular clergy played an extremely important role in prayer for the dead. It was never, however, meant to be an exclusive one. The involvement of both lay women and men in prayer for their families, both living and dead, represents the significance also attributed to individual supplications throughout this period.

Writing perhaps four to six years earlier, the noblewoman Dhuoda advised her son to pray for the past, present and future, not just for himself, but for sixteen other groups of people, including all the clergy, the king, his lord and his father. He should pray for all the dead, including especially his paternal grandparents and godfather. She also asked him to say psalms for himself, his father, and all the dead, and for her, when she was dead, so that she would be amongst the elect and not the damned.[24] Her writings suggest that Frankish nobles regarded such prayers as efficacious, and as part of mainstream lay piety. They remained part of noble lay piety in tenth-century Saxony. We have already seen how Mathilda prayed for sinners and the eternal rest of souls whilst keeping vigil at night, and in one *Life* she is described on her deathbed as handing the *computarium*, in which had been written the names of the family dead, to her grand-daughter, Mathilda, abbess of Quedlinburg, and commending to her the responsibility to pray for the soul of Henry the Fowler, the elder Mathilda's husband, and those of all the faithful whose names were recorded there.[25] Devotion by the living on behalf of the dead also included good deeds as well as prayer. Thus Godila, the widow of the Margrave Liuthar, 'for the sake of his salvation . . . constantly performed as many good deeds as she could'.[26] One Saxon bishop's account makes clearer that such good deeds included prayer, as well as fasting and almsgiving. He describes Werner, margrave of the north Saxon March, as inconsolable at the death of his wife, Liudgard:

> *She had been the faithful guardian of his life and soul, devoting herself to the service of God more for his sake than her own. Above all, she protected him from the plots of the enemy [i.e. the devil] by fasting in the cold, through her constant prayer, and by distributing alms.*[27]

Such selfless devotion cannot, therefore, be regarded as confined to royal wives. Nor are such accounts of wifely devotion confined to the Saxon aristocracy. The hero of the *Ruodlieb*, a Latin romance recorded in an early eleventh-century Bavarian monastery, witnesses the murder of an old man. The murderer is the lover of the victim's much younger wife; the victim's widow repents of her involvement, and learns the psalter, and sings it for the old man's soul, fasts in the day, goes barefoot, and daily visits her husband's tomb to pray, going to church for matins, and returning for Mass and staying until *none*.[28] The *Ruodlieb* is based on a folk tale found all over medieval Europe, but it is evidence that such behaviour had become normative on the part of the widow in Bavaria, at least.

Patrick Geary has suggested that such images of women as intercessors for the family dead are peculiar to tenth-century east Frankia, and that at the same time in west Frankia nobles delegated the task to the clergy.[29] Whilst there is some evidence to substantiate this view, it is impossible to sustain it across the period, for there is evidence for continuation of the practice of lay intercession in twelfth-century Flanders and Burgundy. Writing in the mid-twelfth century, Abbot Hermann of Tournai records how a hermit had a vision of two saints beseeching Mary to punish a certain nobleman for attacking the abbeys of which they were patrons, but Mary refused, saying that the nobleman's wife protected him by repeating the *Ave Maria* sixty times a day, twenty times prostrate, twenty times on her knees, and twenty times standing, either in church or in her room or in some private place.[30] Peter the Venerable, abbot of Cluny (d. 1156) described how his mother confessed her own sins and those of her dead husband at her husband's tomb.[31] These examples of twelfth-century practice should be read as a continuation of the norms of lay piety, as articulated in the ninth century at the council of Mainz, rather than as being an innovation or as the extension of norms of lay behaviour only begun in tenth-century Saxony.[32] Taken together they suggest that prayer for the dead had become a widely accepted feature of widows' behaviour across Europe throughout the period.

Nor can this practice be confined to women. In the words of one eleventh-century English penitential text, which echo those of the Council of Mainz, the penance of a powerful man rich in friends is lightened with their help.[33] The fate of those who died midway through doing penance for their sins clearly provoked anxiety amongst their relations. One tenth-century Anglo-Saxon penitential sought to alleviate their concerns thus:

> *For a good [reconciled] man Mass may be sung on the third day or after seven nights. For a penitent man Mass may be sung after thirty nights or after seven nights if his kinsmen and relations fast for him and make some offering for his soul at God's altar.*[34]

A penitent who had completed his penance and been reconciled should be treated like any Christian, for in monastic practice it had become the norm to remember the dead person at Mass three days, and then a week, and then thirty days after their death. A penitent who had yet to complete his penance should be treated rather differently, but the actions of his relatives could help to speed the process. Punishment for the penitent's sins in the afterlife could thus be alleviated by the actions of his relations as well as the prayers of professional religious. We need, of course, to set references like this one alongside the plentiful evidence that many nobles requested monks, nuns and canons to pray for them. But we also have references to churchmen themselves praying for their own blood relations. Continuity in such practices across the years 900 to 1200 testify to the importance of these practices in Christian devotion, both lay and clerical. Both laymen and women as well as members of the clergy assumed such responsibilities regularly and willingly.

The lay religious life

Up to now we have focused on individual pious actions, and the ways in which lay men and women adopted and adapted monastic models of piety. We turn now to study some of the ways in which lay men and women voluntarily came together for pious purposes, starting with the evidence for those choosing to live a religious life outside the formal structures of regular religion, before moving to that for confraternities. For these forms of collective piety have as much to tell us as those for personal piety about the ways in which groups of lay men and women all over Europe internalised the Christian values inculcated by their pastors.

Whereas Robert advised Countess Ermengarde to live her life in the world, lay people sometimes chose not to join a religious community but rather voluntarily to follow a communal life of personal devotion and prayer in the world. Examples of such informal communities, as we shall see, can be found in tenth-century Spain, where their participants were referred to as *confessi* (the confessed ones), in tenth- and eleventh-century England, where there are various female communities built around noble women, as similarly there were in late eleventh-century France, and finally in late twelfth-century Italy, where there are various examples of groups of lay men and women living religious lives according a rule in their own homes who came to be known as the Humiliati. The Humiliati are usually viewed against a backdrop of the extension of the apostolic life from monasteries to lay households. But this section suggests that these Italian households represent a continuous strand in medieval religious life, and that they are less anomalous and more normative than they seem if treated just in their late twelfth-century context. For these examples of religious households from the tenth to twelfth centuries share two crucial features:

lay men and women chose to follow religious lives either in their own homes or by living with other laymen and women in the lay community; and these households seem to have been ephemeral. They all lacked the institutional structures which allowed them to continue after the death of their founder; instead the lands on which they were based often reverted to the founder's family on their death. There are also, however, differences: the earlier examples are more aristocratic than later ones, reflecting the increased prosperity of later centuries, and the changing socio-religious context. In tenth-century northern Spain lay men and women seemingly made public commitments to lead a religious life; termed *confessi* in the documents, to distinguish them from ordinary lay men and women, they remained living in their own households, rather than joining a monastery. Married couples would even continue to live together, with their children. Sometimes groups of *confessi* might live together. Quite what form their religious life took is unclear. The terminology is not stable. The word *confessa* (a singular female confessed one) was sometimes used interchangeably with terms used for the professed religious: the dowager queen Teresa of Asturias-León, for example, is referred to in different documents as a *confessa*, *ancilla Christi* (maidservant of Christ) and *ancilla ancillarum* (maidservant of maidservants). But Wendy Davies's analysis suggests that the status of *confessa* carried with it rather different resonances because in individual charters *confessa* is sometimes used to distinguish people from those described as *deo vota* (female one vowed to God).[35] *Deo vota* and *ancilla* are terms used throughout the medieval west to refer to a nun or a canoness. Many Spanish *confessi* may therefore be rather similar to the widowed women vowed to God who continued to live on their family's lands found in northern Europe.

In tenth- and eleventh-century England, women similarly chose to live religious lives outside the strictures of institutional regular communities. English widows of high status often adopted the religious life without joining a community, instead living as *nunnan* (Old English for veiled vowesses) on their own lands with other women. Thus the late tenth-century will of the widow Æthelgifu shows she had gathered around her women around her, including Ælfwaru, the daughter of her huntsman Wulfric, and asked that they be freed from their servile status after her death on condition that they say four psalters a week for the first thirty days after her death, and a psalter every week in the year after her death. The conditions attached to her legacy recall monastic practice for the commemoration of the dead, which made much of commemorating the first thirty days, and the first anniversary. In the early 970s a noble widow, Æthelflæd, who is described as a 'famula dei' (servant of God) built herself a house within sight of the door to the abbey church of Glastonbury so that she could serve Lord Jesus Christ day and night. She did not, however, retire completely from the world, and was visited there by King Æthelstan and his retinue when he visited Glastonbury.[36]

A very similar lifestyle to that attributed to Æthelflæd is that ascribed by Guibert of Nogent to his mother. Living a century later, in late eleventh-century northern France, after she became widowed she moved with her household, including two sons, two chaplains, and a tutor, to what was probably the family monastery. There she ordered an old nun to live with her and teach her 'the practices of self-discipline'. Guibert recounts that his mother's holy way of life, and the visions she had of the Virgin Mary, led her to acquire such authority that she was approached by people in the surrounding area, but that she was only consecrated as a *deo vota* three years before her death. Guibert's mother is one example of an anchoress whose way of life gave her importance in the locality; such figures become much better documented in the course of the twelfth and thirteenth centuries. But her behaviour is actually very similar to that ascribed a century and a half earlier to Queen Mathilda who spent a good deal of her prolonged widowhood in retirement in the female house of canonesses she had founded with her husband at Quedlinburg. The only way in which Mathilda's behaviour differed is she chose to spend time in a house of formal religious, rather than to establish her own, albeit temporary, religious household. These informal religious households thus constitute an important background to late twelfth-century developments.

In the late twelfth century a series of communities emerged in the north Italian Po valley, many of which look very similar to the sorts of lay religious groupings which existed earlier in Spain, England, and east and west Frankia. These communities are now known collectively as the Humiliati (the humble ones).[37] They are worth examining in more detail because their history represents the culmination of the two strands of lay devotion which we have considered up to now; that is the ways in which lay people chose to take up aspects of monastic devotion, on the one hand, and the ways in which lay people chose to live the religious life in their own home, on the other.

The early history of the Humiliati is obscure, in part no doubt because they are one of the groups declared heretics by Pope Lucius III at the Council of Verona in 1184, before being received back into the Church by Pope Innocent III in 1201, and in part because their practices fitted so well into the established religious life of northern Italy. They seem to have run foul of papal authority in the late twelfth century because they failed to heed a prohibition on public preaching, and refused to take oaths. Yet notarial records of legal property transactions suggest that the earliest Humiliati houses were built, from 1176 onwards, with the support and approval of local clergy, local bishops and their officers, as well as that of lay communities. These houses thus look very like other orthodox religious communities founded at the time, and like them received legacies from lay families living in the vicinity.

By 1201 they had become more formally organised as follows: the Third Order – married or single lay men and women living a religious life in their own homes, akin to the Spanish *confessi* or English *nunnan* of the tenth century; the Second Order – men and women living a regular life in communities; and the First Order – clerics living a regular life in communities. The way of life of the Third Order approved by Innocent III in 1201 owes much to that of earlier groups of lay religious we have already considered.[38] Their way of life emphasised the importance of humility, and obedience to prelates, but also the importance of penance and living at peace with others. They should not profit from usury. They should pay tithes, not abandon their wives, but rather stay with them, and should fast twice a week, on Wednesdays and Fridays, and when not fasting eat two frugal meals a day. They should say the Lord's Prayer both before and after meals, and observe the seven canonical hours. At the office of prime they must recite the Creed. They should avoid ostentation and wear only sober clothing. They should help those in need. If one of them died, the brethren should all come to the funeral and say the Lord's Prayer and *Miserere mei deus* (Psalm 50) twelve times for the dead person's soul. They should also say the Lord's Prayer three times a day for the living and three times a day for the dead of the fraternity, and once a day for the peace of the Church. They should come together each Sunday to hear the word of God, and one of the brethren might, with the permission of the bishop, exhort others in the group and encourage them in their customs and pious works, but should not speak about doctrine. Clearly they drew on the existing framework for lay piety, itself an extension of monastic ideals.

Their reliance on existing forms of religious life perhaps explains why the Humiliati came to be regarded by many in the last two decades of the twelfth century as not heretical, and why – despite having been formally excluded from the Church in 1184 – they could be reconciled with it so easily seventeen years later. They are testament to the eagerness with which certain members of the laity sought to emulate the religious life, and adopt it for their own purposes. Their way of life combined the tradition of lay people choosing to live the religious life in their own homes which had, as we have seen, a long and vibrant tradition, with that of confraternities, to which we shall now turn.

Confraternities

Another interesting feature of piety in this period is the increasing evidence for voluntary associations of men and women, lay and clerical, coming together for a mix of social and religious reasons, and whose activities focused around a local church, and the cult of its patron saint. Known primarily to modern historians as guilds (*gilda*) or confraternities (*confraternitas*), they are also referred to as consortia (*consortio*), fraternities (*fraternitas)*, rules (*religio*), or charities (*caritas*).[39] As this fluid terminology suggests, these groups were by no means homogeneous, and yet they share so many features that modern scholars have found it easier to lump them together than to try and distinguish between them. Medieval churchmen also often treated them synonymously and found them threatening.[40] There is evidence of such associations from eighth- and ninth-century Frankia and England; Archbishop Hincmar of Rheims, for example, warned priests against participating in the drinking bouts which went on at the feasts held by 'guilds or confraternities'.[41] It is only from the tenth century onwards that evidence for the constitution of such groups survives in the form of charters and statutes. Using the language of brotherhood – 'guild brothers', 'brothers and sisters', 'fraternity' – these texts provide a unique insight into the world in which lay men and women sought an active role in the religious life of their local church, and in the commemoration of the life of fellow members of their group.[42]

It is this mixture of the religious and social – typified by the feasts which Archbishop Hincmar warned his priests to be wary of – together with the link to a local cult in a local church which distinguishes these associations from formal monastic confraternities. Despite sharing the same name, monastic confraternities are very different: organized by the monastic community, they offered members of the laity, the secular clergy, and members from other monasteries the opportunity to be associated with a particular community and remembered in its prayers. They therefore tended to be socially conservative and elitist; membership was restricted to patrons of the monastery. The evidence for these formal communities is rather more profuse than that for lay confraternities; nevertheless enough survives to suggest that lay confraternities focused on local churches played an important part in the religious lives of their lay members.

Lay confraternities reflected the bond which already existed within local communities and served to reinforce them by structuring their meetings around charity, prayer and almsgiving. They also strengthened social ties not just in this life but with those in the next. They enjoyed a broader social membership than monastic confraternities, incorporating not just leading nobles but their followers. For example, sometime in the mid-eleventh century the nobleman Urki and his wife Tole established a guild with its own guildhall at Abbotsbury in Dorset 'to the praise of God and St Peter'.[43] Urki had come with King Cnut to England from Denmark, and been appointed by the new king to the lordship of that area. It has been suggested that he intended the guild to reinforce his lordship in the area by creating a focus for his followers. Its statutes suggest it had a mixture of social and religious concerns, and that they came together in an annual feast and Mass on St Peter's Day (1 August). Each member should contribute a penny or a penny's worth of wax for the lights for the Mass, and bread, wheat, wood and beer for the feast. Feasting and piety combined to celebrate and reinforce ties within the group, centred on the local church. The guild also made provision for looking after its dying and dead: the other members should contribute a penny for the *soulscot* on the death of a member; if any member fell seriously ill within sixty miles, the dying man – or his corpse – should be brought back to Abbotsbury by other members of the guild; they should take the corpse to the church where the other members should pray earnestly for his soul. The demand that the guild bring the dead member back to the church and pay *soulscot* supported the church of Abbotsbury's rights over burial within that area.[44] Yet it is clear that these statutes also encouraged conviviality: the feast had the potential to be an uproarious occasion with fines for those who did not do the brewing satisfactorily, and for those who insulted each other. But members also prayed for their dead fellows; the guild combined social with pious functions. Such feasts, the act of eating and drinking together, created and strengthened existing bonds with local society: members of one twelfth-century Winchester guild were even described as assembling to 'drink their guild'.[45] The dead were also often remembered at these events: we know the names of the dead were to be read out at the annual feast held by the twelfth-century jongleurs guild of Our Lady of Arras.[46] Living and dead thus came together for occasions which combined earthly pleasure with thoughts of the life to come.

But the statutes of many confraternities more usually focused not on feasting but rather on remembrance of, and active prayer for, the dead. Prayer for dead members of the confraternity should not be delegated to professional religious, but rather undertaken by all members, each according to his ability. Although confraternities sometimes included both clerical and lay members, they generally made specific provision for both groups to participate in the remembrance of past members. The fraternity of Sant-Appiano in Valdesa (*c.*1000) in northern Italy, for example, included both churchmen and members of the laity: the orders of priests, deacons, and clerics, lay men and lay women. Its statutes made provision for members of each order to remember the others on a weekly basis, and made special provision for remembrance of dead members: priests should sing three masses each week for their brothers and sisters, and a mass each day for the first thirty days after a fellow member died, clerical members sing the entire psalter each week for their brothers and sisters, and ten psalms a day for a member's soul for the first thirty days after his or her death, and lay men and women should feed three paupers each week for their brothers and sisters, and, upon the death of a fellow member, feed forty paupers for the first forty days and afterwards remember the dead in their prayers and when they pray or give alms. Lay members gave alms rather than undertaking a specific round of prayers, but they should also pray personally for the dead. This is an ambitious programme and suggests a considerable degree of monetary and temporal investment by its members in the fraternity's activities. It points to a vibrant community in which the clergy joined with the laity to remember the living and the dead.

Similar provisions for prayer and almsgiving exist for when a member of the confraternity fell ill.[47] For example, the statutes of one twelfth-century

Italian confraternity from near Bologna provided that if any member fell ill, the other brothers should visit his deathbed with lights and keep vigil over him.[48] When the brother died, members of the confraternity should wash the corpse, and accompany it to the church, and each offer a denarius at the funeral, and have a mass sung for his soul four times a year. The procedures here, as at early eleventh-century Abbotsbury, imitated those for monastic death: the brothers should watch over the dying man, and then participate, through laying out and almsgiving, in the funeral obsequies. In stepping into arrangements for the dead, they make clear that care for the dying should not be confined to family members, nor should it be delegated to professional religious; rather confraternities offered an opportunity for lay people to provide insurance for each other, and to take an active part in their own, and their friends' and associates' salvation. They represent the extension of monastic practice but at the same time they demonstrate their adaptation to a domestic setting.

Alongside care for the dying and prayer for the dead, confraternities also provided a vehicle for supporting the liturgy through payment for lights for the church. Provision of lights is a theme running across many confraternities. The consortium of priests, lay men and women established by Bishop Aldegarius of Ivrea in *c.*940–945 had to meet twice a year, in March and on All Saints Day, and to give a denarius to buy lights for the living and the dead in Lent. But if a member from the parish died, everyone should run to him and bury him with prayers, alms and lights given by the confraternity.[49] The members of the Abbotsbury guild similarly contributed wax for the feast day of their patron, St Peter. The main purpose of the confraternity sometimes even seems to have been to fund the lighting of the church, as, for example, is the case for an eleventh-century list of the names of sixty-five men and forty-four women in a necrology from Modena cathedral who,

> *for fear of God and love of Christ each gave a denarius for the redemption of their souls on lights to illuminate the church of God so that God will illuminate their souls in holy paradise and they promise to do this to help God each year*

to demonstrate their devotion to the Virgin Mary, the patron saint of the cathedral.[50]

In a world in which churches must usually have been rather dark spaces, lights were important both symbolically as well as practically to the enactment of the liturgy: light echoed Christ's message of salvation to the world, and as such deliberate reference was made to light not only in occasional rites, such as Candlemas and Easter, but also in daily evening prayer. Yet both wax and oil were expensive. Funds for light made possible the physical performance of the liturgy in a badly lit space with few windows. By contributing to the practicalities of the liturgy, the lay members of these guilds contributed to the liturgy itself. Their voluntary gifts in this regard are thus evidence of their personal piety.[51]

Some confraternities, such as those of Abbotsbury and S. Cassiano d'Imola, are clearly the personal foundations of lay lords, while others, such as that of Ivrea, have episcopal origins. Taken together they represent not so much the expression of lay autonomous piety but rather the co-operation of different forces within a local community working together. As we have seen, confraternities often had a mixture of purposes, but one that came to the fore only in the twelfth century was the establishment of communities to run hospitals for pilgrims, lepers and the indigent sick.[52] Confraternal in character, these communities used the language and structures of monastic brotherhood. Examples include the leper hospital established at Santa Croce outside Verona in the 1130s, run by a community of brothers and sisters, and that for pilgrims established at Aubrac in southern France in the first half of the twelfth century.[53] The bishop drew up the statutes for the latter in 1162 with the advice of the clerics and laymen, brothers and sisters of the hospital. The members of the community should attend church every morning, unless they were sick, to pray for the brothers and benefactors of the house and the whole Christian population. All the lay brothers and sisters should recite the Lord's prayer at Matins and at the other divine hours. Their lifestyle is akin to that of more formal clerical communities or the informal religious houses which we have seen made up a minor, but constant, feature of the devotional landscape of the medieval west. As this example demonstrates, such hospital communities result from combined clerical and lay initiatives: as such they may represent a continuation of the forces which had led to the establishment of confraternities in both the tenth and eleventh centuries.

The confraternity offered a flexible structure for binding different groups together with a single purpose, and it was one which some churchmen sought to appropriate for their own ends, especially fundraising for building projects, as was the case, for example, of the confraternity founded to finance the construction of the cathedral of Urgel in 1096.[54] Bishop Arnulf of Lisieux (d. 1184) even went so far as to hire certain priests from a neighbouring diocese to establish fraternities and to make collections for the rebuilding of his cathedral in Normandy, but ran into problems when they absconded with the cash.[55]

That churchmen throughout our period repeatedly warned against the dangers to public order posed by the feasts associated with such confraternities points to their ambivalent attitude towards them: on one level they wished to encourage them as an expression of community cohesion and lay piety, on the other they suggest that they remained outside clerical control and as such needed to be monitored carefully.[56] Those organizations which had longer-term success seem to have been ones which emerged from a coalition of local lay and clerical interests. Their increasing presence in the documentary record testifies to their increasing popularity across the years between 900 and 1200. Records of five confraternities associated with local churches and cathedrals survive from tenth- and eleventh-century England, and at least six from tenth- to twelfth-century Italy. The statutes for at least ten further ones survive from twelfth-century Europe, ranging from Flanders to Catalonia.[57] These numbers appear insignificant when compared to those from the later Middle Ages: Gervase Rosser has gone so far as to estimate that in late medieval England there may have been as many as 30,000 guilds.[58] He argues that their numbers grew significantly in the fourteenth and fifteenth centuries as new communities sought socio-religious frameworks for their identity in a period when constraints on parish formation meant there was no alternative outlet through which they could express their feelings. Local communities in this earlier period did have other means for expressing their identity, not least through the formation of parish communities centred on local churches, but it is clear that all over Europe, in both towns and villages, they increasingly sought to establish their own pious associations in local churches.[59]

Conclusions

The evidence assembled in this chapter is necessarily fragmentary; taken together it demonstrates that many members of the laity, especially those at the higher end of the social spectrum, exceeded churchmen's rather minimal religious expectations of lay practice. Seldom content to abdicate religious responsibility, either for themselves or their family and friends, in favour of assiduous observation of the pastoral rites, lay noblemen and women, if not those lower down the social scale, actively prayed both alone and in groups for the salvations of both themselves and those they knew. Rather, the evidence of prayer books, informal religious communities, and confraternities taken together suggests that increasingly across the period between 900 and 1200 many members of the laity went beyond the pastoral expectations laid down by churchmen, and sought voluntarily to direct their own religious lives.

This picture is biased towards the actions of members of the nobility; such conspicuous acts of lay devotion were not open to everyone. They were necessarily mostly confined to the wealthier members of society. But not entirely. Ælfwaru, the unfree daughter of a huntsman, served her mistress, and was sufficiently literate that she could be expected to say four psalters a week for her mistress in the first thirty days after her death. Although unfree, she took part in the movement to live a voluntary religious life which began to reach its late medieval apogee only in the late twelfth century.

We also need to recognise that the seeming rise of active participation by the laity in the religious life is partly a trick of the evidential light; we do not have as much evidence for the earlier period, but this is not, in and of itself, proof that the lay were merely passive vessels for clerically imposed piety in the years before 1200. The evidence for voluntary piety suggests rather that many individuals, acting alone and together, preferred not just to delegate their religious duties to the clergy, but rather to take action themselves. In this they were aided and supported by churchmen. The ways in which they expressed their devotions, collectively and individually, inevitably owed a great deal to clerical, and in particular monastic, practices. Some aspects – such as that of daily prayer – derived from and overlapped with clerical rites. Similarly, the sorts of informal religious communities which culminated in the Humiliati movement in late twelfth-century northern Italy owe a good deal to the customs of regular communities of canons and monks. Both these aspects represent the adaptation of existing clerical norms by devout laymen and women. To this extent lay devotion was highly imitative. But this period also witnessed the emergence of a distinctive, lay-oriented form of piety: mixed confraternities of clerics and lay men and women focused on their local church. The emergence for the first time only in the late tenth century of detailed records of constitutions for such confraternities signals a new trend in lay piety. Centred on the local churches, which we have seen had only recently begun to emerge as the religious centres for many settlements, these confraternities indicate the ways in which the social elite, both spiritual and secular, in local communities began to invest in a collective religious life. The ways in which these confraternities chose to synthesise secular behaviour with spiritual devotion signal the degree to which their lay members had begun to internalise ecclesiastical teaching about the fate of the soul.

We began by asking how typical were the Countess Ermengarde's aspirations to live a religious life; this chapter demonstrates that she shared her wishes with many other lay men and women in this period, and like her, many lived that life in the world. In doing so, they became voluntary directors of their own personal piety, praying for themselves and their dead kin and neighbours, both individually and together. Taking up in different ways the clerical models of personal devotion provided for them, they chose to develop particular aspects of that model, whether acting individually or together. In doing so they acted in company with, and on the advice of churchmen; but that they chose to do so freely indicates the success of the Church's mission across the central Middle Ages.

Notes and references

1 'Sermo domni Roberti de Abrussello ad comitissam Britanniae', *Les deux vies de Robert d'Arbrissel fondateur de Fontevraud. Légendes, écrits et témoignages*, ed. with French and English transl. J. Dalarun, G. Giordanengo, A. Le Huërou, J. Longère, D. Poirel and B. L. Venarde (Turnhout, 2006), c. 17, 474–75.

2 Ibid. cc. 16–23, 472–79; J. Dalarun, *Robert of Arbrissel: Sex, Sin and Salvation in the Middle Ages, trans. B. L. Venarde* (Washington, DC, 2006), 93–101.

3 C. S. Watkins, *History and the Supernatural in Medieval England* (Cambridge, 2007), 103–04, and his citation of *Gilbert of Limerick, Gille of Limerick (c.1070–1145): Architect of a Medieval Church*, ed. J. Fleming (Dublin, 2001), 152–53.

4 B. Hamilton, *Religion in the Medieval West* (London, 1986), 55–56.

5 C. x, *PL* 140, 1000.

6 Hermann of Tournai, *Liber de restauratione monasterii Sancti Martini Tornacensis*, c. 28, ed. G. Waitz, MGH SS XIV, 285; *The Restoration of the Monastery of Saint Martin of Tournai*, trans L. H. Nelson (Washington, DC, 1996), c. 28, 43.

7 Odo of Cluny, *Life of St Gerald of Aurillac*, I.xi, *PL* 133, 649–50; trans. G. Sitwell, *St Odo of Cluny Being the Life of St Odo of Cluny by John of Salerno and the Life of St Gerald of Aurillac by St Odo* (London, 1958), I.xi, 104–05.

8 William of Malmesbury, *Gesta regum anglorum* I, 492–93; Hermann of Tournai, *Liber de restauratione*, c. 23, 283, trans. *Restoration*, c. 23, 38.

9 Byrhtferth of Ramsey, *Life of St Oswald*, c. 4 in Byrhtferth of Ramsey, *The Lives of St Oswald and St Ecgwine*, ed. M. Lapidge (Oxford, 2009), 16.

10 Adriaan Gaastra, 'Between Liturgy and Canon Law: A Study of Books of Confession and Penance in Eleventh- and Twelfth-century Italy' (Ph.D. thesis, University of Utrecht, 2007), n. 634.

11 Translated in *Saints and Cities in Medieval Italy*, ed. and trans. D. Webb (Manchester, 2007), 55.

12 Peter Damian, *Epistolae*, ed. K. Reindel, *Die Briefe des Petrus Damiani*, 4 vols, MGH Briefe der deutschen Kaiserzeit 4 (Munich, 1983), I, 167; trans. O. J. Blum, *The Letters of Peter Damian, 1–150*, 5 vols (Washington, DC, 1989–), I, 158, cited by R. Fulton, *From Judgment to Passion: Devotion to Christ and the Virgin Mary, 800–1200* (New York, 2002), 224.

13 Donizo of Canossa, *Vita Mathildis celeberrimae principis Italiae*, Königin II. 20, *PL* 148, 1035, cited by R. Fulton, *From Judgment*, 225.

14 Widukind of Corvey, *Rerum gestarum Saxonicarum libri tres*, MGH SRG 60 (Hannover, 1935), III.74, 150–51; *Vita Mathildis Posterior*, c. 10, *Die Lebensbeschreibungen der Königin Mathilde*, ed. B. Schütte, *MGH SRG* 66 (Hannover, 1994), 163–67; trans. in S. Gilsdorf, *Queenship and Sanctity: The Lives of Mathilda and the Epitaph of Adelheid* (Washington, DC, 2004), 101–03.

15 Thietmar of Merseburg, *Chronicon*, IV. 48, 186.

16 M. McC. Gatch, 'Piety and Liturgy in the Old English Vision of Leofric', in M. Korhammer, ed., *Words, Texts and Manuscripts* (Cambridge, 1992), 159–79.

17 P. J. E. Kershaw, 'Eberhard of Friuli, a Carolingian Lay Intellectual', in P. Wormald and J. L. Nelson, eds, *Lay Intellectuals in the Carolingian World* (Cambridge, 2007), 77–105 at p. 99.

18 H. M. Thomas, 'Lay Piety in England from 1066 to 1215', *Anglo-Norman Studies* 29 (2007), 179–92 at p. 189.

19 S. Hamilton, 'Most Illustrious King of Kings': Evidence for Ottonian Kingship in the Otto III Prayerbook (Munich, Bayerische Staatsbibliothek, Clm 30111)', *Journal of Medieval History* 27 (2001), 257–88.

20 B. J. Muir, 'The Early Insular Prayer Book Tradition and the Development of the Book of Hours', in M. M. Manion and B. J. Muir, eds, *The Art of the Book: Its Place in Medieval Worship* (Exeter, 1998), 9–19 at p. 19.

21 D. Webb, 'Domestic Space and Devotion in the Middle Ages', in A. Spicer and S. Hamilton, eds, *Defining the Holy: Sacred Space in Medieval and Early Modern Europe* (Aldershot, 2005), 27–47 at p. 31.

22 Duffy, *Marking the Hours*, 55.

23 C, 26, *MGH Concilia III: Concilia aevi Karolini 843–859*, ed. W. Hartmann (Hannover, 1984), 173–74, translated by Paxton, *Christianizing Death*, 166.

24 *Dhuoda, Manuel pour mon fils*, ed. P. Riché, trans. B. de Vregille and C. Mondésert, Sources Chrétiennes 225 (Paris, 1975), VIII.2, VIII.8–16, XI.1.

25 *Vita Mathilda Antiquior*, c. 13, 137–38; trans. Gilsdorf, *Queenship*, 85–86.

26 Thietmar, *Chronicon*, VI.86, 377–78, trans Warner, 294.

27 Ibid. VI.85, 377; trans, Warner, 294.

28 *Waltharius and Ruodlieb*, ed. and trans. D. M. Kratz (New York, 1984), 151.

29 P. Geary, *Phantoms of Remembrance: Memory and Oblivion at the End of the First Millennium* (Princeton, NJ, 1994), 60–61; compare Karl Leyser's argument that the noblewomen of tenth-century Saxony had an almost institutional role as spiritual protectors of their menfolk, both dead and alive, through their own good works and prayers: *Rule and Conflict in an Early Medieval Society* (Bloomington, IN, 1979), 72–73.

30 Hermann of Tournai, *Liber de restauratione*, c. 57, 298–300; trans, *The Restoration*, 79.

31 *The Letters of Peter the Venerable*, ed. G. Constable, 2 vols (Cambridge, Mass. 1967), no. 53, I.153–73 at p.161 cited by Iogna-Prat, *Order and Exclusion*, 153.

32 See Patrice Corbet's argument that the author of the *Vita Antiquior* of Mathilda viewed her prayers for the dead as good lay practice rather than as a mark of her sanctity: *Les saints ottoniens* (Sigmaringen, 1986), 141.

33 *Old English Handbook for the Use of a Confessor*, Cambridge, Corpus Christi College, Ms 201, p. 124, ed. and trans. A. J. Frantzen, *The Anglo-Saxon Penitentials: A Cultural Database* (http://www.anglo-saxon.net/penance, accessed 17 August 2012); cf. Council of Mainz (847), c. 26, *MGH Concilia III*, ed. Hartmann, 173–74 (cited in n. 23 above).

34 The *Scriftboc*, Oxford, Bodleian Library, Junius 121, fol. 96v, ed. and trans. A. Frantzen, *The Anglo-Saxon Penitentials: A Cultural Database* (http://www.anglo-Saxon.net/penance/index.html) (accessed 19th August 2012).

35 W. Davies, *Acts of Giving: Individual, Community and Church in Tenth-century Christian Spain* (Oxford, 2007), 107–08, 177–80.

36 S. Foot, *Veiled Women II: Female Religious Communities in England, 871–1066* (Aldershot, 2000), 93–97, 183–86.

37 F. Andrews, *The Early Humiliati* (Cambridge, 1999).

38 G. G. Meersseman, *Dossier de l'ordre de la pénitence au XIIIe siècle*, Spicilegium Friburgense 7 (Freiburg, 1961), 276–82; English translation, R. M. Stewart, *De illis qui faciunt penitentiam: The Rule of the Secular Franciscan Order: Orgins, Development, Interpretation*, Bibliotheca Seraphico-Capuccina (Rome, 1991), 365–71.

39 S. Reynolds, *Kingdoms and Communities in Western Europe 900–1300* (Oxford, 1984), 67–78 at p. 69.

40 P. Michaud-Quantin, *Universitas: Expressions du mouvement communautaire dans le moyen-age latin* (Paris, 1970), 179.

41 Hincmar of Rheims, *Capitula I*, c. 16, *MGH Capitula Episcoporum II*, ed. R. Pokorny, M. Stratmann, W.-D. Runge (Hannover, 1995), 43–44.

42 Meersseman, *Ordo fraternitatis*, 50, 61, 64.

43 *EHD* I, 559–60.

44 Blair, *Church*, 454, 466.

45 M. Biddle, ed., *Winchester in the Early Middle Ages* (Oxford, 1976), 1: 34, 335, cited by G. Rosser, 'Going to the Fraternal Feast: Commensality and Social Relations in Late Medieval England', *Journal of British Studies* 33 (1994), 430–46 at p. 431.

46 C. Symes, 'The Lordship of Jongleurs', in R. F. Berkhofer, A. Cooper and A. J. Kosto, eds, *The Experience of Power in Medieval Europe 950–1350: Essays in Honour of T. N. Bisson* (Aldershot, 2005), 237–52.

47 G. G. Meersseman, *Ordo fraternitatis: confraternite e pietà-dei laici nel medioevo* (Rome, 1977), 60–64.

48 S. Cassiano d'Imola (*c.*1160) near Bologna, ibid., 66–67.

49 Ibid. 96–97.

50 Ibid. 98–99.

51 D. Postles, 'Lamps, Lights and Layfolk', *Journal of Medieval History* 25 (1999), 97–114.

52 D. le Blévec, 'Fondations et oeuvres charitables au Moyen Âge', in J. Dufour and H. Platelle, eds, *Fondations et oeuvres charitables au moyen âge* (Paris, 1999), 7–21.

53 M. Miller, 'Toward a New Periodization of Ecclesiastical History: Demography, Society, and Religion in Medieval Verona', in S. K. Cohn Jr

and S. A. Epstein, eds, *Portraits of Medieval and Renaissance Living: Essays in Memory of David Herlihy* (Ann Arbor, 1995), 233–44 at p. 240; L. le Grand, *Statuts d'hotels-Dieu et de léproseries: Recueil de textes du XIIe au XIVe siècle* (Paris, 1901), 16–21. See also the statutes of the mid-twelfth-century leper house in Montpellier drawn up by the bishop which decreed that those entering the house who were unlearned (illiterate) must go to church daily for the office, and pray for their benefactors and the sins of all, and recite the *Our Father* each time a member of the community died; the literate should recite the seven penitential psalms each day and read the whole psalter at the death of a brother; ibid., 181–84.

54 Meersseman, *Ordo fraternitatis*, 109–110.

55 *The Letters of Arnulf of Lisieux*, ed. F. Barlow, Camden Society 3r ser. 61 (London, 1939), trans. *The Letter Collections of Arnulf of Lisieux*, trans. C. P. Schriber (Lewiston, NY, 1997), no. 63.

56 E. Coornaert, 'Les ghildes médiévales (Ve–XIVe siècles: definition et évolution', *Revue historique* 199 (1948), 22–55, 208–43; on twelfth- and thirteenth-century attempts to prohibit guilds as a source of public disorder in France, German and the Low Countries, see V. R. Bainbridge, *Gilds in the Medieval Countryside: Social and Religious Change in Cambridgeshire c.1350–1558* (Woodbridge, 1996), 1–21.

57 Bedwyn, Exeter I, Abbotsbury, Cambridge, and Exeter (England); Ivrea, Modena, Sant'Appiano in Valdesa, Santa Felicità, Verona, Sancta Croce, Verona, S. Cassiano d'Imola (Italy); Arras, Toulouse x 2, Lisieux, Béthune (E. Guibert, *Histoire de l'antique confrérie des charitables de Saint-Eloi de Béthune fondée en l'an 1188* (Béthune, 1934), Urgel. For an estimate of fifteen autonomous corporations from the eleventh- and twelfth-century Southern Low Countries, of which four were associated with parish churches, and eight with monasteries, see A.-J. Bijsterveld, 'Looking for Common Ground: From Monastic Fraternitas to Lay Confraternity in the Southern Low Countries in the Tenth to Twelfth Centuries', in E. Jamroziak and J. Burton, eds, *Religious and Laity in Western Europe 1000–1400* (Turnhout, 2006), 287–314.

58 Rosser, 'Going to the Fraternal Feast'; idem, 'Communities of Parish and Guild in the Late Middle Ages', in S. J. Wright, ed., *Parish, Church and People: Local Studies in Lay Religion 1350–1750* (London, 1988), 29–55.

59 For the argument for expansion in the tenth and eleventh centuries in the Latin West, see: P. Horden, 'The Confraternities of Byzantium', in W. J. Sheils and D. Wood, eds. *Voluntary Religion*, Studies in Church History 23 (Oxford, 1986), 25–45.

chapter 7

Local piety: Saints' cults and religious movements

Suger, the twelfth-century abbot of Saint-Denis, told the following story to explain how his house came to establish a priory at Champ, Essonne in the Île-de-France. Reports came to the monks at Saint-Denis that local people living near the site of an abandoned chapel on the monastery's land at Champ had witnessed candles burning in it every Saturday, although the roof of the building had long since collapsed and the altar was so covered in plants that sheep and goats were grazing on it. The miraculous light gradually drew the attention of the sick of the area, who came there in hope of a cure. Suger explained the miracle thus: the chapter was dedicated to the Virgin Mary, and Saturday was the day of the week dedicated to the Virgin. The Mother of God thus made it known, through the miraculous light, her desire for the chapel to be brought back into use. Suger therefore sent two monks 'to re-establish religion there', and the chapel later became the site of the priory.[1] According to Suger, the Virgin revealed her presence initially not to the clergy but to the common people, first through light, then through cures. The clergy took over the cult subsequently, which is suggestive of a belated attempt to regulate and control this expression of lay piety. But, crucially, Suger relied on the evidence of popular cult as testimony to explain how and why the monastic community at Saint-Denis came to establish a priory at this particular site.

Tales such as this one highlight the importance of local topography and local lay audiences in the establishment of a new site for a cult, and the construction of a new building in which to house it. As such they provide a contrast to most surviving writings about cults, be they *Lives*, miracle accounts, or accounts of translation, which tend to reveal much more about the interests of the community who acted as custodians of the site or relics of the cult, than about those of their audience. Suger's narrative is not, however, unusual in linking a saint's cult, in this case that of the Virgin Mary, to both a popular religious revivalist movement and the rebuilding of a church in a locality. Accounts of such movements often made much of their popularity with the laity, and associated them with the reconstruction of church buildings; at the same time the surviving physical remains of local chapels, churches, priories, monasteries and cathedrals serve as powerful witnesses to the hopes and investments of the wider community in centres dedicated to the cult of a particular saint. For one of the most interesting features of this period is the role awarded in clerical writings to the agency of lay groups in the establishment of the sites for the cult of saints and the building of churches to accommodate particular cults. This chapter seeks to explore this aspect of the evidence for saints' cults further.

Suger's tale also points to the tensions between clergy and laity inherent in such cults, as churchmen sought to direct popular enthusiasm by bringing such sites under their control. For the focus for religious cult and expression was never just confined within the walls of the local church or local monastery: rather natural features throughout the landscape of Europe, such as springs, wells and trees, and other sites, were suffused with religious associations. The cults associated with such natural sites have long been viewed as evidence of lay popular religion, and their popularity as due to the opportunities they provided for the laity to beseech the aid and support of particular saints directly. The cult of the saints from this perspective points at one and the same time to the remnants of pre-Christian pantheistic cults, in which particular places had associations with particular spirits, and to the projection of contemporary views of intercessory lordship on to the court of heaven; just as earthly men and women would approach their earthly ruler with a request via an intermediary, so medieval people approached the heavenly Lord via His intermediaries, the saints. For saints had known what it was to be human, but attained their place in heaven either through their steadfastness to the faith in death (martyrs) or in life (confessors): they thus provided the ideal intercessor between the earthly and heavenly spheres. Where they existed it was their relics which acted as vectors between heaven and earth, that is their physical remains, be it their bones, their clothes or other objects associated with the saint, such as books written or owned by them. But, as Suger's story demonstrates, cults did not always require relics to be successful: the association of the saint with a particular site, when combined with miraculous events, sufficed to attest to its holiness.

Tales such as Suger's have usually been read as attempts by churchmen to take over the direction of existing popular devotions. Yet the evidence for such lay popular cults only survives largely because clerical communities, such as that at Saint-Denis, sought to control and promote them. The laity's role as initiators of the cult is embedded within a wider narrative of monastic authority. This familiar tension between rhetoric and reality is played out in other churchmen's writings too: for the popularity of a cult served as a tool through which clerical communities promoted their authority within a local area. Lay popularity functioned as both a rhetorical trope which churchmen relied upon in their accounts to suggest widespread support for the cult, and as the physical means through which communities of professional religious sought to interact with other communities, both lay and clerical, living in the locality.[2] It cannot therefore be dismissed as a literary device: the very success of cults depended on lay support.

Taking up these tensions, this chapter will explore the limitations and potential of the evidence for local lay piety. Beginning with the nature of the evidence for local saints' shrines, it will then extend its focus to consider some of the other ways in which clerics used saints' cults to attract and harness popular support for movements to support reform, promoting both peace and, later, the rebuilding of churches. Investigating the problems posed by the literary conventions governing such accounts allows us to examine the degree to which lay people rather than religious communities used these local movements to shape their own religious lives.

Local saints' cults

As mentioned above, saints' cults were never confined just to ecclesiastical shrines, be they in cathedrals, monasteries or local churches. Shrines to saints peppered the European landscape: many springs, wells, trees and caves became associated with individual saints and were often attributed with healing properties. In England, for example, a healing spring at Clent, Worcestershire became linked to St Kenelm, a young ninth-century

Mercian prince murdered on the orders of his sister by her lover. His eleventh-century *Life* records two legends associated with the site: first that a spring sprung up on the site of his grave, and secondly that the ash tree there had sprouted from the staff planted in the ground by the boy just before his death.[3] Similarly the healing well at Binsey near Oxford had become associated with the cult of St Frideswide, an early eighth-century Anglo-Saxon princess, by the time her *vita* came to be written in the early twelfth century.[4] Not all shrines were confined to the natural realm. Local churches also often became the site of local cults, usually of the founder or patron, like that of St Milred, an eighth-century bishop of Worcester, whose cult was maintained only at Berkswell in Warwickshire, or St Wulfric, a tenth-century hermit, whose cult was located only at the minster he founded at Holme in Norfolk.[5] Yet the documentation for the majority of these local shrines is fragmentary, and usually late. In some areas with poor records for the central Middle Ages, such as Cornwall, the only evidence of local cult is the mention of otherwise unheard of saints in place names.[6] Such names are powerful testimony to what Julia Smith has described as a 'landscape of intense religious particularism' reflecting local interests and traditions.[7] They are the result of the processes of early medieval Christianisation and seek to commemorate the figures behind the foundation of local churches, but the mechanisms by which such sites became associated with particular cults are, for the most part, unrecorded. These *lacunae* mean we need to ask how far these local cults owe their origins to lay enthusiasm or whether they are, as in tales like that of Abbot Suger, the result of clerical attempts to harness and direct local piety? Eleventh- and twelfth-century accounts of these cults suggest the latter but they are a product of their time, and cannot be used as evidence for the forces at work when the cult first began in, say, the eighth century.

Such sites – be they local features or local churches – are interesting because they are not always associated with the possession of the physical relics of a saint, as was the case for the great central medieval shrines built in monastic or cathedral churches. Rather they owed their reputation to oral traditions linking the saint to that particular place as, for example, Julia Smith shows to have been the case for several local Breton cults. As such they are testimony to vibrant traditions of local piety. The clergy of Quimper removed the relics of St Corentin, the patron saint of this Breton see, to inland France in the face of Viking attacks in the ninth century, and distributed them to other monasteries in Paris and the Loire. His cult in central medieval Brittany therefore could not be based on his physical remains, which were now elsewhere, but rather on his association with certain local features in the landscape. For example, St Corentin's healing spring at Kerfeunteun, which is known from a thirteenth-century account of a man who had the temerity to fish in it, had a chapel associated with it which regularly attracted crowds of local people. As the presence of this chapel suggests, such local cults may not have been established independently of the clergy but rather in conjunction with them. Such an alliance of lay and clerical interests is clearly reported as at work in another example, this time from an eleventh-century account of the origins of a particular cult site in Lille in northern France. It occurs in a text recording the miracles worked by the relics of St Ursmer when the monks of Lobbes toured Flanders and northern France in the mid-eleventh century. The townspeople of Lille, we are told, set up a cross at the crossroads where the monks had set down the relics of St Ursmer when they visited the town; the cross later became a site for miracle cures. Relics, monastic initiative and lay support all contributed to the establishment of this particular site of divine power within the local urban landscape.[8]

The story of why this particular cross became the site for local piety does not survive, and its omission from the monks' miracle account points to a wider problem with the evidence for local cults. Detailed contemporary written documentation in the form of saints' lives, accounts of the translation of their relics, and posthumous miracle collections, is limited to those cults under the control of religious communities anxious to defend their cults in particular circumstances. Thus there is an inherent evidential bias in the written record in favour of the conclusion that lay piety came under the control of religious communities rather than existing as an autonomous phenomenon. The clergy of the cathedral at Quimper, for example, only recorded the miracle which took place at the spring at Kerfeunteun because of the attempt to violate the spring's claim to holiness, and to treat it like any other spring as a source of fish rather than recognising its distinctive status.[9] Other communities' accounts of the successful miracles worked at their shrines also sought, in their different ways, to promote and protect the interests of their custodian communities, demonstrating the efficacy of their patron in the wake of challenges to their property and jurisdictional privileges. They are evidence for clerical ambitions and interests, rather than for those of the lay audience for the cult. Such narratives are also formulaic and often drew on literary tropes and earlier textual precedents. At the same time they demonstrate the attempts made by religious communities to reach out to establish authority over, and make links with, the wider lay communities alongside whom they lived. Moreover, as we shall see, their authors often had reasons for portraying support for these cults as numerous, socially diverse and voluntary.

Such accounts usually record the crowds which attended the cult. As we have already seen, in thirteenth-century Brittany crowds attended the healing spring at Kerfeunteun. But such crowds are a common trope within the literature. In tenth-century Winchester 'more and more of the faithful', as well as the clergy, attended the translation of the relics of St Swithun from his grave to the minister church in 971, joining the clergy in an all-night vigil by the tomb, having kept a three-day fast, before witnessing the translation of the relics to the cathedral the following day.[10] Each person from Winchester, of all ages, and both sexes, free and unfree, was ordered to process barefoot three miles outside the city to meet a crowd (*turba*) accompanying a new gold and silver reliquary, commissioned by the king for the relics of St Swithun, from its place of manufacture on a royal estate; a relic of St Swithun had already been placed in the new reliquary, and when the two groups met they accompanied the relic into the city.[11] The language of the account echoed that of the Gospel's description of Christ's entry into Jerusalem on Palm Sunday when he was met by a crowd.[12] Thus the presence of the laity is an essential feature of a text describing St Swithun's triumphant entry into the town, and through its language links St Swithun to Christ. Yet, clerical hyperbole also refers to such crowds sometimes getting out of hand. Writing in *c.*1030 in south-western France, Adhemar of Chabannes, recorded how the crowd (*multitudine populi*) attending the night vigil at the tomb of St Martial in Limoges some twelve years earlier had been so large that more than fifty people, men and women, were trampled to death in the crush.[13] A century later, Abbot Suger described the crush which had built up in the old church of Saint-Denis on feast days, as the density of the crowds of men and women who came 'to worship and kiss the holy relics, the Nail and the Crown of the Lord' meant no one 'could do anything but stand like a marble statue, stay benumbed or, as a last resort, scream'.[14] In all four of these cases the crowd's presence serves to demonstrate the cult's popularity, and also, at least in Suger's case, the need to rebuild the church. It also allows writers, and readers, to echo the language of the Gospels and thus to reinforce, in their audience's mind, the link between Christ's mission and the appeal of their own saint. Popularity in all these accounts is essential testimony to the cult's success.

The writers of such accounts looked to stress not only their popular appeal, but also the universality and generally voluntary nature of the audience for the cult. Their saint should attract support from across the social spectrum, ranging from kings and nobles to merchants and peasants, from the free to the unfree. Writing in the late ninth century, for example, Adrevald recorded how the beneficiaries of miracles worked by the relics of St Benedict at the monastery of Fleury in the Loire valley ranged from the viscount of Tonnerre to an unnamed poor man.[15] He carefully emphasised how, although the relics were housed in the church within the monastic enclosure, and thus out of bounds to all women, the abbot and monks listened to the pleas of women and nobles to be allowed access to them, and set up a pavilion

> *outside the gate of the monastery . . . [to which] the relics of the saints were brought at a certain time, that is on the vigil of the Lord's day, and remained there under the reverent guard of both monks and clerks until the same hour on the Lord's day, when they were taken back to the sacred building. When this was done, multitudes of common people, not only from the neighbourhood, but from faraway places, flocked there to seek remedy for body and soul.*[16]

Half a century later, Odo of Cluny took up the same theme when he recorded in a sermon on St Benedict that the miracles worked by that saint's relics meant that 'Not just country folk (*pagenses*), but even people (*plebs*) from the city, a mingling of noblemen and distinguished clerics' came together to seek the saint's patronage not just on the feast of his translation but also on other feasts dedicated to him.[17]

Yet later in our period the imagined constituency for these cults became less socially diverse. Modern scholars investigating the audience for eleventh- and twelfth-century cults in France and England have suggested that clerics in this period began to target very particular groups within the community. Pierre André Sigal's analysis of the miracle collections generated by fundraising tours in northern France and Flanders and southern England in the eleventh and twelfth centuries, for example, suggests that 65 per cent of miracles were experienced by members of the bourgeoisie rather than the clergy.[18] Simon Yarrow has similarly noted that many beneficiaries of twelfth-century English miracle collections were members of the new, and growing, urban communities.[19] Their researches suggest that this bias towards townspeople reflects the attempt by their monastic authors to recognise the burgeoning power and influence of the new urban elite.[20] The old certainties of a world dominated by nobles, at one end of the spectrum, and peasants at the other, were giving way to a new one in which townspeople had much greater independence. Monks trod their way carefully in this new world, but used established methods, promoting their authority over this increasingly important social group through their particular saint's miracle-working powers.

Such accounts thus tell us much more about the needs and aspirations of their custodian clerical communities than about those of their clientele. Nowhere is this more clear than in the miracle story, found in many collections, in which a pilgrim is described as visiting many other shrines unsuccessfully, before being cured at that particular shrine. A version of it is recorded in an account written in the Loire monastery at Micy in the late eleventh century. It records how a man called Henry, who suffered severe pain, had a vision in which he was told to 'search for the tomb of St Maximinus . . . You will return to health there through God's mercy'. He set out for the tomb going first to Trier, but despite keeping vigil there at the tomb of their St Maximinus, was not cured, and thence to St Maximinus of Chinon, near Tours, where he was also unsuccessful, before visiting Micy where he was cured on the saint's feast day.[21] This text demonstrates the problems covered by shrines dedicated to saints with the same name, and seeks to assert Micy's primacy. Sometimes the accounts demonstrate the shrine's superiority to more recent rivals which might challenge its influence within a particular area; for example, a late twelfth-century collection of miracles worked at Durham by the seventh-century monk and hermit, St Cuthbert, mentions the cure of four sick men who had first visited the nearby shrine of the twelfth-century hermit Godric of Finchale, some four miles away, but had been referred to St Cuthbert by Godric himself.[22] Nor need rivals come from within the immediate vicinity: further miracles in the same account assert St Cuthbert's superiority over the new shrine of St Thomas at Canterbury in Kent.

Their monastic authors composed these texts with multiple audiences in mind. The primary one was usually the clerical community which served as guardians of that particular shrine, but many miracle accounts seem to have been composed with a much wider audience in mind, judging from the didactic agenda behind many of these stories. Punishment and vengeance miracles are a frequent feature of such accounts, especially in the tenth and early eleventh centuries. Such miracles generally seem to be part of an attempt to defend the community's claims to property against those of rival lay claimants. Thus the eleventh-century collection of miracles for the shrine of Ste Foy at Conques, in south-western France, included the following miracle:

> *In the province of Quercythere was a noblewoman . . . [who] obsessively coveted the holy martyr's lands that adjoined her own fields. Therefore she subjected the farmworkers ploughing the monks' field to a great deal of abuse and succeeded in driving them away. The next day she arranged to have this field ploughed with her own ploughshare, and she dared to make it part of her own property. And so divine power brought it about that, while she was ordering that her property line be extended to include the field and insisting strenuously, her whole body shrivelled instantly and she croaked and hissed horribly as she sent her miserable soul down to Orcus [Hell]. The ploughmen were terrified by her horrendous death and fled the field, leaving the plough behind. Out of breath and completely distraught, they scarcely managed to tell their lord what had happened. He grieved over his wife's death, sent for her body, and had it buried. And after she was destroyed in this way, the holy martyr's land was henceforth safe from all who had designs on it, and remained afterwards the property of the monks.*[23]

This account works on several levels and points to several different audiences. First, this miracle may have been intended for preaching to an audience of lay nobles who might, otherwise, have been similarly tempted to maintain their claims to lands owned by the monastery. Monastic charter collections are full of disputes between monasteries and their lay neighbours about the ownership of particular properties. It also therefore spoke to monks who felt vulnerable to attack, and in its written form the tale presumes a learned audience; it is likely that only highly educated churchmen would recognise the reference to Orcus, a Roman god of the underworld and punisher of perjurers. The manuscript evidence supports this assumption, for the collection is found in the libraries of several northern French institutions. But for the occurrence of the miracle to have been witnessed, and thus a record of it made, the ploughmen also needed to be there. The tale therefore required, and spoke to, a varied audience. The whole process of reporting, recording and listening to this tale points to the socially diverse constituency for this particular miracle.

Healing miracles, which are an even more dominant feature of such accounts, similarly testify to the complicity of the wider community in the process, for they too require independent witnesses to the occurrence of the miracle. Sick people seldom visited shrines alone and unsupported: rather accounts in collections from both England and France suggest friends and family usually accompanied them. Lantfred's late tenth-century account of the miracles worked by St Swithun after the translation of his relics to the new church at Winchester records, for example, how a London man, who was paralysed in all his limbs, having heard of the miracles taking place at St Swithun's tomb, 'was taken – in accordance with his wishes – by his kinsmen to Winchester . . . [where] he was cured on the night of his arrival by heavenly agency'.[24] In the mid-eleventh century the parents of a paralysed man from the Agenais took him to the shrine of Ste Foy in Conques, where he was cured.[25] In the late twelfth century Edilda of Canterbury, who was paralysed from the knee down, was carried to the shrine of St Thomas by three women, where she was cured; Robert, a blacksmith from the Isle of Thanet, who was blind for two years, journeyed to the same shrine with the guidance of his wife and daughter, where he was cured after daubing his eyes in St Thomas's blood.[26] These travelling companions served as witnesses; that they usually comprised family or neighbours conjures up a world in which a much wider community participated in one individual's experience. Both punishment and healing miracles thus promoted a similar message about the judgment of the omniscient Lord, and the possibility of redemption for all. In order to ensure this message's pastoral success, however, such miracles had to be depicted as taking place in familiar contexts, in the field, or at the shrine but with the support of family and friends.

At the same time as many clerical authors sought to universalise the audience for their cults, by recording their wide appeal, as well by recording the size of the crowds which attended particular shrines, some also described the very specific lay practices followed at the shrine. Can such accounts be used as evidence for the nature of popular devotion? Or are they too part of a clerical rhetoric in support of the shrine's popularity? What are we to make of stories such as that told by Bernard of Angers about how the pilgrims to Ste Foy chose to worship at her shrine? A northern Frenchman, Bernard visited the monastery of Ste Foy at Conques in south-western France and compiled two books of miracles worked at her shrine in *c.*1010. In them he records his shock at witnessing how the local peasants kept their vigils in their own ways:

> *It has been the custom since the old days that pilgrims always keep vigils in Ste Foy's church with candles and lights, while clerics and those who are literate chant psalms and the office of the vigil. But those who are illiterate relieve the weariness of the long night with little peasant songs and other frivolities. This seemed to ruin utterly the solemn dignity and decency of the sacred vigil.*[27]

Bernard went on to describe how he had preached about this 'detestable and absurd custom' to the monks of the custodian community in chapter. They, however, had defended the practice, saying that they had previously tried to forbid 'the unsuitable commotion made by the wild outcries of the peasants and their unruly singing, but they were unable to enforce silence', and had decided to shut the doors to the church at night so that the peasants could not attend the vigils but that, when shut out, the pilgrims had stood outside the monastery begging to be let in, and whilst the monks were sleeping, the bars of the doors of the church had opened of their own accord, so that when the monks rose for matins, they 'found the church so full of people keeping the vigil that each one of us had difficulty forcing his way forward to his station' in choir. In the light of this miracle, the monks, and subsequently Bernard of Angers, reconsidered their initial dismissal of the peasants' songs. In the words of Bernard:

> *I am satisfied that on account of the simplicity of those people, an innocent little song, even a peasant song, can be tolerated somehow. For it may be that if this custom were abolished, the crowds that frequent the sanctuary would also disappear. Nevertheless, we should not believe that God rejoices over a little song; it is the hardship of keeping vigil and the good will of simple people that please Him . . . these peasants are permitted to sing the songs that they know while their celebration is directed towards the One God Himself.*

Bernard self-consciously constructed the peasants' practices as different: he defended them not because he accepted the validity of an alternative 'lay liturgy' but because he wished to make the point that God is interested in the intentions of all Christians, not just those of 'high learning'.[28] He thus made a rhetorical distinction between the rites of the learned monks and those of the peasant audience in order to support his arguments about universality and intention.[29] Knowledge of this strategy need not, however, prohibit us from accepting it as having some relationship to 'popular' practice, for his tale would probably not have convinced his readers if it did not.

Accounts from other shrines similarly testify to lay practices at the shrine which are independent of the liturgical rites conducted by the custodian clergy. Their authors recounted each of them for a different reason but taken together they suggest a very clear and distinctive image of lay devotions independent of those of the clergy. The author of a sermon, '*Veneranda dies*', which survives now in a twelfth-century manuscript of various materials about the cult of St James of Compostella, records the practices of the pilgrims of diverse nationalities who made the journey to Compostella:

> *Whoever sees these choruses of pilgrims keeping vigil around the venerable altar of Blessed James marvels with extreme delight: Germans remain in one area, French in another, Italians in a throng in another, holding burning candles in their hands from which the whole church is lit up like the sun on the brightest of days. Each one sagaciously carries out his vigils by himself with his countrymen. Some sing with lutes, some with lyres, some with drums, some with flutes, some with pipes, some with trumpets, some with harps, some with violas, some with British or Gallic wheels, some with psalteries. Some keep vigil by singing to the various kinds of music; some lament their sins; some read psalms; and some give alms to the blind.*[30]

Whilst the author's main aim is to convey the international nature of the pilgrimage, he also suggests the active devotion of the laity, through portraying their participation in a liturgy independent of that of the clergy of the church of Compostella. This codex also contains a collection of miracles which includes an account of the pilgrimage by the count of Saint-Gilles and his brother from Provence. When the two arrived the count requested permission to keep the vigil in front of Saint James's tomb, but the clergy refused his request as it was the custom to close the gates of the oratory from sunset until sunrise. The count returned to his lodgings and 'said to all those present that he wanted to go to Saint James with those of a similar mind accompanying him, if, by chance, the place should deign to open for them all by itself'. A large group of some two hundred people thus approached the church with lamps, and as they did so they prayed to Saint James to allow them in to keep the vigil; as they did so the locks and chains on the gates became undone 'by an invisible power', allowing them to enter, just as the doors of the church in Conques had opened to allow the laity to keep the vigil by Ste Foy's relics in their own manner.[31] The trope of the miraculously opening doors thus testifies to the voluntary nature of the cult, as well as its popularity. Similarly, other accounts report pilgrims making up their own songs. The collection of miracles compiled for the shrine of Our Lady of Rocamadour (1172–73) describe how it was the custom of a minstrel, Peter Ivern, on arrival at churches to 'pour out his prayers to the Lord, after which he would play upon the strings of his lute and sing the Lord's praises'. He followed this practice when he came to the shrine of the Virgin Mary at Rocamadour, and after a while he asked the Virgin that she grant him a piece from the measures of waxes hanging there, perhaps as *ex voto* offerings, if his playing and singing pleased her, and 'as he played and sang in this way, and in the full view of those who were present, a little piece of wax dropped onto his instrument'. This upset the guardian of the church, the monk Gerard, who put the valuable wax back on the altar, but Peter carried on singing and the wax dropped down again, and Gerard again restored it to its proper place; it happened a third time, and amazed all those present. Peter then returned the wax to the altar, praising God, and throughout the rest of his life gave an annual offering of a pound of wax to the shrine.[32] Here the tale of lay devotion is used to account for, and promote, gifts to the shrine, as well as indicating the importance of each praising the Virgin in his or her own way. No doubt this account of the tension between Gerard and Peter captures something of the complicated nature of relations between custodians and pilgrims at such shrines. All three accounts – those from Conques, Compostella and Rocamodour – share the idea that the laity had their own way of celebrating the saint with their own chants. The extent to which they are a portrait of a specific lay experience is harder to judge, for the popularity of, and popular features of, these cults are both a necessary part of their authors' argument.

But these texts contain other hints which suggest that the clergy were anxious to ensure their shrines appealed to a lay audience. In many collections miracles seem to have been deliberately pitched to reflect the concerns of the laity in the immediate vicinity of the shrine: thus in the Auvergne and Rouergue Ste Foy freed local knights imprisoned by their enemies, reflecting the acrimonious politics of that region in the eleventh century; men and women from Winchester, Hampshire and the Isle of Wight formed the main constituency for the cult of St Swithun; and the townsmen and women of Oxford feature prominently amongst the beneficiaries of miracles at the shrine of St Frideswide in the late twelfth century, although others came from further afield.[33] The gaudy nature of many reliquaries no doubt appealed to lay as well as clerical taste. Bernard of Angers defended the inhabitants of the Auvergne, Rouergue and Toulouse against the charge of idolatry because they erected gold statues to their saints, decorated with precious stones:

> *The image [of Ste Foy] represents the pious memory of the holy virgin before which, quite properly and with abundant remorse, the faithful implore her intercession for their sins.*[34]

The metalwork required considerable investment: Ste Foy's crown was donated by a Carolingian prince; in England King Edgar commissioned the reliquary of St Swithun from a goldsmith. Such examples of elaborate metalwork reflect an attempt to make the shrine distinctive and to reflect the esteem in which the faithful held the saint.

But how far did the services at such shrines offer the laity a different religious experience to that provided by their own local church? It is clear that local communities might be expected to attend the shrine itself on feast days, especially if their usual local church lay on the estates of the guardian community for the shrine. One miracle in the Rocamadour collection, for example, describes how one priest took his parishioners to the shrine of Our Lady of Rocamadour every year on the feast of the nativity of the Virgin.[35] Is this because of the nature of the religious experience or is it a statement of the monks' authority within the area? Given how little we know about the liturgy on offer in local churches, it is impossible to establish how far the liturgy of popular shrines might be designed to appeal to the laity more than that of their home church.[36] Rather such evidence as we have presents the shrine as a complement to existing local religious services.

The success of shrines such as Rocamadour and Conques manifests itself in the churches built and rebuilt to house them. The considerable financial support they received from pilgrims made them possible. That at Conques, for example, was rebuilt in the second half of the eleventh and twelfth centuries in the Romanesque style. Abbot Suger rebuilt that at Saint-Denis in the mid-twelfth century in the new Gothic style. Both churches were extended to accommodate pilgrim congregations, and ambulatories were built so that pilgrims could progress around behind the high altar where the shrine was located. They manifest in stone the popularity of these cults.

But pilgrims left more mundane traces too. The popularity of such shrines is also testified to by the extent to which these sites became market centres. The author of the *Veneranda dies* sermon lists the range of goods on sale in the market place outside the church in Compostella – food, medicines, belts and other leather goods, cloth, and candles – before warning of the dangers pilgrims might face from merchants anxious to make a profit from them.[37] Lesser shrines also attracted markets. The Cluniac priory of Bromholm in Norfolk acquired a relic of the True Cross sometime in the late twelfth century; it soon became the centre of a local cult. Recent archaeological investigation has uncovered evidence that markets were regularly held within the precincts of the monastery itself, presumably to cater for the pilgrims who came to the church.[38] It is useful evidence of the role that such cults played within their local environment.

The laity's presence at such shrines thus served several different functions within the rhetoric of different authors' accounts. The ways in which lay supporters are depicted therefore have a good deal to tell us about the ambitions of the clerical custodians of these cults. Whilst the laity's participation is usually cited to attest to the success of a particular cult, the specific demographic features which writers chose to emphasise – the age, class, and gender of lay participants – indicate the ambitions of the clerical guardians of the cult rather than the nature of the actual audience. By focusing on the people of Winchester and Hampshire, for example, Lantfred tells us more about how the community at Winchester cathedral wished to assert its authority over the town and its lands than the devotional preferences of people living in that area. Similarly the focus of many of the Ste Foy miracles on local landowners suggests the importance of that particular constituency for the support of the monastic community guarding her shrine at Conques in the Rouergue. It might be thought that the local loyalty of Hampshire people to their local saint, St Swithun, could be relied upon, but, as Simon Yarrow has shown in his study of English twelfth-century cults, the allegiance of local communities could be more fickle. The canons of Laon visited the town of Christchurch in Dorset, for example, as part of their fundraising relic tour of southern England to support the rebuilding of their cathedral; the clergy of Christchurch minster refused them hospitality but the burghers of the town took them in, giving them support and lodging. In this case the canons of Laon benefited from an otherwise unknown dispute between the townspeople of Christchurch and the established clergy.[39] This story hints at what may have been more widespread tensions, and the fact that local support could not be presumed helps explain why churchmen invested so much energy in defining and recording the constituency for their particular cult. But they cited lay devotion for other reasons as well: to justify the locus of a particular local cult, as that of the Virgin Mary at Champ, Essonne or St Ursmer at Lille; to endorse the practice of giving very specific gifts to the shrine, such as that of wax to Our Lady of Rocamadour; to attest to the importance of the voluntary nature of such cults, as in the miraculously opening doors at Conques and Compostella; and to substantiate the theological argument that God is mindful of all Christians, not just educated ones, as in the case of Bernard of Anger's account of the 'peasant' liturgy to Ste Foy. Cumulatively, all these different tropes point to the underlying importance of lay popularity to written accounts of such cults. The laity's presence at such shrines had become a rhetorical necessity. It was also a physical reality. The survival of elaborate reliquaries wrought in precious metal, of substantial church buildings built to accommodate considerable crowds of visiting pilgrims, and the mundane remains of markets at such shrines all testify to the actuality of lay involvement. But such participation could not be presumed, it had to be fought for and won. Consequently the surviving evidence for cults often testifies to the tensions between churchmen and laity, but such anxieties and wranglings are, in themselves, evidence of ways in which particular ecclesiastical and lay communities came together to provide particular local focuses for their devotions.

Local religious movements: Peacemaking and rebuilding

It is only by understanding the ways in which monks thought about the laity that we can begin to understand one of the newer features of the three centuries between 900 and 1200, that is the various reports of the appearance of mass popular movements of lay people, all of which focused upon the renewal and promotion of Christian values which constitute one of the newer features of central medieval religious thought. Men and women are reported as coming together in groups which transcended class for very specific religiously inspired purposes, namely the promotion of peace and the physical rebuilding of specific churches. These movements are all reported from the French-speaking world of France, Flanders and southern England in the eleventh and twelfth centuries. Two, focused on peacemaking, originated in the south-west of France: the Peace of God movement which began in the late tenth century, and the Capuciati peacemaking brotherhood established in the Auvergne in the 1180s, almost two centuries later. The movements which originated in the north focused instead on church rebuilding: they comprise the fundraising relic tours for church rebuilding from the second half of the eleventh and early twelfth centuries, and the 'Cult of the Carts' from the 1140s. Each of these movements, taken on its own, is suggestive of new developments in popular piety and of growing enthusiasm for religious causes amongst the laity. Large groups of people came together for pious purposes, apparently on their own initiative, testifying to the successful internalisation of Christian values.

These movements are usually treated in isolation from each other as autonomous movements, which makes it easy to neglect their many shared features. Scholars have long acknowledged the debts these movements owed to the cult of the saints. Churchmen are described as using ritual elements drawn from the liturgical commemoration of the saints to direct these lay assemblies: the public display of relics; mass meetings of the laity; collective vows and prayers. It is thus not surprising to discover that clerical accounts of these movements are themselves heavily indebted to hagiographical conventions, as we shall see. But like the reports of saints' cults, the descriptions of these popular movements can tell us a good deal about the ways in which the clergy interacted with the laity on these occasions. Exploring the relationship between church and people on such occasions allows us to ask, on the one hand, how far the clergy harnessed lay support for particular cults to promote particular messages about reform and renewal and, on the other, the extent to which lay communities actively participated in such movements and employed features of the cult for their own ends. By investigating the parallels these movements share with each other and with features of the cult of the saints more generally we can reconsider their apparent novelty and ask how far they instead represent a continuum of ideas and practices across these centuries. They thus offer another prism through which it is possible to explore the tensions in the relationship between clergy and laity surrounding saints' cults.

We will treat them in chronological order. The earliest example of a popular movement in this period is the series of some twenty-six councils collectively known to modern scholars as the Peace of God movement. In recent years some scholars have suggested these councils represent a unique alliance of the clergy and the laity in favour of reform ideals. As we shall see, the written accounts built on existing conventions surrounding lay support for cults and, at the same time, paved the way for those for other movements. Beginning in south-western France – in Poitou, the Limousin and the Berry – in the late tenth century, these councils, attended by bishops, abbots, and secular magnates, sought to restrict violence against churchmen and ecclesiastical property, and against others unable to defend themselves: peasants and women. Those attending these councils swore oaths to abstain from such attacks on pain of anathema, the worst ecclesiastical sanction in the episcopal spiritual armoury. From 1027 the direction of the movement began to evolve into what is now known as the Truce of God as those present swore an oath to keep the peace on certain days of the week for certain periods. At the same time the movement itself began to spread outwards from south-western France into northern France, Flanders, the German Reich and central Italy.[40]

The evidence for these councils survives in a variety of different forms, but the authors of narrative accounts are anxious to depict them as mass occasions attended by large audiences of lay people. In the words of Rodulfus Glaber:

> *At the millennium of the Lord's Passion . . . the bishops and abbots and other devout men of Aquitaine first summoned great councils of the whole people (*ex uniuersa plebe*) to which were borne the bodies of many saints and innumerable caskets of holy relics. The movement spread to Arles and Lyons, then across all Burgundy into the furthest corner of the French realm. Throughout the dioceses it was decreed that in fixed places the bishops and magnates of the entire* patria *should convene councils for restoring the peace and celebrating the institution of the holy faith. When the entire*

> *populace heard this, great, middling and poor, they came rejoicing and ready, one and all, to obey the commands of the clergy no less than if they had been given by a voice from heaven speaking to men on earth.*[41]

Other reports testify to the 'crowds of common people without number of every age and both genders [who] hurried' to the site of the council, where monks brought their relics.[42] It is clear that these reports built on the universalist rhetoric which we have seen is a feature of the literature surrounding saints' cults; yet a contemporary critic of the movement, Andrew of Fleury, cited the rabble's involvement as one of his reasons for disliking the movement, suggesting that real phenomena underlay these descriptions.[43]

Recent scholars, however, have emphasised that the individual councils should be seen as much as a response to specific events or particular political contexts as part of a self-conscious movement.[44] They have acknowledged how the councils are less about the alliance of the Church with the masses than about the reassertion of local authority, both secular and ecclesiastical, in what was a far from peaceful world with weak royal rule. In the ninth century it had been the duty of Frankish kings to defend the persons and property of the poor and the weak, including clerics, peasants, widows and orphans, from attack; in the late tenth and eleventh centuries local lords assumed these duties, and in doing so enhanced their own lordship. In the words of the eleventh-century chronicler of much of this movement, at the council of Limoges in 994 the nobles present 'took peace oaths in the presence of both the duke [William V of Aquitaine] and of the assembled masses on the relics of the saint'.[45] The duke held a similar council at Poitiers almost two decades later at which both spiritual and secular penalties were invoked against those who disregarded the duke's authority, and refused to submit disputes to his court.[46] Maintenance of the peace constituted an essential component of early medieval Christian models of rulership; espousing the promotion of peace at a time of weak royal rule thus helped nobles in the construction of their own authority. Nobles such as the duke of Aquitaine therefore used these councils to assert their authority and lordship in areas where it was well established, or where they wished to establish it.[47] For secular nobles played a significant role in orchestrating and directing such councils, often because, as we have already seen in Chapter 3, they cannot be easily distinguished from the ecclesiastical leadership. Geoffrey Greymantle, count of Anjou, and advocate of the

Sainte-Croix convent in Poitiers, was also the brother of Guy, bishop of le Puy, who held a council in *c.*975 which is sometimes seen as a precursor to the 'first' peace council of Charroux in 989; Guy was in turn also related to Archbishop Gunbaldus who presided on that later occasion. And nobles frequently used their title of lay abbot to expand their authority in the region: Duke William used the title of lay abbot of the college of Saint-Hilaire in Poitou in his charters, for example.[48] That these councils continued to be directed at the nobility, rather than the wider populace, is clear from Adhemar of Chabannes' account of the council of Limoges in 1031 in which he records how Bishop Jordan addressed the *milites* specifically, calling on them to restore what they had stolen from the church and the poor, citing the example of Zacchaeus, a repentant sinner who is described in Luke 19.1–10 as a rich prince who submitted to Christ, returned what he had unjustly taken from the poor, and was saved.[49] The choice of subject here suggests the importance of a noble audience to this council.

Although it is possible that there was a popular lay presence at many of them, the Peace of God councils must therefore be viewed within the context of noble politics. Although clerical accounts of such occasions referred to popular participation, they adopted this feature from hagiography to testify to the success of these councils. They seem therefore to be movements of the elite, grounded in earlier ideas of the role of nobles in preserving the peace, rather than mass movements of the populace.

The next movement to appear in the records is comprised of the various accounts of the wide support given to particular communities of churchmen when they took the relics of their particular patron saint on a tour in order to raise funds for the rebuilding of the saint's church. Such accounts survive only from the late eleventh century onwards, but in all some eighteen accounts of successful fundraising relic tours conducted by existing religious communities exist from the late eleventh and twelfth centuries.[50] In their reports, churchmen depict the rebuilding of particular churches as being accompanied by popularist religious revival movements. It is difficult for modern scholars to know what to make of such descriptions and whether they can be trusted: how far are their descriptions of large crowds turning out to witness the miracles wrought by the relics of the saint merely the result of the continuation of the rhetoric of a universal Church which was, as we have already seen, such a common component in accounts of particular saints' miracles? Or are they, rather, evidence for the importance churchmen attributed to lay support for providing essential funds to underpin the costs of such reconstructions? And how far can we read across such accounts to distinguish clerical motives from those of the lay communities they encountered: can we use these descriptions to identify the extent to which these tours met the concerns and needs of those lay communities which chose to take part? Or do they tell us only about those of the guardians of these relics? Further investigation of two specific accounts allows us to begin to answer these questions.

The earliest reported example of such a movement dates to 1060 when some monks from the community at Lobbes took the relics of their founder, St Ursmer, on a tour around Flanders.[51] The tour took place against a backdrop of a recent outbreak of plague, which had led many of Lobbes' surviving peasant tenants to flee their lands, and recent wars between the German emperor and count of Flanders which had led to the loss of various of the community's lands in Flanders. At the same time the monastery's church had been, we are told, reduced to being 'a decrepit ruin'. The tour thus had two objectives: to raise funds for the rebuilding of the church, and to obtain comital support for the restoration of their lands. At each place they visited, the monks set down the relics of St Ursmer, and used the occasion to call the feuding nobility together and to ask them to make peace with each other by swearing on the relics of St Ursmer. A revivalist Christian message thus accompanied fundraising but the focus of the tour was on the nobility rather than the peasantry. Here the universalist aspects of the account seem secondary to the more specific interests of the Lobbes community.

Other accounts, however, suggest some clerical promoters were alert to the money-raising potential of appealing to a socially broader audience. In his detailed study of twelfth-century saints' cults, Simon Yarrow demonstrates how the canons of Laon cathedral sought to translate the universalist rhetoric into specific support from both the urban bourgeoisie and the peasantry. They undertook a tour of relics of the Virgin Mary around central France and southern England in 1112 and 1113. Two records of the tour survive: that by Hermann, former abbot of Tournai, who wrote up his account in the mid-1140s, but seemingly based it on the canons' own records, and that by Guibert of Nogent, who wrote a more critical account in *c.*1115.[52] The tour took place in the wake of an uprising by the citizens of Laon against the bishop which had resulted in his murder, and a fire which severely damaged the cathedral and twelve other churches within the city. Hermann records how the canons raised some 120 marks, plus gifts of textiles and ornaments, on the English leg of the trip; this precision suggests his account is based on earlier records kept by the canons on tour.[53] As noted above, Hermann also records how the canons occasionally encountered objections from the clergy of churches in towns which they visited, as at Christchurch in Dorset. There the visiting canons were able to take advantage of the local townspeople's grievances against the local ecclesiastical elite to attract support for their cause.[54] But, as Hermann makes clear, the laity did not just provide funds for the rebuilding work; they also sometimes played an active part in it. He records how two cripples were cured when the canons visited the castle of Issoudun, and then joined those working on rebuilding the cathedral, encouraging the people by carrying stones and water, and preparing mortar. When the work on the church had been completed, one man went home, whilst the other joined the staff of the hospital in Laon as a servant. The implication is that although the men lacked the financial resources to contribute to the rebuilding fund, they could contribute in other ways.[55] It seems, given the specificity of Hermann's account, that the Laon canons deliberately set out to attract support from new constituencies. In this the requirements of the canons' ambitions met those of members of the laity who had become dissatisfied with current ecclesiastical provisions in new ways. Again the initiative came from the clergy but the laity were crucial to its success.

The involvement of peasants like those from the castle of Issoudun in the rebuilding of a church anticipates the next mass religious movement to be reported: that now known as 'the cult of the carts'.[56] This movement began in northern France in the 1140s as laymen and women came together as an act of physical devotion to drag the carts of materials needed for ecclesiastical rebuilding projects. Although this practice may have earlier origins, as we shall see, it seems to have begun at Chartres in 1144, where two reports survive which describe how men and women began to drag carts of stone and beams by hand for the construction of the new cathedral.[57] The words of one account emphasise how this activity was not confined to the lower orders:

> *Whoever saw, whoever heard in all the generations past [of such a thing], that kings, princes,* potentates, *puffed up with honours and riches, men and women of noble birth, should bind bridles upon their proud and*

> *swollen necks and submit them to wagons (*plaustris*) which, after the fashion of brute beasts, they dragged with their loads of wine, grain, oil, lime, stones, and beams, and whatever else is necessary to sustain life or for the construction of churches, even to Christ's abode.*[58]

Haymo, abbot of the Norman house of St Pierre-sur-Dives, wrote this account in a letter addressed to his house's priory at Tetbury in Staffordshire promoting the practice. He goes on to describe how priests oversaw the work. Each priest presided over a 'cart of Christ' exhorting those taking part to penance, confession, lamentation and the resolution of a better life; at each halt they preached peace and forgiveness, and those who refused to join in the peacemaking were cast out from the group, and their offering removed from the cart as unclean. When the carts arrived at the church of Notre Dame in Chartres, those taking part submitted to flagellation from their priests, and, stripping off their clothes, lay on the ground, and crawled to the high altar to pray to the Mother of God, and patron of Chartres, for the answer to their prayers. This led to a mass healing of all the sick and infirm.

This rite spread from Chartres to Normandy where it became associated with churches dedicated to Mary; in Normandy, too, much was made of the need for those taking part to confess their sins, and to make peace with their enemies.[59] The written account of the rebuilding of the cathedral of Châlons-sur-Marne, composed between 1162 and 1171, also owes much to Haymo's account.[60] The cult seems to have been revived again at Chartres when the cathedral was rebuilt again in 1194.[61] Abbot Suger described similar lay efforts in his account of how devoted neighbours, both noble and ignoble, joined the abbey's men to haul classical columns out of a quarry for the rebuilding of the church of Saint-Denis.[62] The old church had grown too small to accommodate increasing numbers of pilgrims; Suger thus made an explicit link between the need for a new church to house visiting pilgrims, and the rebuilding which was itself accomplished owing to the miraculous involvement of the laity. Suger wrote in *c.*1145 about events which had taken place before 1140; it is unclear whether events in Chartres and Normandy influenced his account, or whether it represents an earlier example of this practice.

All these accounts, but Haymo's in particular, bring together many of the elements found in accounts of both earlier mass movements and of lay devotion to the saints. The universalism of crowds of laymen and women from every class coming together for a common purpose was fundamental to descriptions of all these movements. The role of mutual peacemaking amongst participants had been integral to accounts of both the Peace of God councils and those of some fundraising campaigns, like that of the Lobbes community. The religious value attributed to physical work had an immediate precedent in the Laon community's funding campaign, but its emphasis on the salutary effects of manual labour also drew upon the importance attached to such efforts in the rules for monastic life. As we saw in Chapter 4 the value that monastic orders such as the Cistercians placed on manual work led them to offer new opportunities to the laity to enter the religious life as labourers, *conversi*. But the significance they attribute to labour had its roots in the Rule of Benedict. The 'cult of the cart' thus seems to represent the extension of these general monastic values more widely to the laity. But the ways in which monastic writers like Haymo understood such contributions also owed something to earlier hagiographical traditions. For the significance they attributed to the practice also has its roots in the ways in which earlier churchmen understood distinct lay Christian practices as evidence for God's acceptance of the importance of the intentions of all Christians. Just as Bernard of Angers accepted the peasants' own ways of praising Ste Foy, so his successors came to value the physical contributions of twelfth-century men and women. Haymo built on earlier elements in his account of the 'cult', but he also identified a new element which is not mentioned in accounts of earlier mass religious movements: penance. Participation in the cult is treated as a form of penance: the participants confess their sins, undertake strenuous, demeaning work as a form of penance, and thus, renewed, vow to live a better life. Participation led to personal reform. Individual efforts collectively led to the rebuilding of the Church. Thus personal and institutional initiatives joined together in a single movement for the renewal of the Church itself.

As this analysis indicates, Haymo's account is a very self-conscious piece of ecclesiastical rhetoric. It seems unlikely, given the number of different examples, that the 'cult of the carts' was merely a literary trope, but it is worth noting that the accounts we have are also heavily influenced by earlier texts, starting with the Bible. The Latin word for cart, 'plaustra', is the term used in the Vulgate to refer to the vehicle on which the Ark of the Covenant was carried back to Jerusalem by King David, accompanied by singing and music, where it was housed in the temple built by his successor,

Solomon. Conventional medieval biblical exegesis interpreted the Ark of the Covenant as presaging Jesus Christ, and linked the drawing of the ark especially to church building.[63] The decision to promote the drawing of cults and link them to these building campaigns thus found powerful biblical resonances. Previous authors had made this link. A fifth-century Greek text, Mark the Deacon's *Life of St Porphry*, bishop of Gaza, describes the faithful as dragging columns from the beach to build the cathedral in Gaza in 402–07.[64] A copy of this text certainly existed in eleventh-century Italy which may explain why the chronicler of Monte Cassino recorded in 1066 the faithful carrying the first column of the new abbey church 'on the strength of their necks and arms'.[65] Suger seems to have drawn on the Monte Cassino material for his own account. Monte Cassino may also have been the inspiration for the early twelfth-century account composed by a Belgian abbot, Roger of Saint-Trond, who described how the faithful contributed to the rebuilding of the abbey church between 1055 and 1082: they purchased building materials at their own expense and carried them on their shoulders and on carts, and dragged up columns without the use of carts.[66] Both biblical and earlier precedents lie behind surviving accounts of the efforts of participants in the 'cult of the carts'.

These accounts are self-conscious and highly literary creations. It is far from clear how far large numbers of lay men and women, motivated by the hope of forgiveness of their sins, and thus of increasing their chances of future salvation, took part in the 'cult of the carts' but the chances are that some of them did. It is a big leap from seeing the accounts as influenced by earlier texts to viewing them as fictional. Although it is impossible to identify the motives of lay participants except through the prism of clerical reporters it is important to recognise that the use of this rhetoric suggests that churchmen thought it important to portray this ecclesiastical rebuilding movement as the product of lay aspirations and effort.

Up to now we have focused on the ways in which clerical authors constructed their accounts of mass popular religious movements, and the reasons they might have had for portraying such movements as popular and socially diverse. In all the examples we have considered so far the clergy seem to have been firmly in control, albeit sometimes in conjunction with the secular elite, as is the case for the Peace of God councils. Seen through their eyes, the laity responded enthusiastically to clerical direction but did not initiate these new expressions of personal devotion. Sometimes, however, as in our final example of the Capuciati, the sources allow us to investigate the interplay of relationships between the clergy and the laity in greater depth, and to begin to uncover the degree to which the clerical control only came to be applied rather belatedly to cults which had their origins in lay popular devotion.

The Capuciati is a more short-lived peacemaking movement which began in southern France in the late twelfth century. The accounts of it, some supportive, some much more negative, suggest that unlike the Peace of God movement a century and half earlier it began within the lower echelons of the lay community before being taken up by the local ecclesiastical hierarchy. Like the earlier peace movement, it used elements from saints' cults to promote its message. It started in the Auvergne in 1182 when a carpenter called Durand Dujardin had a vision of the Virgin who was holding a picture of herself with the Christ child in her arms which bore the inscription 'Lamb of God who takes away the sins of the world, grant us peace'. This text, the *Agnus dei*, was recited by the priest in the Mass during the breaking of the Host, and would thus have been familiar to both the laity and the clergy. The Virgin told Durand to go to the bishop of Le Puy and to set up a brotherhood to maintain the peace. This he did, and the brotherhood quickly became established; reports of it soon reached Saint-Denis and Laon in northern France and Canterbury in England.[67] Members of the brotherhood wore a uniform of a small white hood, from which hung two bands of cloth, one at the back, and one over the breast, and a pewter badge of the Virgin and Child with the words 'Lamb of God' on it. Each year at Pentecost members swore to go to Mass, and not to gamble, blaspheme, frequent taverns, wear foppish garments, or carry weapons; in other words they were to behave in a similar way to that expected of the secular clergy. In choosing this dress and way of life, members of the brotherhood sought to mark themselves off from their enemies, the brigands, against whom they swore to take action. They also swore to maintain the peace amongst themselves, even when one member of the brotherhood killed the relative of another. They even adopted the structures of a religious confraternity, paying an annual membership fee. The movement quickly spread from the Velay and the Auvergne, to Berry, Burgundy, Aquitaine and Provence.

Although the movement initially seems to have received the support of the churchmen in the area, within two years the brotherhood had come to be perceived as a challenge to lordly authority in the area, and the brotherhood is instead presented as a form of peasant rebellion against the excessive demands of lordship:

> *There was in Gaul a widespread enthusiasm which impelled people to revolt against the powerful. Though good at the outset the movement was nothing else than the work of the devil, disguised as an angel of light. The league of the sworn of Puy was only a diabolic invention. There was no longer fear or respect for superiors. All strove to acquire liberty, saying that it belonged to them from the time of Adam and Eve, from the very day of creation. They did not understand that serfdom is punishment of sin! The result was that there was no longer any distinction between great and small, but a fatal confusion tending to ruin the institutions which rule us all, through the will of God and the agency of the powerful on this earth . . . this formidable pestilence began to spread in most parts of France, especially in Berry, Auxerre and Burgundy. The adherents of the sect reached such a height of folly that they were ready to take by force the fights and liberties they claimed.*

This account goes on to describe how the newly appointed bishop of Auxerre, Hugh of Noyers (1183–1206) took armed action against members of the brotherhood, fining them and taking away their hoods, commanding them to go bareheaded for a year.[68] It is a panegyric to Bishop Hugh; what is portrayed by others as a pious, disciplined movement has become in this text a challenge to the social order by a mob which only the bishop was able to deal with effectively.

The earliest accounts to be written are by contrast much more supportive of the Capuciati, stressing the movement's order and organisation. They also emphasised its social diversity. Although founded by a carpenter, they report how bishops, counts and people of the middling sort as well as the poor all joined the sect. They clearly subscribe to the universalising norm which we have seen was usual in approving accounts of religious movements. It is thus not surprising that critics chose to invert these traits, portraying the movement as a rabble of 'stupid and undisciplined persons' who had the temerity to issues orders to their social superiors.[69] The rapid shift within one year from clerical approval to condemnation may hint at the failure of clerical attempts to prevent the radicalisation of a genuinely popular movement, or at their frustration of not being able to control it.

The movement clearly shared some features with the Peace of God councils two centuries earlier: participants swore to preserve the peace actively, and drew on the features of saints' cults for their origin and group identity. Yet, unlike the Peace of God meetings, the movement owed its inception to the actions of laymen. Whilst one account suggests that a canon of Le Puy had deceived Durand and acted as his puppet master, this report comes from a writer hostile to the Capuciati, and perhaps sought to explain away how it initially received clerical support by blaming it on one renegade priest.

The ways in which different churchmen chose to report the activities of the Capuciati point to the different tensions which clearly existed within the movement. The clergy never comprised a unity, but rather a series of rival groups, and the different accounts hint at the tensions between canons and bishop, and between different sees: the bishop of Le Puy authorised the movement, the bishop of Auxerre suppressed it. At the same time, the way in which a movement founded by a layman made use of the increasingly popular cult of the Virgin Mary, and adopted its structures and constitution from existing ecclesiastical organisations, points to the ways in which such devotion was never the monopoly of the clergy either.

Saints, and their cults, allowed the laity direct contact with the divine. Access to shrines, and participation in movements associated with saints' cults, thus offered individuals and local communities the chance to move beyond the contact mediated through the official rites of the Church presided over by clerics and monks.[70] Such opportunities help to explain their popularity, and their diversity.

But the evidence for such cults is highly problematic. As we have seen, the popularity of particular cults is a textual construct of their clerical custodians, anxious to promote individual shrines for their own purposes. Churchmen adduced examples of lay support and lay piety to create their claims for the importance of movements and cults in which they had an especial interest. In doing so they drew on a wealth of earlier textual precedents. Although we must acknowledge this, we also need to recognise that popularity is never an empty topos: rather clerical writers, as we have seen, chose to use it for very specific purposes. The examples of saints' cults and popular religious movements considered here, for example, are often treated in isolation, yet taken together they suggest the extent to which clergy could harness lay support for saints' cults to promote their own messages about the reform and renewal of the Church through the changes wrought on the individual. At the same time they hint that lay communities often bought into such movements for their own, to us generally unknown, reasons.

Control of particular cult sites or religiously inspired movements could be contested and, as we have seen, often was. It is an important feature of our source material that it is often only when the authority of their clerical custodians became challenged in some way that we learn about such cults. It is thus important to recognise how many other successful cults probably went unrecorded because no one contested them. Those we know about probably represent a rather atypical sample of those on offer to the people living in the medieval west. These problems notwithstanding, it is also clear that such cults served as an important focus for the piety for both the laity and the clergy living near them.

Notes and references

1 *Abbot Suger on the Abbey Church of St Denis and its Art Treasures*, ed. and trans. Erwin Panofsky (Princeton, NJ, 1946), 9–10.

2 In general, see P. Brown, *The Cult of Saints: Its Rise and Function in Latin Christianity* (London, 1981); J. Howard-Johnston and P. A. Hayward, eds, *The Cult of Saints in Late Antiquity and the Early Middle Ages* (Oxford, 1999); S. Yarrow, *Saints and their Communities: Miracle Stories in Twelfth-century England* (Oxford, 2006); J. M. H. Smith, 'Saints and Their Cults', in Noble and Smith, eds, *The Cambridge History of Christianity: Early Medieval Christianities c.600–c.1100*, 581–605.

3 *Vita et Miracula S. Kenelmi*, in *Three Eleventh-century Anglo-Latin Saints' Lives: Vita S. Birini, Vita et Miracula S. Kenelmi and Vita S. Rumwoldi*, ed. R. Love (Oxford, 1996), 50–73; on places and landmarks associated with the saint recorded in later writings, see J. Blair, 'A Saint for Every Minster? Local Cults in Anglo-Saxon England', in A. Thacker and R. Sharpe, eds, *Local Saints and Local Churches in the Early Medieval West* (Oxford, 2002), 455–94 at p. 483, n. 81.

4 Yarrow, *Saints and Their Communities*, 169–88.

5 Blair, 'A Saint for Every Minster?', 473, 477; idem, 'A Handlist of Anglo-Saxon Saints', in Thacker and Sharpe, eds, *Local Saints*, 495–565 at pp. 545–47, 562.

6 O. J. Padel, 'Local Saints and Place-names in Cornwall', in Thacker and Sharpe, eds, *Local Saints*, 303–60.

7 J. M. H. Smith, 'Oral and Written: Saints, Miracles and Relics in Brittany, *c.*850–1250', *Speculum* 65 (1990), 309–43 at p. 337.

8 'The Miracles of St Ursmer and His Journey through Flanders', c. 3, ed. and trans. G. Koziol in Head, *Medieval Hagiography*, 346.

9 Smith, 'Oral and Written', 329.

10 Wulfstan of Winchester, *Narratio metrica de S. Swithuno*, i. v, in M. Lapidge, *The Cult of St Swithun* (Oxford, 2003), 455–61 at p. 457.

11 Ibid., ii. i, 492–97.

12 Matt. 21.8–9.

13 Adhemar, *Chronicon*, III.49, 169.

14 *Abbot Suger*, ed. and trans. Panofsky, 87–89.

15 *Les miracles de Saint Benoit*, ed. E. de Certain (Paris, 1858), I. 31, I. 32, 68–69.

16 Ibid., I. 28, 64–65.

17 'Sermo de S. Benedictio', *PL* 133, 722, translated by T. Head, *Hagiography and the Cult of the Saints*, p. 136.

18 P.-A. Sigal, 'Les Voyages de reliques aux onzième et douzième siècles,' in *Voyage, quête, pèlerinage dans la litterature et la civilisation médiéale* (Paris, 1976), 75–103.

19 Yarrow, *Saints*, 216–18.

20 Ibid.

21 *The Miracle of St Maximinus*, trans. T. Head in Head, *Medieval Hagiography*, 287–92.

22 Reginald of Durham, *Libellus de Admirandis Beati Cuthberti Virtutibus*, Surtees Society (London, 1835), cc. 113, 121, 124, 126, pp. 254–55, 266–68, 270–72.

23 Trans. P. Sheingorn, *The Book of Sainte Foy* (Philadelphia, 1995), 165–66.

24 Lantfred, *Translatio et miracula s. Swithuni*, c. 11, in Lapidge, *The Cult of St Swithun*, 297.

25 *Liber miraculorum sancte Fidis*, IV.13, trans. Sheingorn, 200–01.

26 J. C. Robertson, *Materials for the History of Thomas Becket, Archbishop of Canterbury*, Rolls series 67 (London, 1876), vol. II, 61–62, 65.

27 *Liber miraculorum sancte Fidis*, trans. Sheingorn, 61–62, 65, 137–38.

28 *Liber miraculorum sancte Fidis*, II. 12, trans. Sheingorn, 138.

29 On the importance of recognising the popular-elite distinction as a self-conscious one made by medieval authors in support of their argument, see Yarrow, *Saints and Their Communities*, 5–16.

30 'Veneranda dies', trans. in T. F. Coffey, L. K. Davidson and M. Dunn, eds, *The miracles of Saint James* (New York, 1996), 18–19; *Liber Sancti Jacobi: Codex Calixtinus*, ed. W. Muir Whitehill *et al.*, 3 vols (Santiago, 1944). On the text, see the sceptical note by Christopher Hohler, 'A Note on the Jacobus', *Journal of Warburg and Courtauld Institutes* 35 (1972), 31–80.

31 'The Miracles of Saint James', no. 18, in Coffey *et al.*, *The Miracles of Saint James*, 89–90.

32 M. Bull, *The Miracles of Our Lady of Rocamadour: Analysis and Translation* (Woodbridge, 1999), I. 34, 122–23.

33 B. Abou-el Haj, 'The Audiences for the Medieval Cult of Saints', *Gesta* 30 (1991), 3–15; K. M. Ashley and P. Sheingorn, *Writing Faith: Text, Sign and History In the Miracles of Sainte Foy* (Chicago, 1999); Yarrow, *Saints and their Communities*, 177–89; H. Mayr-Harting, 'Functions of a Twelfth-century Shrine', in idem and R. I. Moore, eds, *Studies in Medieval History Presented to R. H. C. Davis* (London, 1985), 193–206; Lapidge, ed., *The Cult of St Swithun*.

34 *The Book of Sainte Foy*, trans. Sheingorn, 79.

35 Bull, *The Miracles of Our Lady of Rocamadour*, I.2, 101–02.

36 Cf. Colin Morris, 'Introduction', in Morris and Roberts, eds, *Pilgrimage*, 9.

37 Cited by Birch, *Pilgrimage*, 118–20.

38 T. Pestell, 'Using Material Culture to Define Holy Space: the Bromholm Project', in A. Spicer and S. Hamilton, eds, *Defining the Holy: Sacred Space in Medieval and Early Modern Europe* (Aldershot, 2005), 161–86.

39 Yarrow, *Saints and Their Communities*, 63–99.

40 In general on this movement and its importance, see T. Head and R. Landes, eds, *Peace of God: Social Violence and Religious Response in France around the Year 1000* (Ithaca, NY, 1992); on the number of councils held between 989 and 1038, see R. I. Moore, *The First European Revolution c.970–1215* (Oxford, 2000), 9. For those who think the level of popular participation in the councils has been exaggerated: D. Barthélemy, 'Le Mutation féodale, a-t-elle eu lieu?', *Annales* 47 (1992), 767–77, and his 'Le Paix de Dieu dans son contexte', *Cahiers de civilisation médiévale* 40 (1997), 3–35; Janet L. Nelson, review of T. Head and R. Landes, eds, *The Peace of God* in *Speculum* 69 (1994), 163–69.

41 Rodulfus Glaber, *Histories*, IV.14, 194–95.

42 *De diversis casibus cenobii Dervensis et miracula S. Bercharii*, c. 27, *Acta sanctorum ordinis sanctis Benedicti*, 9 vols, ed. L. D'Achéry and J. Mabillon (Paris, 1668–1701), II, 859, trans. in T. Head and R. Landes, 'Introduction', in Head and Landes, eds, *The Peace of God*, 5–6.

43 K. Cushing, *Reform and the Papacy in the Eleventh Century: Spirituality and Social Change* (Manchester, 2005), p. 51; Andrew of Fleury, *Miracula s. Benedicti*, trans. Head and Landes, *Peace of God*, 339–42.

44 J. A. Bowman, 'Councils, Memory and Mills: The Early Development of the Peace of God in Catalonia', *Early Medieval Europe* 8 (1999), 99–129; T. Head, 'The Development of the Peace of God in Aquitaine (970–1005)', *Speculum* 74 (1999), 656–86; T. Head, 'Peace and Power in France around the Year 1000', *Essays in Medieval Studies* 23 (2006), 1–17.

45 Adhemar of Chabannes cited by C. Taylor, *Heresy in Medieval France: Dualism in Aquitaine and the Agenais, 1000–1249* (Woodbridge, 2005), 29.

46 Taylor, *Heresy*, 30, citing D. F. Callahan, 'William the Great and the Monasteries of Aquitaine', *Studia Monastica* 19 (1977), 321–42.

47 J. Martindale, 'Peace and War in the Early Eleventh-century Aquitaine', in C. Harper-Bill and R. Harvey, eds, *Medieval Knighthood IV: Papers from the Fifth Strawberry Hill Conference* (Woodbridge, 1992), 147–176.

48 Head, 'The Development of the Peace of God'; idem, 'Peace and Power'.

49 M. Bull, *Knightly Piety and the Lay Response to the First Crusade: The Limousin and Gascony, c.970–c.1130* (Oxford, 1993), 44–45.

50 R. Kaiser, 'Quêtes itinerantes avec des reliques pour financer la construction des églises (XIe–XIIe siècles)', *Le moyen âge* 101 (1995), 205–25; P.-A. Sigal, 'Les voyages des reliques aux onzième et douzième siècles', in M. A. Cuer, ed., *Voyage, quête, pélerinage dan la Littérature et la civilisation medièvale* (Aix-en-Provence, 1976).

51 'The Miracles of St Ursmer on His Journey through Flandrers', trans. Koziol; G. Koziol, 'Monks, Feuds and the Making of Peace in Eleventh-century Flanders', in Head and Landes, eds, *The Peace of God*, 239–58.

52 *De miraculis beatae Mariae Laudunensis*, *PL* 156, 961–1018; Guibert of Nogent, *Monodiae*, III.12–13, *PL* 156, 937–42; trans. Archambault, *A Monk's Confession* 173–81. For modern accounts, see: J. S. P. Tatlock, 'The English Journey of the Laon Canons', *Speculum* 8 (1933), 454–65; B. Ward, *Miracles and the Medieval Mind: Theory, Record and Event, 1000–1215* (Aldershot, 1982), 133–42; Yarrow, *Saints and their Communities,* 63–99.

53 Yarrow, *Saints*, 81–84.

54 Ibid., 89–92.

55 *PL* 156, 968D; Yarrow, *Saints*, 84.

56 Carl F. Barnes, Jr, 'Cult of the Carts', *Dictionary of Art*, ed. J. Turner (London, 1996), 8: 257–59.

57 A. Kingsley Porter, *Medieval Architecture: Its Origins and Development with Lists of Monuments and Bibliographies*, 2 vols (1909; repr. New York, 1969), II, 156–57.

58 Ibid., II, 154.

59 'Letter of Archbishop Hugh of Rouen to Bishop Theodorich of Amiens', c. 114, ibid., II, 157.

60 Barnes, 'Cult of the Carts', 258.

61 Ward, *Miracles*, 153.

62 *Libellus alter de consecratione ecclesiae sancti Dionysii*, in *Abbot Suger*, ed. and trans. Panofsky, 92–93.

63 II Samuel 6.3; I Chronicles 13.7–8.

64 Barnes, 'Cult of the Carts', 257.

65 *Chronica monasterii Casiensis*, trans. C. Davis-Weyer, *Early Medieval Art 300–1150* (Englewood Cliffs, NJ, 1971), 136; *Abbot Suger*, ed. and trans. Panofsky, 214.

66 Rodulf of Saint-Trond, *Gesta abbatum Trudonensium*, ed. D. R. Koepke, *MGH SS* X (Hannover, 1852), 234–35.

67 A. Luchaire, *Social France at the Time of Philip Augustus*, trans E. B. Krehbiel (London, 1912), 13–19. See also J. Perrel, 'Une révolution populaire au moyen âge: le mouvement des Capuchonnés du Puy, 1182–84', *Cahiers de la Haute-Loire* (1977), 61–79; G. Dickson, 'Religious Enthusiasm in the Medieval West and the Second Conversion of Europe', in his *Religious Enthusiasm in the Medieval West: Revivals, Crusades, Saints* (Aldershot, 2000), I, 14–15; J. H. Arnold, 'Religion and Popular Rebellion, from the Capuciati to Niklashausen', *Cultural and Social History* 6 (2009), 149–69.

68 Luchaire, *Social France*, 17; *Historia Episcoporum Autissiodorensium*, *Recueil des historiens des Gaule et de France*, ed. M. Bouquet *et al.*, rev. L. Delisle (Paris, 1904), XVIII, 729–30.

69 Arnold, 'Religion and Popular Rebellion', 158–62.

70 J. M. H. Smith, 'Saints and Their Cults', in Noble and Smith, eds, *The Cambridge History of Christianity: Early Medieval Christianities c.600–c.1100*, 581–605 at 582.

chapter 8

Extraordinary piety: Pilgrimage and the crusades

Sometime in the late tenth century a nobleman from Provence called Bobo set out on his annual pilgrimage to the shrines of SS. Peter and Paul in Rome, but he died before he got there at the town of Voghera, near Pavia in northern Italy.[1] His own grave became the centre of a long-lived cult within that town, for Bobo was no ordinary pilgrim. According to his *vita*, composed sometime in the first half of the eleventh century, Bobo's way of life marked him out from his fellow nobles. Born of noble parents, in due course he inherited the family estates, which soon came under regular attack from the 'pagans' – Moslem pirates who had established a secure base for their activities at Fraxinetum, at the mouth of the Rhône. Ranging over land and sea, they attacked those living in western Provence as well as those travelling to and from Italy, capturing both rich and poor, and leading many away into captivity. Anxious to defend his people and to lead a campaign against the pirates, he encountered a major difficulty: the pirates' base had very good natural defences, with mountains on one side and the sea on the other. Bobo therefore vowed

> *that if God permitted him to suffocate the enemies of Christ attacking him, he would lay down his arms, take up the care of orphans and widows, and journey each year to the threshold of SS Peter and Paul.*[2]

Christian victory followed, he defeated the Moslem army and their king converted to Christianity, because, in the words of the *vita*, what Bobo 'sought from God he obtained, and he fulfilled what he had vowed faithfully'. He gave up arms, and chose instead to look after the weak and the vulnerable, and to make an annual pilgrimage to Rome. There is nothing very exceptional about his vow. Its terms echo the ideals of ninth-century royal ministry, and Bobo is depicted as behaving like a good early medieval Christian prince, defending his lands and people, promoting peace, and protecting the poor, widows and orphans. But he departed from noble convention because his victory over the pirates was followed by a more substantial personal conversion, in which he is depicted as imitating Christ even more overtly. Thus we are told that he forswore taking vengeance against his brother's murderers, just as Christ had enjoined his followers to love their enemies, that he rode the mule of a peasant rather than the horse befitting his noble status, just as Christ had entered Jerusalem on an ass, and that he mortified his body and carried a cross, again in imitation of Christ. And he marked this new way of life by making an annual pilgrimage to Rome, which he continued in fulfilment of his oath until his death in *c.* 986.

Bobo's life embodies the themes of this chapter which will examine the acts of extraordinary piety displayed by individuals which led them outside their quotidian existence. It is these acts of passivity and humility which marked Bobo out from his fellow nobles. The conduct of his campaign against the pirates and the terms of his vow identify him as a member of the Christian nobility, subscribing to existing values associated with Christian rulership, but the seriousness with which he took his vow, and the personal conversion which accompanied it, led him to forsake the customs of his rank, forsaking the trappings of wealth, and the social norms which expected him to take action against his brother's murderers rather than pardon them. At the same time his annual pilgrimage regularly took him outside the constraints of his ordinary life. But it is his exemplary life as Christian soldier and lord which justified his claim to sanctity rather than his regular pilgrimage.

Up to now our investigation into the laity's experience of the Church has focused on the impact which it had on their daily lives. But one of the most obvious novel features of lay piety in this period is the increase in those making long-distance pilgrimages to Rome, the Holy Land and shrines on the periphery of Christendom. Increasing numbers of individuals left their local communities to voyage far afield for religious reasons. Examination of pilgrimage accounts, the context in which individuals decided to undertake such journeys and the reasons they did so thus provides a fresh perspective on the nature of the laity's religious experience in this period.

Unlike the pastoral rites demanded of all Christians, and which came under the control of the clergy, the decision to go on pilgrimage was generally voluntary. It is usually presented as a personal decision, made independent of clerical guidance, as a response to personal circumstances, as in the case of St Bobo. There are hints that in many cases such journeys might have been subject to wider social and political pressures. In such circumstances it becomes impossible to distinguish the actions and motives of particular lay individuals from those of the collective, and investigation of the motives of the individual can stand for those of the group. The emphasis on personal conversion in many pilgrimage accounts, for example, results from their authors' desire to compare their subject to Christ. *Imitatio Christi*, as in the example of St Bobo, is viewed as evidence of sanctity. The focus on the individual is therefore as much a consequence of clerical authors' ambitions as a reflection of trends in personal piety. Yet whilst historians must recognise the rhetorical constraints imposed on their sources by genre, they must also acknowledge that in order for such tales to resonate with their audiences they required a grounding in reality.

We begin this investigation of lay pilgrimage with an examination of the changes which occurred in the nature of long-distance pilgrimage across this period, before asking why it became so popular. Tracing the reasons for the fluctuations in the popularity of different destinations, we examine in detail the evidence for pilgrimage to the Holy Land, Rome and Compostela. We then turn to investigate the role pilgrimage came to play in narratives of lay conversion. It is against this background of changes in the conduct of pilgrimage and depictions of it that we then turn to explore how far the First Crusade represents a new development in lay piety, or whether it is rather the consequence of existing trends.

The increase in long-distance pilgrimage

By 900 pilgrimages to distant shrines, such as Jerusalem, the site of Christ's Passion and Resurrection, or Rome, the home of the popes and the site of the martyrdom and burial of two of Christ's apostles, SS Peter and Paul, had become a well-established feature of Christian piety. But the following three centuries witnessed a significant increase in the evidence for long-distance pilgrimages, not just to the Holy Land and Rome, but to shrines on the periphery of Christendom, such as those of the apostle St James (Santiago), whose relics came to light at Compostela in western Galicia in Spain in the ninth century, of the archangel St Michael at Monte Gargano in Apulia and Mont St-Michel off the Norman and Breton coasts, both of which were visited by pilgrims en route from northern Europe to Jerusalem from at least the ninth century onwards, as well as those of well-established saints, such as that of the Roman soldier St Martin at Tours, in the Loire valley.[3]

The next section investigates, through three case studies, the evidence for the increasing numbers of Christians setting out on difficult and time-consuming journeys, which took them away from their familiar surroundings, friends and family for prolonged periods, by asking *who* undertook such journeys; *how* they went – how they financed the journey, what routes they followed, where they stayed, how they knew what to look for, and how they understood what they saw – and *what* acts they performed when they got to their destination; and *why* individuals chose to make such arduous journeys away from their home.

Pilgrimage to the Holy Land

As the site of Christ's life, passion, and resurrection, the Holy Land had long had great importance for medieval Christians; indeed, the earliest accounts of journeys there from the Latin West date to the fourth century, and the pilgrimage had a continuous history throughout the early medieval period. Yet it seems that the years 900 to 1200 witnessed a significant increase in the numbers visiting Jerusalem. The Burgundian chronicler, Rodulphus Glaber, writing in the 1030s, observed that at the time of the millennium of Christ's passion,

> *an innumerable multitude of people from the whole world, greater than any before could have hoped to see, began to travel to the Sepulchre of the Saviour at Jerusalem. First to go were the petty people, then those of middling estate, and next the powerful, kings, counts, marquesses, and bishops; finally, and this was something which had never happened before, numerous women, noble and poor, undertook the journey.*[4]

Rodulphus self-consciously structured his account around commemorating the events surrounding the two millennial years of Christ's Incarnation in 1000 and Passion in 1033 in order to demonstrate that all that happened in the world could be attributed to God, and to God's concern to offer all of mankind the opportunity to save themselves from sin. For Rodulphus, the pilgrimage in 1033 had been one of the times when people from all ranks took up that opportunity. But it also needs to be placed in the context of other evidence which suggests the number of nobles travelling to Jerusalem from all over Europe grew over the course of the tenth and eleventh centuries.

This evidence is haphazard but points to increased pilgrimage from all over the medieval west, from Saxony and England in the north, to southern France and Italy in the south. These pilgrims included the counts of Ardèches (south central France), Vienne (western France), and Verdun (Lorraine), Hilda, countess of Suabia, who died en route in 969, the count of Anhalt (Saxony), and the count of Gorizia (north-east Italy).[5] Marcus Bull's detailed study of the piety of the nobility of Gascony and the Limousin suggests that pilgrimage to Jerusalem became reasonably widespread there throughout the late tenth and eleventh centuries. In 986, for example, Gerald of La Valène gave much of his property to the Limousin monastery of Tulle before setting out on the journey to Jerusalem; Viscount Guy I of Limoges went on pilgrimage to Jerusalem, with his brother Bishop Hilduin, in the 990s; two brothers, Gerard Cabrols and Ranulf of Chazarein, gave property to Tulle before making the journey sometime between 1053 and 1084; as did Sancho Auriol to the monks of the Gascon house of St-Savin, Lavedan sometime between 1060 and 1080. The Limousin Viscount Boso I of Turenne died at Jerusalem in 1091.[6] Studies of the charter and chronicle evidence for other areas reveal a similar picture. In north-western France Fulk Nerra, count of Anjou (987–1040) is reported to have gone on pilgrimage to Jerusalem three times: in 1003, 1010 and towards the end of his life in 1038 or 1039. Robert I, duke of Normandy, died on his way home from the pilgrimage in 1035. Svein Godwinsson went with a party of Englishmen in 1052 but died in Anatolia. Count Theodoric of Trier set off in 1068.[7] Whilst the western crusader armies which captured Jerusalem in 1099 introduced a new element to such journeys – the opportunity to go on armed pilgrimage – straightforward pilgrimage remained popular throughout the twelfth century. The

Englishman Saewulf, for example, left a detailed account of his itinerary in 1102; Godric of Finchale, a merchant from the north of England, went twice in the early twelfth century, and in the late twelfth century an Italian cobbler from Piacenza, Raimondo Palmario, visited the Holy Land with his mother.[8]

These men seldom travelled alone, and Rodulphus Glaber's description of people from all the social strata leaving for the Holy Land in 1033 is thus not mere hyperbole. In 1026 the northern French and Flemish monastic reformer Richard of Saint-Vannes, with the support of Richard, duke of Normandy, who 'provided him with all the expenses for the journey, for he was generous with alms, expansive in charity, notable in honour', led a group said to number 700 to the Holy Land; according to the Aquitainian chronicler, Adhemar of Chabannes, the party included William, count of Angoulême, Odo du Berry, the lords of Déols, and Géraud Fanesin, as well as two other abbots and a great troop of nobles.[9] In 1035 Robert, duke of Normandy, made the journey 'with a great many of his people'.[10] The pattern of mass pilgrimage continued in the later eleventh century: in 1064–65 three different German accounts record how Bishop Gunther of Bamberg led 'many reputable men, both clergy and laity from eastern Francia as well as from Bavaria' overland to the Holy Land. Theirs was a particularly difficult journey in which the pilgrims were attacked, although they were rescued by the Moslem governor of Ramleh who was concerned that the attacks might put people off from making the pilgrimage, which provided an important source of revenue for him and his people.[11]

As this remark suggests, going on pilgrimage was an expensive business for those who went, as well as a profitable one for those living in the Holy Land. The research of Jonathan Riley-Smith and Marcus Bull shows how the lesser nobility of France financed such journeys by selling or pledging their property to religious communities. They and their families often already had existing relationships of patronage and affiliation with these communities.[12] In such cases the Jerusalem pilgrimage represents the extension of existing patterns of devotion. The personal pilgrimage of one individual had ramifications for other members of their family, and the decision to go helped reinforce and strengthen its ties with that religious community. In the late eleventh century William of Bort, for example, surrendered his fifth-share in a property which his father, the monks claimed, had given to Tulle earlier, and persuaded his four other brothers to surrender their claims, in return for thirty *solidi*.[13] But of the five brothers only William went. It is worth remembering that going on pilgrimage, whilst becoming more common, remained exceptional. The Limousin chronicler, Adhemar of Chabannes, goes so far as to report how the body of one pilgrim who died during his journey back from Jerusalem performed miracles. Like St Bobo, the very act of pilgrimage helped to mark out this man, a local castellan, and led him to be regarded as a saint in the locality.[14] Such extraordinary travels had meaning for those left behind as well as for those who went.

Even for those who survived, the journey was long and hazardous. Count William IV of Angoulême's journey in 1026 took nine months, and Saewulf's journey to and from England must have taken nearer two years: he begins his account when he left Bari in southern Italy in July 1102, returning to Constantinople fourteen months later in September 1103, where his account breaks off, to which one must add the time to travel from and back to England. Saewulf travelled by sea from southern Italy, travelling slowly through the Greek islands, and thence to Cyprus before reaching the port of Jaffa.[15] It has been suggested that Saewulf's journey may be atyptical because he had left it relatively late in the season to travel: the main pilgrim fleets usually left southern Italy in March and travelled to the Holy Land more directly. He is proof that although the overland route down through the Balkans, across the Bosphorus, and through Asia Minor to the eastern Mediterranean coast became feasible after the conversion of the Hungarians at the beginning of the eleventh century, many still continued to go by sea. The sea route from southern Italy had been popular throughout the eleventh century. Eighty years before Saewulf left, Adhemar of Chabannes reported how fighting in southern Italy had disrupted the 'via Hierosolimae' making it impossible for people to make the pilgrimage to the Holy Land.[16] By 1070 the route had become so profitable that the merchants of the Campanian port of Amalfi built a hospital in Jerusalem dedicated to St John the Almsgiver.[17]

Once pilgrims reached the Holy Land they encountered a world accustomed to such visitors. The early eleventh-century saint Symeon of Trier (d. 1035) was a Byzantine who lived out his final years as a hermit enclosed in the Roman gate of the city of Trier, but earlier in his life he had spent seven years as a professional guide to pilgrims to the Holy Land.[18] The need for such guides is made clear in the written accounts we have from the twelfth century of individuals' visits, such as that of Saewulf, which reveal the detailed itineraries they undertook of the sites associated with Christ's life. Indeed, in the words of the Russian abbot Daniil, who visited the Holy Places in 1106:

> *Without a good guide and a translator it is difficult to examine and see all the Holy Places. I gave the little I possessed to those who knew the city and the surrounding area well in order that they might show me everything.*[19]

Daniil wrote his guide in Old Russian, but at least twelve guides to the Holy Land written in Latin survive from the twelfth century, which compares to three from the eighth and ninth centuries. These new works met the demand for information in the west from those unable to travel east as much as that of those who did. This demand reflects the considerable increase in the popularity of the pilgrimage to the Holy Land in the years after the First Crusade when Jerusalem and the other places associated with Christ's life came under Frankish rule.[20] One such guide to the Holy Places, that written by the German monk Theodoric after his visit, probably in 1169, makes clear how the popularity of the pilgrimage led to considerable overcrowding at pilgrimage sites. He describes how the porters manning the doors to the shrine of Christ's sepulchre

> *will not allow less than six or more than twelve to go in, for the place is too cramped to receive more. Furthermore they compel the people, after they have worshipped, to go outside the door.*

Such was the demand that porters strictly rationed time spent inside in order to avoid the dangers of overcrowding. He again referred to this problem when he reported how the porters at the doors of the church on the site of Calvary

> *allow as many pilgrims to enter as wish to, unless there is a very big crowd. This is often apt to happen here, and if this is the case someone might get crushed or be in danger of death. From that vestibule one ascends by three steps through another door into a chapel preeminent in sanctity and holiness beyond all other places under the sun.*[21]

Such accounts provide powerful support for the success of the Jerusalem pilgrimage in the twelfth century.

But why did these people choose to go on pilgrimage? Various explanations have been offered for the growth in the numbers of those willing to make the considerable sacrifice in terms of time and money needed for the journey to Jerusalem. The first is that the Jerusalem pilgrimage might be undertaken as a form of penance for a crime so heinous that it was beyond the powers of normal ecclesiastical authority to forgive; pilgrimage therefore acted as a form of punitive exile. Robert, duke of Normandy, for example, went to atone for his involvement in the murder of his brother. Fulk Nerra, count of Anjou (987–1040), made his second pilgrimage in 1010 in the wake of his involvement in the assassination of King Robert the Pious's favourite, Hugh of Beauvais, an event so contentious that it led to threats of excommunication.[22] Fulk's retreat in such circumstances may have been a strategic retirement from what had become a highly contentious political scene. But Fulk's other two pilgrimages cannot be so easily explained; the first time he went, in 1003, he was in Rodulfus Glaber's words, 'driven by fear of hell to go to our Saviour's sepulchre at Jerusalem' because he had shed so much blood in many battles. The third time in 1038 or 1039 seems to have been for devotion.[23] Fulk is exceptional in visiting so often but his experience suggests that penance for a specific sin only constituted the primary motive in a minority of cases.

Devotion, and concern about one's general sinfulness, rather than penance for a specific sin, seems to have been the prime motive for the majority of pilgrims, in so far as we can tell. They set out explicitly to visit the location of those events from the Old and New Testament which are central to the narrative of Christian salvation. Through such journeys Christians linked their concern for the fate of their own soul in the afterlife to the metanarrative of Christian history. Saewulf's early twelfth-century account reveals that he regarded his entire journey as a pilgrimage. For him his whole voyage through the eastern Mediterranean resonated with New Testament associations. He thus reports on the spiritual significance of the various stops in the Greek islands his party made en route, including Patras where they prayed at the shrine of St Andrew the Apostle, Corinth where St Paul had preached, Pathmos, the home of St John the Apostle, Myra, the see of Nicholas, and Cyprus where all the Apostles had met after Christ's Ascension, before arriving at Jaffa, where St Peter had preached. From Jaffa, Saewulf travelled inland to Jerusalem, which he entered through the gate of King David, before going straight to the edicule of the

Holy Sepulchre in the Byzantine rotunda.[24] This most holy of all the Christian sites was a complex of churches and sites, all of which had resonances with the events of Christ's passion. Saewulf tells us he visited the prison where Christ was confined; the place where Helena, the mother of Constantine, discovered the cross on which Christ had been crucified; the marble column against which Christ had been scourged and near which spot the soldiers had mocked Christ, stripped him of his garments, clad him in purple and crowned him with thorns; the Mount of Calvary, the site of Abraham's attempted sacrifice of his son Isaac, and of Christ's crucifixion, and below this Golgotha, where Adam was said to have been first raised to life, and near there the church of St Mary on the site where Christ's body had been anointed, and wrapped in a shroud prior to burial; the site where Christ appeared to the women in the garden, and the edicule of the Holy Sepulchre, where Christ had been buried, itself. Saewulf's description testifies to the extent to which pilgrims sought to give a concrete reality to the New Testament accounts by visiting the sites of Christ's life and those associated with him. He later visited the temple, built by Solomon, where Christ had sat amongst the doctors as a child, had cast out the moneylenders as an adult, and had protected the woman taken in adultery from stoning; he visited the tomb of Christ's mother, Mary, in the valley of Josephat; the garden of Gethsemane where Judas betrayed Christ; the Mount of Olives, where Christ preached and gave his apostles the text of the Lord's Prayer, and the church built on the site of the house where the Last Supper was held, and where Christ later appeared to Doubting Thomas. And then he left Jerusalem to visit Bethlehem, the scene of Christ's birth; Hebron, the burial site of the Old Testament patriarchs; Nazareth, the site of Christ's childhood; the site of the marriage at Cana, and the Sea of Galilee where Christ first preached.[25] He thus focused largely on sites associated with the New Testament rather than the Old.

Other pilgrims did not content themselves with just visiting the places associated with Christ's life; they also sought, through the re-enactment of various episodes, to enter into the drama of Christ's life. Theodoric's guide reports how pilgrims had themselves flogged at the pillar where Christ himself had been flogged:

> *After he had asked him many questions, Pilate caused him to be led to the judgement hall, and he sat down, by way of a judgement-seat, in the*

> *place that is called the Pavement, which is situated in front of the Church of St Mary, on Mount Sion, in a high place near the city wall. Here is a holy chapel dedicated to our Lord Jesus Christ, in which stands a great column round which the Lord was bound by Pilate and ordered to be scourged after he had been condemned by him to be crucified. There pilgrims are scourged in imitation of him. In front of the church, on a stone cut in the likeness of a cross, these words are inscribed: 'This is the place called the Pavement, and here the Lord was judged'.*[26]

Elsewhere, other decorations reinforced the message of the link between Christ's life, the present and future judgement: engraved on the cornice of the shrine in the church of the Holy Sepulchre, which the Frankish rulers rebuilt in the twelfth century, were the words:

> *Christ being raised from the dead will never die again; death no longer has dominion over him.*[27]

The pilgrimage to the Holy Land thus brought home to pilgrims the physical reality of Christ's life and his humanity in a very literal way and at the same time signalled the importance of his sacrifice to their own lives.

It is part of a contemporary movement within the eleventh- and twelfth-century western Church which emphasised Christ's humanity, as opposed to his divinity. Giles Constable's analysis of monastic writers in this period suggests that:

> *The ideal of imitating Christ in all respects deepened in the eleventh century into a passionate devotion to His humanity, which increasingly excluded other models and established Christ as the supreme exemplar for devout Christians.*[28]

The desire to imitate Christ led to the wish to imitate his physical suffering, and ran alongside the interest amongst both laymen and churchmen in a return to the literal re-enactment of the principles of the apostolic life. In earlier chapters we have examined the impact which the *vita apostolica* had on the lifestyles of clerics, monks, and some communities of lay men and women. But the preoccupation with Christ's life and suffering had an even wider impact on religious cultures, particularly those of prayer and art. Depictions of Christ on the cross moved from portraying him in Majesty, victorious over death, to suffering and being vulnerable, and prayers and other devotional texts began to emphasise how great was God's love for man that He became man and died for the sake of humankind.[29] The experience of pilgrims to Jerusalem, who participated in a very literal way in Christ's human life, is at once both a reflection of this shift in piety, and an engine for it, fuelling the popularity of the *imitatio Christi* as well as *vita apostolica* in contemporary piety.

This connection between Christ's life and the changing nature of the Christian devotion is spelt out very clearly in the early thirteenth-century *Life* of Raimondo 'Palmario' of Piacenza (d. 1200). It records how, on the death of his father, this Italian cobbler went on pilgrimage to the Holy Places with his mother. His visit is recorded in highly emotional terms: he and his mother, we are told, wept at the treachery of the Jews, meditated on the immense love of God, visited and prayed at the church of the Holy Sepulchre and that of the nativity in Bethlehem, where the Lord was born a helpless child, as well as other sites, and then decided to return home to

> *share all the marvels they had seen with pious and religious men and inflame the cold hearts of worldly men and women with divine love.*[30]

Back in Piacenza Raimondo married, but continued to live a religious life, studying scripture, preaching to his fellow workers but, being a layman, not in public because 'that was the office of priests and learned men'. He fasted, gave alms, prayed, attended divine office, made regular confession, and wore only modest clothes. His exemplary life served as a model for lay piety. On his wife's death he left Piacenza to go on pilgrimage again, first to Compostela, then various shrines in southern France and northern Italy, before reaching Rome where he had a vision of Christ who enjoined him in the following terms not to go on pilgrimage to the Holy Land but rather to return to Piacenza and take up Christ's work:

> *I want you to engage in occupations more pleasing to me and more beneficial to you: I mean works of mercy. You are not to think that I shall be thinking principally of pilgrimage and works of piety of that kind when at the time of judgement I say, 'Come, O blessed of my Father, take possession of the kingdom of Heaven, for I was hungry and you gave me food; I was thirsty, and you gave me drink; I was naked and you clothed me; I was sick and you visited me; I was in prison and you ransomed me, I do not want you, my son, to wander any more around the world, but to*

> *return to your homeland, Piacenza, where there are so many poor people, so many abandoned widows, so many sick and overcome by various misfortunes who call upon my mercy and there is no one to help them.*

Raimondo returned to Piacenza where he set up a hospice for the needy. He came to be regarded as a holy man within the city, acting as peacemaker, and when he died the people of the city rushed to his deathbed to take pieces of his clothing as a relic of his sanctity.

The author of his *Life* described Raimondo as 'Palmario', that is the one who had been on pilgrimage. This tag presumably dates from his lifetime: his numerous pilgrimages had distinguished him from his peers. But it is his embodiment of Christian virtue rather than his journeys to specific holy places which underlay the claims made for his sanctity. His charitable activities in Piacenza, combined with his ascetic lifestyle and pious devotions, reflected the adoption of the apostolic life by a relatively humble man, a cobbler. His way of life rather than his travels marked him out from his fellows, and served as a model to them. The parallels with St Bobo two centuries earlier are marked: like Bobo, Raimondo 'Palmario' sought to imitate Christ in the conduct of life and to implement His teachings. But the differences are equally significant. A nobleman and warrior, Bobo's actions owed much to early medieval ideals of the duties of Christian rulers. The author of Bobo's *Life* based his claim to sanctity not only on the way he sought to imitate Christ in his daily actions but on his annual pilgrimage to Rome. The author of Raimondo's *Life* by contrast regarded pilgrimage as merely a precursor to his adoption of an exemplary life. The changes reflect most clearly the democratisation of pious ideals between the tenth and late twelfth centuries, and the role of pilgrimage in this process. As Bobo's *Life* demonstrates, the principles of the apostolic life had not been forgotten in the early Middle Ages but the social and economic changes of the central Middle Ages, and in particular the increases in commerce and urbanisation, allowed people from a wider social class to adopt them. The success of the Jerusalem pilgrimage reflected these developments in Christian piety and benefited from them; it did not create them.

Pilgrimage to Rome

Pilgrimage to Rome, like that to Jerusalem, had been popular throughout the early Middle Ages. Bobo's vow to visit 'the shrines of the Apostles Peter and Paul once a year, and more if he could, for the rest of his life' in the tenth century, and Raimondo's visit in the twelfth century testify to Rome's continued significance as a centre for personal devotion. Raimondo even had his inspiring vision of Christ whilst sleeping with other poor pilgrims on the steps of St Peter's in Rome. The city owed its high status amongst other shrines to its role in early Christian history, particularly as the place that witnessed the martyrdom of the apostles Peter and Paul as well as that of various early Christians. The tombs of these early Christian martyrs served as cult centres. As well as shrines dedicated to the apostles SS Peter and Paul, they included ones to SS Agnes and Cecilia, and those of various other martyrs.

Rome served as a centre for devotional pilgrimage throughout the years 900 to 1200. Marcus Bull's case study of one region demonstrates its significance in the piety of the Aquitainian nobility of the tenth and eleventh centuries. Like the Provencal Bobo, St Gerald of Aurillac is reported to have visited Rome regularly, seven times in all, and to have 'made it a rule to go every second year . . . to gaze spiritually on the two lights of the world, Peter and Paul'.[31] Gerald is also reported to have visited the shrines of St Martin at Tours and St Martial at Limoges.[32] In the late tenth century, Viscount Guy I of Limoges visited Rome as well as Jerusalem. In the later eleventh century a lesser noble from Gascony, Fort Sancho of Godz, pledged his share of the family church to the Gascon church of St Mont in return for the money to go to Rome.[33] What marks both Bobo and Gerald out is not so much their pilgrimage to Rome as the ways in which they repeated the journey.

But Rome did not just serve as a centre for devotional pilgrimage: its distance from much of northern Europe, combined with the presence of the papacy, explain why, like Jerusalem, it became an important centre for penitential pilgrimages. Legislation from the ninth century onwards criticised the laity for thinking that they could sin with impunity and bypass local structures for imposing penance by appealing to the pope in Rome. The Council of Seligenstadt (1023), for example, enjoined against the

> *many people [who] are so deceived by the foolishness of their minds that they do not wish to accept the penance laid down upon them by their priests for capital crimes and believe firmly that the pope can absolve all their sins if they go to Rome.*[34]

They should only go to Rome *after* having completed the penance enjoined upon them by their priest, and having obtained the permission of their bishop who should give them a letter to take to the pope outlining the circumstances of their sin. Master copies of such letters survive from late tenth- and eleventh-century England testifying to the relative normality of such a practice in cases of heinous sins such as parricide.[35]

The pilgrimage to Rome from northern Europe possessed a well-developed infrastructure. In the city, hostels had been established to cater for Anglo-Saxon, Lombard, Frisian and Frankish pilgrims from the mid-eighth century onwards.[36] Hospices also existed along the road (the *Via Francigena*) from the Great Saint Bernard Pass down through Lombardy and Tuscany to Rome. They were necessary: so great a person as Archbishop Sigeric of Canterbury stopped at seventy-nine stages on his way back from Rome in 990.[37] Nevertheless it constituted a dangerous journey: Saracen raiders killed two large parties of Anglo-Saxon pilgrims in the Alpine passes in 921 and 923, whilst Abbot Maiolus of Cluny was kidnapped for ransom by Saracens in July 972. These very real dangers help explain why part of St Bobo's claim to sanctity was that he protected Roman pilgrims in the late tenth century.[38]

Pilgrims continued to make the journey from northern Europe for much of the eleventh century. Yet Debra Birch's analysis of the French charter evidence suggests that pilgrimage to Rome from France declined in the twelfth century, relative to the popularity of Jerusalem and Compostela. This decline may in part be due to the political vicissitudes of Rome at the time, as contested claims to the papal throne led to various papal schisms.[39] Although it is possible such schisms may have undermined the faithful's belief in papal penitential authority, it is unlikely as the twelfth century as a whole witnessed a great increase in appeals to the papal curia to adjudicate in difficult ecclesiastical disputes. Rather the twelfth-century decline in the Roman pilgrimage reflects the change in Christological devotion which, we have already seen, explains the increased popularity of the Holy Land pilgrimage. Rome had long been a centre for pilgrimage, and a source of saints' relics; in the eighth and ninth centuries it became a source of Roman martyr relics for Frankish pilgrims to take back to their own churches in northern Europe, but the twelfth century witnessed a renewed emphasis on tangible relics of the apostles and of Christ himself, a development to which Rome only slowly adjusted.[40] It did so by the end of the century. When

King Philip Augustus of France visited in 1191, for example, the pope took him to see not just the heads of the apostles Peter and Paul in the Lateran, but the Veronica, the cloth which bore the imprint of Christ's face, in the Vatican. The relic collection of the pope's private chapel, the *Sancta Sanctorum*, housed in the Lateran palace, became especially important to pilgrims in the later twelfth and thirteenth centuries; it included various testaments to Christ's humanity and passion including a phial of His blood, a portion of the crown of thorns, the Virgin Mary's clothes, her milk, and the bones of John the Baptist, who presaged Christ's coming.[41] Rome, like Jerusalem, can therefore be seen to be adapting to the renewed interest in Christ's humanity.

Pilgrimage to Compostela

When compared to Jerusalem and Rome in the central Middle Ages, the shrine of St James (Santiago) at Compostela in Galicia in north-western Spain is a much more recent cult centre. Medieval people believed that St James the Great, one of Christ's apostles, preached in Spain before returning to martyrdom in Jerusalem, after which his disciples chose to bury his body in Spain. His remains were only discovered at Compostela in the ninth century. Nevertheless the tomb soon attracted pilgrims from southern France and Catalonia, including Bishop Gottschalk of Le Puy in 951, Archbishop Hugh of Rhemis in 961, and at around the same time Raymond II, count of the Rouergue.[42] By the early eleventh century Compostela had become a leading destination for devout members of the Aquitainian nobility, second only to Rome in its popularity. Adhemar of Chabannes reported how Duke William V of Aquitaine (d. 1030) made an annual pilgrimage to Rome or, if that was impracticable, he 'compensated' by going to Compostela.[43] By the late eleventh century pilgrims are recorded as travelling there from England and north-eastern France. Hugh of Die, archbishop of Lyons and papal legate (d. 1106), for example, led a large party of lay and clerical pilgrims there in the late eleventh century. Duke William V's great great grandson, Duke William X, died in the cathedral there whilst making the pilgrimage on Good Friday in 1137.[44] By the early twelfth century those clerics in charge of the cult had become anxious to emphasise the diversity of its appeal, recording how those coming to the shrine comprised the Franks, Scots, Normans, Lorrainers, Romans, Apulians, Frisians, Dacians, Bithinians, Bulgarians, Cappadocians, and the impious inhabitants of Navarre.[45] Universality, as we saw in Chapter 7, is a trope of such works but there is a good deal of evidence to suggest that over the course of the tenth, eleventh and twelfth centuries, Compostela came to rival Rome as an important destination for Christian pilgrims from across the medieval west.

Pilgrims found the journey to Compostela, like those to Rome and Jerusalem, to be long, arduous and potentially dangerous. They had to cross the Pyrenees, and until the late eleventh century the route across Spain ran close to the Moslem frontier. Yet it soon developed its own traditions and infrastructure, which are recorded in the guidebook for pilgrims – the fifth and final book of the twelfth-century collection now known as the *Liber sancti Jacobi* (*LSJ*).[46] It is a problematic text and did not circulate widely; one historian has even suggested it may represent a parody of such literature.[47] Even if this is the case, it suggests that such guides did exist. It begins by outlining the four main routes from France to Compostela, starting from Saint-Gilles in Provence, Le Puy in the Limousin, Vézelay in Burgundy, or Tours in the Loire valley, the stopping places and towns en route, and the obstacles which face the pilgrim: the dangerous rivers; the nefarious people who haunt the route, telling lies to travellers, encouraging them to let their horses drink bad water, and levying unjust tolls; the saints' shrines which should be visited en route, and even sometimes describes the customs to be undergone at each of these shrines. At Arles in Provence, for example, it instructed pilgrims to visit the cemetery of Alyscamps, where they should intercede for the dead with prayers, psalms and alms; if a layman had a mass celebrated in one of the seven churches on the site, or if a cleric recited the Psalter, then 'he may be certain to have those pious deceased lying there intercede for his salvation in the presence of God at the final Resurrection'.[48] As with the journey to the Holy Land, prayer en route is as significant as that at the destination. The guide concludes with a description of the city of Compostela itself, and the reception given there to pilgrims. Like Rome and Jerusalem it came to have hostels to accommodate pilgrims. Other texts also testify to the bustle of the town itself. The author of the *Veneranda dies* sermon, which is also found in the *LSJ*, condemns the traders in the market outside the cathedral shrine for being far from honest, and out to profit from the sale to the pilgrims of food, medicines, belts and other leather goods, cloth, and candles.[49]

Like Rome, Compostela was the site of the shrine of an apostle: like Rome it lacked the direct connection to Christ's life embodied by the Holy Land sites. Why then, unlike Rome, did its attraction grow exponentially in the course of the eleventh and twelfth centuries? Like other distant shrines, the journey there was too arduous to attract the sick. Instead pilgrims went out of devotion, and for penance. Like Rome, like Jerusalem, Compostela became a centre for penitential pilgrimages.[50] Its place in the hierarchy of penitential shrines is highlighted in Peter Damian's account of the penances he imposed as papal legate on all the clergy of the Church of Milan whom he found guilty of simony in 1059. In addition to penance, the archbishop of Milan promised to send them all on pilgrimage, either to Rome or to St Martin of Tours, and proposed himself to visit Compostela. The archbishop's own penance was the most severe because he had failed to root out the sins of simony and nicolaitism; it was to last a hundred years although he was allowed to commute it to an annual payment. His pilgrimage should therefore be longer and more onerous than that of his clergy. The arduousness of the pilgrimage contributed to its attraction as a form of penance.[51] Like Rome, like Jerusalem, Compostela owed its popularity to the increased consciousness amongst medieval Christians of their own sinfulness for, whilst some pilgrims went because they were told to do so, many more went out of devotion to alleviate their sense of their own guilt.

The role of pilgrimage in personal conversion narratives

Yet long-distance pilgrimage remained the exception rather than the norm for most people in this period. Its exceptional nature explains why it is portrayed as an important instrument in several narratives of personal conversion: put simply, going on pilgrimage helped to lead some men to change their way of life. For example, in *c.*1079 five knights from Laon in north-eastern France went on pilgrimage to Compostela, and on their return entered the newly established monastery of La Sauve-Majeure, fifteen miles east of Bordeaux, at the behest of its founding abbot, Gerald of Corbie, who had encouraged them to make their pilgrimage.[52]

In two accounts of twelfth-century individuals' conversions to the religious life pilgrimage is portrayed as more overtly penitential. Pilgrimage indicates the start of a process whereby the subjects signified their regret and atonement for their previous sinful way of life. St Gerlac (d. *c.*1170) began his life as a soldier and lover of tournaments but, on hearing of the death of his wife, gave up his sword and, seeking to atone for his previously sinful life, went to the pope in Rome to seek penance for his way of life; the pope imposed upon him a penance of ministering to the poor in Jerusalem for seven years, which he did before returning home to live as a hermit in an oak tree on his estates.[53] Pons of Léras decided in 1132 to give up his former life as a brigand, attacking and stealing the property of various people. As we saw in Chapter 4, he signified his regret by undertaking a very public penance in the square of his local town, and making restitution of livestock and property which he had stolen to its owners. He then went on went on pilgrimage to Compostela, and returned home via other shrines at Mont-St-Michel, St Martin of Tours, St Martial of Limoges and St Leonard of Noblat. He completed his penance by establishing a monastery at Silvanès, in southern France, where he served out his days as a humble lay brother.[54] His pilgrimage, like that of Gerlac, marked an important stage in the narrative transition from sinful to religious life.

In other examples of personal conversion, pilgrimage is more clearly devotional but constituted an important transitional stage. Such is the case for the hermit Godric of Finchale (d. 1170). Born in Norfolk, Godric began his career as a pedlar before graduating to becoming part-owner of a ship. In the course of his work he made pilgrimages to Rome, St Andrew's in Fife, Jerusalem, Santiago de Compostela, Saint Gilles in Provence, and Rome. After going to Rome for a third time he decided to become a hermit, and after two years, made a second pilgrimage to Jerusalem; on his return to England (*c.*1113) he established a hermitage at Finchale, near Durham, with the support of the bishop, where he became well regarded as a holy man amongst the local community, and closely associated with the monks of Durham. His numerous pilgrimages are portrayed by the author of his life as shaping his turn away from the world.[55] Pilgrimage plays a similar role, as we have seen, in the life of Raimondo 'Palmario' of Piacenza, who was first moved to live an exemplary life as a layman, preaching to fellow members of his confraternity, and studying scripture only after his return to Jerusalem, and who, upon being widowed, and after an extensive pilgrimage tour involving both Compostela and Rome, became moved to establish a hospice to care for the poor and the sick.

In portraying pilgrimage as an agent for personal conversion, clerical authors played on the special status of the pilgrim. One of the ideals of early medieval rulership is the protection of the poor and vulnerable, including pilgrims, and this element of St Bobo's vow, as we have seen, owed much to ninth-century ideals of secular rulership: pilgrims, like widows and the poor needed protection. They often (but not always) travelled weaponless in unfamiliar territories for reasons of piety; they thus became a popular object of charity, hence the founding of hostels for pilgrims. The dangers of making a journey into unfamiliar territory meant that by the eleventh century a special rite had been developed to bless the scrips (leather bags) and staffs of those about to set off on pilgrimage to Rome. The emergence of a formal liturgy marked pilgrims out as a separate group distinguished by their dress and equipment. Earlier medieval liturgical books contain blessings for those setting out on a journey, but the rite found in an eleventh-century pontifical from Mainz is the earliest evidence for blessing what it described as the 'signs of pilgrimage': the scrip and the staff. The prayers ask the Lord not only to bless these insignia of a pilgrim's status, but to protect the pilgrims from all secular dangers.[56] By the early twelfth century the rite for blessing pilgrims had become listed among the duties a parish priest could be expected to perform, suggesting pilgrimage's increased popularity at parochial level.[57] Indeed the *Life* of Raimondo 'Palmario' reports pilgrims by the time of its composition as being marked out by the fixing of a sign: it describes how he and his mother took leave of their friends and family before receiving a blessing from the bishop of Piacenza who 'fixed a red cross on their breasts and said "This is the sign which will guard you from all danger. May the most merciful Saviour lead you and bring you back safely."'[58] The absence of earlier evidence for this rite suggests it to be a new development, and perhaps a consequence of the growth in its popularity.

Various explanations have been offered to explain why pilgrimage became more prevalent in this period. One is that pilgrimages acted as the objects of cults which sought to unify societies; the Compostela pilgrimage is, for example, seen as emerging in the context of the Christian fight against the Muslims in Spain; the cult of Ste Foy, examined in Chapter 7, became the local focus for the piety of knights within the relatively lawless Rouergue. Another is that pilgrimage is a 'liminal' experience which took people outside their normal life and created a new community of individuals freed from the ties of daily life.[59] The former explanation has found rather more favour than the latter: just as monks used saints' cults to promote their authority over those living on their lands, pilgrimages helped unify communities. As the evidence gathered here suggests, despite the emphasis of conversion narratives, pilgrimage seems seldom to have been a life-changing rite; the evidence for pilgrims being regarded as a separate *ordo* is late, and instead the evidence of pilgrims' experiences suggests it was, in Colin Morris's words, 'incorporated within the normal structures of social aspiration'.[60] Groups of nobles often travelled together, as did the founders of La Sauve Majeure, or the group led by Richard of Saint-Vannes which made the mass pilgrimage to Jerusalem in 1026. Families might adopt the practice and regard it as normative, as did successive members of the same family, that of the dukes of Aquitaine. Pilgrimage thus became for nobles 'a public demonstration of piety appropriate to their social standing'; it rarely, despite the prevalence of this trope in *vitae*, acted as a catalyst to a change of life.[61] Most pilgrims returned home and to their existing responsibilities: Raimondo 'Palmario' represents the exception, not the rule. Indeed, one of pilgrimage's attractions seems to have been that, unlike monasticism, it did not require a fighting man to change his way of life, or give up his family.[62]

The First Crusade

On 15 July 1099 an army of Latin Christians captured Jerusalem which had been under Moslem control since 638. The collective forces which left Western Europe for the Holy Land in 1096 came from Flanders, the Rhineland, Italy, England and especially France; modern estimates suggest they may have comprised as many as 100,000 at a time when the population of England has been estimated at somewhere between 1.5 and 2.25 million.[63] These forces were far from homogeneous. The first wave left in the spring of 1096; led by several nobleman, both French and German, later chroniclers, writing after its defeat by the Turks in Asia Minor, nevertheless dismissed it as being a rabble of ill-equipped peasants who left for the Holy Land with chiliastic expectations. The main armies left in the late summer, led by Count Raymond of Toulouse, Duke Godfrey of Lorraine, Duke Robert of Normandy and Prince Bohemond of Taranto, in southern Italy, and included some 6,000–7,000 knights. Less than three years later they had taken control of the holiest city in the Christian faith.

Their journey to Jerusalem took just under three years; it had taken Count William IV of Angoulême less than nine months to go there and back, seventy years earlier in 1026. As this comparison suggests, the crusaders encountered a number of practical and military obstacles whilst crossing Asia Minor and travelling down the eastern Mediterranean seaboard. They had to fight the Turks in Asia Minor. They had difficulty finding food and fodder in the Anatolia, and horses and pack animals died, so that knights were reduced to riding oxen. They then spent almost eight months besieging the city of Antioch, and once they had captured it, became entrapped in the citadel in turn by a Moslem relief army. They broke out of this siege only after receiving a morale boost from the miraculous discovery of the Holy Lance which they believed had pierced Christ's side. Less than a month after travelling on from Antioch, and capturing Jerusalem on 15 July 1099, they had to deal with an attack from Egypt. As this brief account suggests, the Christian armies faced major difficulties. They thus quickly came to see their success in taking Jerusalem from Moslem control for the first time in over four hundred years as the will of God. As Jonathan Riley-Smith has demonstrated, the crusaders' very success against such insurmountable odds helped to reinforce their idea of this as a new, and divinely inspired enterprise.[64]

This campaign became known as the first of the crusades and constitutes a new manifestation of extraordinary lay piety. It shared many features with pilgrimage. Like pilgrimage, going on crusade did not require its participants to make any lasting or major changes to their way of life. Like pilgrimage it led them to travel far away from home, initially east across the Mediterranean to fight in the Holy Land, and later to fields in the Baltic and southern Europe. Like pilgrimage, participation seems to have been governed by existing ties of kinship and lordship. As these similarities suggest, crusading built a good deal on the foundations laid previously by devotional and penitential pilgrimages. But medieval commentators attributed the success of the first expedition to its novelty. Writing in *c.*1115, the north French writer Guibert of Nogent wrote of it:

> *God had established holy war in our day so that the order of knights and their followers . . . can find a new way of attaining salvation. Now they need not abandon secular affairs completely by choosing the monastic life, or any other religious profession, as was once customary. Now they can to*

> *some degree win God's grace while pursuing their own way of life, with the freedoms, and in the dress to which they are accustomed.*[65]

Old and new factors combined together to explain the movement's success. Before the First Crusade most ecclesiastics regarded all warfare as sinful even though they accepted St Augustine's thesis that a war is just if fought on the orders of a just prince in a just cause, that is in defence of the Church and the kingdom. But they believed all warfare to be a cause of moral contamination. For example, Burchard of Worms in his early eleventh-century canon law collection prescribed a penance of three annual forty-day fasts if someone killed a man whilst fighting in defence of the peace on the orders of a legitimate prince. He regarded all killing as sinful, and participation – even in a just war – as inherently polluting. The penance rose to fasting for forty days on bread and water for seven consecutive years for someone who killed in battle *without* the orders of a legitimate prince.[66] Burchard merely embodied earlier legal traditions, and records suggest that several bishops sought to implement this general precept. The ordinance drawn up by the west Frankish bishops after the battle of Soissons in 923 between two claimants to the west Frankish throne enjoined a three-year penance on all those who had taken part; it went into detail about the fasts which should be observed, unless prevented by illness or military service.[67] The pragmatism displayed here by the west Frankish bishops points to a world anxious to maintain ecclesiastical support for war, at the same time as preserving the principle that homicide is always sinful. The ordinance drawn up by the Norman bishops after William the Conqueror's victory at Hastings in 1066 a century and a half later enjoined a seven-year penance on those who taken part, and killed, for personal gain, which they reduced to three years to those who had fought for justice.[68] Although both ordinances relate to contentious battles over rival claims to kingship, they signal a world in which active fighting necessarily raised real ethical problems for those who undertook it. Where the crusades departed from earlier practice is in offering a way for knights to atone for past sins not by rejecting the secular life, but by doing what had previously been regarded as intrinsically sinful: fighting.

It is not clear what Urban II intended when he preached his sermon at Claremont, for no contemporary record of it has survived: all the chroniclers wrote their accounts after the successful capture of Jerusalem, and only private notes made by those in attendance at the council itself survive, such as this one:

> *For anyone who, out of devotion alone, and not for the sake of honour or wealth sets out to free the Church of God in Jerusalem, that journey shall be considered as equal to all penance.*[69]

Yet the earliest chroniclers of crusading took up the ideas outlined in this text, suggesting that it represents a widespread understanding within the movement of its purpose. The author of the earliest account, the *Gesta Francorum* (*c.*1100 × 1103), attributes the following speech to Urban II:

> *Whoever wishes to save his soul should not hesitate humbly to take up the way of the Lord, and if he lacks sufficient money, divine mercy will give enough . . . The Franks upon hearing such reports forthwith caused crosses to be sewed on their right shoulders, saying that they followed with one accord the footsteps of Christ, by which they had been redeemed from the hand of hell.*[70]

As this language suggests, in many ways the First Crusade represented a continuation of earlier practices: the idea of going on pilgrimage to Jerusalem as a penance for previous sins, as we have already seen, is not new. Letters written by Pope Urban II soliciting support for the expedition, and those written by participants en route, used the language of both pilgrimage and war to describe the movement, referring to it variously as an *iter* (journey), a *via* (a route), a *peregrinatio* (a pilgrimage), and an army (*exercitus*).[71] Popes had sanctioned wars before: Leo IX absolved the sins of those fighting in his army in 1053, and Gregory VII called on all Christians to go to the aid of the eastern Christians in 1073. But Pope Urban II's call to all lay Christians to go to the aid of the Christians in the east differed from these earlier calls, not least because of the large-scale nature of the response he received. The very success of the First Crusade, improbable given the likelihood of a western army achieving what the Byzantines had failed to do for four centuries, helped to meld existing ideas about warfare, penance and pilgrimage into a developing crusading doctrine.

The emergence of a crusading doctrine is not, however, the entire answer as to why people joined the First Crusade. Investigation of the charter collections of French monasteries by Jonathan Riley-Smith and Marcus Bull has demonstrated the extent to which existing connections influenced whether individuals decided to go or to stay at home. The patronage of one's lord constituted an enormously important factor: certain nobles, for example, took their entire household, down to their huntsman.[72] Leading subjects accompanied great lords such as Stephen, Count of Blois. Kinship played an equally important role: Count Baldwin I of Guines in Flanders left for the east with his four sons, whilst at a lower level three members of the Bernard family of Bré in the Limousin went on crusade; Riley-Smith has identified over forty families from which two or more members took the cross. Individuals lacked the autonomy to decide to take part. Crusading cannot therefore be interpreted as a manifestation of personal piety; rather it represents the collective decisions of local associations and families.

But how did such groups learn about the call, and then arrive at the decision to leave on crusade? Here individual monasteries with which families already had existing ties played a crucial role. It seems likely that individual monks preached about the benefits of going on crusade to their lay patrons. Certainly many monasteries provided crucial financial support which allowed individuals to take part. Charters record the sale of properties in return for money to go to Jerusalem, and the loans made to those going to Jerusalem in return for the use of the property. They also document nobles abandoning their claims to rights over which they were in dispute with monasteries in return for funds to go on the crusade. Such decisions necessarily involved the participation of those staying at home, as well as those leaving, and charters record the agreement of all members of the family who might have a claim to the property against such transactions. Crusading resulted from a collective familial decision.

That crusading armies were recruited through pre-existing ties of family and lordship may perhaps explain one of the features of the movement which is often forgotten. Whilst participants in the First Crusade came mainly from Flanders, the Rhineland, Italy, England and especially from modern-day France, some eminent churchmen and writers of the time in those regions failed to refer to it in their writings, suggesting that the movement's influence may have been more limited to certain pockets of Latin Europe than many writers at the time, or since, would suggest.[73]

In many ways the crusade represents a continuation of existing trends. Although instigated by the ecclesiastical leadership, it is these earlier foundations which allowed it to become a popular movement so rapidly. Whilst it is unclear quite what the pope originally intended, the fact that the idea of crusading grew so quickly is a consequence of the enthusiasm for an idea which developed its own momentum. The experience of the First Crusade itself was so adverse that the crusaders believed, and the Church came to preach, that participation in the crusade could lead to absolution of all sins and that the end object of the crusade was Latin control of the Holy Land where Christ had lived and died and been resurrected. It thus incorporates elements of both devotional and penitential pilgrimage. Crucial to the movement's success were existing social ties: kin, lords, and monasteries all helped promote the doctrine of penitential piety and provided the financial support needed to go on crusade. The very popularity of the First Crusade itself testifies to the increase in lay enthusiasm for religion over the previous two centuries.

Conclusions

Visits to distant saints' shrines and the places associated with the life of Christ, and those of his associates, offered opportunities for medieval Christians to engage with the holy in ways outside the norms of their ordinary daily lives. Indeed, it was not just the visit to the shrine itself, but rather the fact of having gone on such an arduous and difficult journey which marked people out as special: to that extent there seems to be little difference between the claims made for the extraordinary piety displayed by Bobo and that demonstrated by Raimondo 'Palmario' two centuries later. Both men had been, as we have seen, also inspired to care for their fellow men by Christ's teaching; such active piety represented an extension of current norms of lay piety, but, combined with their commitment to pilgrimage, marked them out as extraordinary. At the same time, the mechanisms which allowed Christians to go on pilgrimage, and supported them, meant that pilgrimage should be seen as an extension of their lives, enmeshed as they were in the demands of lordship and family: it was extra-ordinary, but not abnormal.

Such piety, as we have seen, had its grounding in the desire to imitate the life of Christ and his apostles. Raimondo 'Palmario' may have been inspired to take up his life of Christian charity by the preaching of clerics inspired by the *vita apostolica*, such as members of the Vallombrosan order. He anticipates the revival of such ideals by Francis of Assissi and Waldes of Lyons. Bobo, however, lived at the same time or very slightly earlier than one of the earliest proponents of the *vita apostolica* in the medieval west, Romuald of Ravenna, and his *Life* was written in the first half of the eleventh century which is when the earliest formal orders inspired by the apostolic life are first recorded. The lives of both men therefore suggest that apostolic ideals circulated amongst laymen at the same time as they did amongst churchmen: they did not spread from the clergy to the laity. Both laity and clergy lived in the same milieu.

Such an explanation does not, however, encompass the penitential overtones of some pilgrimages. Penitential pilgrimage for heinous crimes such as murder of a bishop or parricide had a long tradition. Thus when Arduin, marquis of Ivrea was sentenced to live as an itinerant pilgrim for the killing of the bishop of Vercelli in 997, when Robert, Duke of Normandy left for Jerusalem to atone for the death of his brother in 1035, and when Count Theoderic of Trier went barefoot to Jerusalem in 1066 to atone for the murder of the archbishop of Trier, they all took part in a well-established custom: the exile of the sinner from the community.[74] But such offences and such sentences never constituted the norm, and cannot, in and of themselves, explain the growth in pilgrimage to distant shrines. The development of a more general penitential awareness of their own sinfulness which guided the travels of many pilgrims, the concern with their own personal salvation and deliverance at the Last Judgement, prevailed amongst pilgrims to Compostela, Rome and Jerusalem, concern not so much with heinous sins but with the consequences of daily life, and of the inherent sinfulness of the noble way of life. The experiences of men such as Pons and Gerlac who turned away from their past lives as knights and brigands to adopt a religious life came to exemplify and articulate the concerns of 'ordinary' lay nobles. Such men might not go to such extremes as these exemplary figures but pilgrimage offered a way for them to make their own contribution to ensuring their soul's fate. The growth in pilgrimage and crusading thus represents not so much the extension of old ideas of penitential punitive exile, but rather the extension of awareness of and concern for their own salvation.

Notes and references

1 *Vita S. Bobonis*, *Acta sanctorum*, *Mai V*, 184–91; Claude Carozzi, 'La vie de Saint Bobon: un modèle clunisien de sainteté laïque', in M. Lauwers, ed., *Guerriers et moines: Conversion et sainteté aristocratiques dans l'occident médiéval (IXe–XIIe siècle)* (Antibes, 2002), 467–91.

2 *Vita S. Bobonis*, 185. The fall of Fraxinetum is dated to 972.

3 F. Avril and J.-R. Gaborit, 'L'*Itinerarium Bernardi monachi* et les pèlerinages d'Italie du Sud pendant le haut moyen-age,' *Mélanges d'archéologie et d'histoire* 79 (1967), 269–98; J. C. Arnold, 'Arcadia Becomes Jerusalem: Angelic Caverns and Shrine Conversion at Monte Gargano', *Speculum* 75 (2000), 567–88; Bernard the Monk, a late ninth-century pilgrim to Jerusalem, ends up at Mont-Saint Michel.

4 Rodulfus Glaber, *Histories*, IV.18–21, 198–201.

5 S. Runciman, 'The Pilgrimages to Palestine before 1095', in K. M. Setton (gen. ed.), *A History of the Crusades, I: The First Hundred Years*, ed. M. W. Baldwin (Madison, Milwaukee and London, 1969), 68–78.

6 Bull, *Knightly Piety*, 208–17.

7 B. S. Bachrach, 'The Pilgrimages of Fulk Nerra, Count of the Angevins 987–1040', in T. F. X. Noble and J. J. Contreni, eds, *Religion, Culture and Society in the Middle Ages: Studies in Honour of Richard E. Sullivan* (Kalamazoo, MI, 1987), 205–17; *Gesta Normannorum Ducum of William of Jumièges, Orderic Vitalis and Robert of Torigni*, ed. E. van Houts (Oxford, 1995), II, 79–85; A. Williams, 'Swein, earl, d. 1052', *Oxford Dictionary of National Biography*; for evidence of pilgrimage to Jerusalem from Bas-Rhône: Bernold of Constance, *Chronicon*, ed. G. Pertz, *MGH SS* V, a. 1066, a. 1073, 428–30; C. Blanc, 'Les pratiques de pieté des laïcs dans les pays du Bas-Rhone aux XIe et XII siècles', *Annales du midi* 72 (1960), 137–47.

8 *Peregrinationes tres: Saewulf, Iohannes Wirziburgensis, Theodericus*, ed. R. B. C. Huygens with J. H. Pryor, CCCM 139 (Turnholt, 1994), 59–77; English translation: 'The Travels of Saewulf AD1102 and 1103', J. Wilkinson, J. Hill and W. F. Ryan, trans, *Jerusalem Pilgrimage 1099–1185*, Hakluyt Society 2nd series 167 (London, 1988), 94–109; Reginald of Durham, *Libellus de vita et miraculis S. Godrici heremitae de Finchale*, ed. J. Stevenson, Surtees Society (London, 1847); *AASS* Julii VI, 645–57, trans. D. Webb, *Saints and Cities in Medieval Italy* (Manchester, 2007), 65–92.

9 Hugh of Flavigny, *Chronicon, MGH SS VIII*, II.18–24, 393–98; Adhemar, *Chronicon*, III.65, 184–85.

10 See n. 7 above.

11 *Vita Altmanni episcopi Pataviensis*, *MGH SS* XII, 230; Lambert of Hersfeld, *Annales*, *MGH SS* V, 168–71.

12 Bull, *Knightly Piety*, 210–17; J. Riley-Smith, *The First Crusaders, 1095–1131* (Cambridge, 1997).

13 Bull, *Knightly Piety*, 212.

14 Adhemar, *Chronicon*, III.48, 167–68.

15 *Peregrinationes tres*, ed. Huygens *et al.*, 59–77; J. Wilkinson *et al.*, *Jerusalem Pilgrimage 1099–1185*, 94–109.

16 Adhemar, *Chronicon*, III.55.

17 D. Pringle, *The Churches of the Crusader Kingdom of Jerusalem: A Corpus*, 4 vols (Cambridge, 1993–2009), III, *The City of Jerusalem*, 192–93.

18 M. C. Ferrari, 'From Pilgrim's Guide to Living Relic: Symeon of Trier and his Biographer Eberwin', in M. W. Herren, C. J. McDonough and R. G. Arthur, eds, *Latin Culture in the Eleventh Century: Proceedings of the Third International Conference of Medieval Latin Studies*, Cambridge, September 9–12 1998, 2 vols, Publications of the Journal of Medieval Latin 5 (Turnhout, 2002), I, 325–43.

19 Cited by Ferrari, 'From Pilgrim's Guide', 325.

20 S. Schein, *Gateway to the Heavenly City: Crusader Jerusalem and the Catholic West (1099–1187)* (Aldershot, 2005), 76.

21 *Peregrinationes tres*, ed. Huygens *et al.*, 148, 155; trans. Wilkinson *et al.*, *Jerusalem Pilgrimage 1099–1185*, 279, 285.

22 Rodulfus Glaber, *Histories*, III.7, 106–09; Fulbert of Chartres, *Letters*, 26.

23 Rodulfus Glaber, *Histories*, II.5, 60–61; Bachrach, 'The Pilgrimages of Fulk Nerra'.

24 On this complex site, see Pringle, *The Churches*, III, 10–14.

25 *Peregrinationes tres*, ed. Huygens *et al.*, 59–77; trans. Wilkinson *et al.*, *Jerusalem Pilgrimage.*

26 Theoderic, c. 25, *Peregrinationes tres*, 172; trans. Wilkinson *et al.*, *Jensalem Polgrimage*, 41; Schein, *Gateway*, 67.

27 B. Hamilton, 'The Impact of Crusader Jerusalem on Western Christendom', *Catholic Historical Review* 80 (1994), 695–713 (citing Theodoric at p. 707).

28 G. Constable, 'The Imitation of the Humanity of Christ', in his *Three Studies in Medieval Religious and Social Thought* (Cambridge, 1995), 169–93 at p. 179. See also his 'The Imitation of the Body of Christ', ibid., 194–217.

29 R. Fulton, *From Judgement to Passion: Devotion to Christ and the Virgin Mary, 800–1200* (New York, 2002), 142–92; S. Lipton, 'Images in the World: Reading the Crucifixion', in M. Rubin, ed., *Medieval Christianity in Practice* (Princeton, NJ, 2009), 173–85; eadem, 'The Sweet Lean of His Head: Writing about Looking at the Crucifix in the High Middle Ages', *Speculum* 80 (2005), 1172–208.

30 C. 2, *Acta Sanctorum* Iulii VI, 648–49; trans. Webb, *Saints and Cities*, 69.

31 Odo of Cluny, *Life of Gerald of Aurillac*, II. 17, *PL* 133, 680; trans. Sitwell, 146–47.

32 Ibid. II. 22, *PL* 133, 683; trans. Sitwell, 150.

33 Bull, *Knightly Piety*, 208, 214.

34 C. 18, *PL* 140, 1062.

35 *C&S* I, 230–37.

36 H. W. Dey, 'Diaconiae, Xenodochia, Hospitalia and Monasteries: 'Social Security' and the Meaning of Monasticism in Early Medieval Rome', *Early Medieval Europe* 16 (2008), 398–422 at 409; R. Krautheimer, *Rome: Profile of a City, 312–1308* (Princeton, NJ, 2000), 80–83.

37 R. Stopani, *La via francigena in Toscana*, 2nd edn (Florence, 1984); V. Ortenberg, 'Archbishop Sigeric's Journey to Rome in 990', *Anglo-Saxon England*, 19 (1990), 197–246.

38 S. G. Bruce, 'An Abbot Between Two Cultures: Maiolus Of Cluny Considers the Muslims of La Garde-Freinet', *Early Medieval Europe* 15 (2007), 426–40.

39 D. Birch, *Pilgrimage to Rome in the Middle Ages: Continuity and Change* (Woodbridge, 1998), 150–202.

40 Julia M. H. Smith, 'Old Saints, New Cults: Roman Relics in Carolingian Francia', in J. M. H. Smith, ed., *Early Medieval Rome and the Christian West: Essays in Honour of Donald A. Bullough* (Leiden, 2000), 317–39.

41 Birch, *Pilgrimage*, 110–112.

42 R. A. Fletcher, *Saint James's Catapult: The Life and Times of Diego Gelmirez of Santiago de Compostela* (Oxford, 1984), 53–101; Special issue of *La Corónica: A Journal of Medieval Spanish Language and Literature* 36 (2008).

43 Adhemar, *Chronicon*, III.41.

44 Bull, *Knightly Piety*, 230–35.

45 The 'Veneranda dies' Sermon in *Liber Sancti Jacobi: Codex Calixtinus*, ed. W. M. Whitehill, G. Prado and J. C. Garciá, 3 vols (Santiago, 1944); trans. in *The Miracles of Saint James*, ed. and trans. T. F. Coffey, L. K. Davidson and M. Dunn (New York, 1996), 8–56 at 18–19.

46 *Liber Sancti Jacobi*, ed. Whitehill; W. Melczer, trans., *The Pilgrim's Guide to Santiago de Compostela* (New York, 1993).

47 C. Hohler, 'A Note on the Jacobus', *Journal of the Warburg and Courtauld Institutes* 35 (1972), 31–80.

48 Melczer, trans., *The Pilgrim's Guide*, 97–98.

49 'Veneranda dies', trans. Coffey *et al.*, *The Miracles of Saint James*, 41–49.

50 U. Berlière, 'Les pèlerinages judiciares au moyen âge', *Revue bénédictine* 7 (1890), 520–26; H. Platelle, 'La violence et ses remèdes en Flandre au XIe siècle', *Sacris Erudiri: Jaarboek voor Godsdienstwetenschappen* 20 (1971), 101–73; C. Vogel, 'Le Pèlerinage pénitentiel', *Revue des sciences religieuses* 38 (1964) 113–53; repr in idem, *En Rémission des péchés: recherches sur les systèmes pénitentiels dans l'église latine*, ed. A. Faivre (Aldershot, 1994), no. VII.

51 Ep. 65, *Die Briefe des Petrus Damiani*, II. 228–47; S. Hamilton, *The Practice of Penance, 900–1050* (Woodbridge, 2001), 186–88.

52 M. Bull, 'The Confraternity of La Sauve-Majeure: A Foreshadowing of the Military Order', in M. Barber, ed., *The Military Orders: Fighting For the Faith and Caring for the Sick* (Aldershot, 1994), 313–19.

53 *AASS Januarii I*, 307–08.

54 B. M. Kienzle, 'The Works of Hugo Francigena: 'Tractatus de conversione Pontiide Laracio et exordii Salvanensis monasterii vera narratio; epistolae' (Dijon, Bibliothèque municipale MS 611)', *Sacris erudiri* 34 (1993), 273–311; 'The Tract on the Conversion of Pons of Léras and the true account of the beginning of the monastery at Silvanès', trans. B. M. Kienzle, in Head, ed., *Medieval Hagiography*, 499–513.

55 Reginald of Durham, *Libellus de vita et miraculis S. Godrici heremitae de Finchale*, ed. J. Stevenson, Surtees Society (London, 1847); V. Tudor, 'Godric of Finchale', *New Oxford Dictionary of National Biography.*

56 *PRG* II.362.

57 J. Fleming, *Gille of Limerick c.1070–1145. Architect of a Medieval Church* (Dublin, 2001).

58 *Acta Sanctorum* Julii VI, 647.

59 For a review of the anthropological literature, see J. Eade and M. J. Sallnow, eds, *Contesting the Sacred: the Anthropology of Christian Pilgrimage*, 2nd edn (Urbana and Chicago, IL, 2000).

60 Colin Morris, 'Introduction', in C. Morris and P. Roberts, eds, *Pilgrimage*, 7.

61 Webb, *Medieval European Pilgrimage*, 107.

62 Webb, *Pilgrims*, 20.

63 J. France, *Victory in the East: A Military History of the First Crusade* (Cambridge, 1994): 'The main force of the People's Crusade was of the order of 20,000. . . . A total of 70,000–80,000 reached Asia Minor at one time or another. Thousands more must have died on the road to Constantinople, or turned back before they got there', 142. England's population: Barlett, *England*, 290–92; E. Miller and J. Hatcher, *Medieval England: Rural Society and Economic Change 1086–1384* (London, 1978), 28–33.

64 J. Riley-Smith, *The First Crusade and the Idea of Crusading* (London, 1986).

65 *Guibert of Nogent, Gesta dei per Francos* cuted by A. Jotischky, *Crusading and the Crusader States* (Harlow, 2004), 30.

66 Hamilton, *Practice*, 190–96; Burchard, *Decretum* VI.23, *PL* 140, cols 770–1.

67 Mansi, *Concilia*, XVIIIA, 345–46.

68 *C&S* I, no. 88, 581–84.

69 R. Somerville, *The Councils of Urban II*, vol. 1: *Decreta Claromontensia* (Amsterdam, 1972), 74; 'The Council of Clermont (1095) and Latin Christian Society', *Archivum Historiae Pontificiae* 12 (1974), 55–90.

70 *Gesta Francorum et aliorum Hierosolimitanorum*, ed. R. Hill (London, 1962).

71 Riley-Smith, *The First Crusaders*, 67.

72 J. France, 'Patronage and the Appeal of the First Crusade', in J. Phillips, ed., *The First Crusade: Origins and Impact* (Manchester, 1997), 5–20. Riley-Smith, *The First Crusaders*; Bull, *Knightly Piety*, 274–80.

73 S. Edgington, 'The First Crusade: Reviewing the Evidence', in Philips, ed., *The First Crusade*, 57–77.

74 Vogel, 'Le Pèlerinage'.

part 3

Church and people

chapter 9

Discipline and belief

For we can see that many matters of importance to the Catholic faith are canvassed by the feverish restlessness of heretics, and the result is that they are more carefully examined, more clearly understood, and more earnestly propounded, with a view to defending them against heretical attack, and thus an argument aroused by an adversary turns out to be an opportunity for instruction.

Augustine, *De Civitate Dei*, XVI.2[1]

Many of the narrative accounts written between 900 and 1200 are peppered with accounts of lay opposition to ecclesiastical authority, lay resistance to clerical attempts to impose the norms of religious practices, lay expressions of blasphemy and disbelief, and cynicism about some of the less rational aspects of theological teaching. People who dare to mock the powers of a particular saint or to challenge the authority of the custodians of her cult are thrown to the ground or lose their minds; dreadful things happen to those who have the temerity to refuse to take communion at least once a year at Easter. Such tales have much to tell us about the messages which their clerical authors wished to convey to their fellow churchmen and their lay flocks; their interest in defending clerical authority and in articulating correct practice and belief testify to the importance of both these issues to their readers.

At the same time such incidents provided churchmen with opportunities to develop and articulate their own visions of how lay Christians should behave and what they should believe. To that extent tales of dissent and disbelief often serve a function within a particular text and it is tempting to dismiss them as literary convention. But in what follows it is worth remembering that if such behaviour had not occurred it is unlikely these accounts would have taken the forms they did. What would be the point of recounting miracle stories about the dreadful things which happened to those guilty of such behaviour, if the audience for these anecdotes did not include churchmen and lay men for whom encounters with such scepticism, apathy and dissent constituted a real phenomenon?[2] At the same time, such incidents provided churchmen with opportunities to develop their own vision of how lay Christians should behave and what they should believe. Students of such accounts of lay dissent and apathy need to bear in mind Augustine's axiom, cited above, that real encounters with heresy provide an 'opportunity for instruction'. Although his text is part of a widely known work, it is not yet clear whether medieval churchmen knew this particular passage better than modern historians. Recent scholars of medieval heresy and lay piety have, however, reached the same conclusion as Augustine did almost sixteen hundred years ago, albeit by different paths: such incidents provided ecclesiastics with an opportunity to instruct their flock as to how Christians should behave (orthopraxy) and what they should believe (orthodoxy). Dominique Iogna-Prat has gone so far as to suggest that the twelfth-century abbot of Cluny, Peter the Venerable (1122–1156), helped create a new sense of Christian order through his critiques of heresy, Judaism and Islam.[3] But Peter's writings failed to circulate widely outside Cluny; they tell us about the views of his monastic circle rather than those of clerics in the wider pastoral Church.

It is therefore worth investigating in more detail than Iogna-Prat was able to do whether Peter's approach is not part of a wider trend in pastoral and theological writings across the years 900 to 1200. How far was his attempt to promote a vision for Christianity outlining what it should be – by establishing what it was not – shared more widely amongst other writers? This chapter investigates a sample of accounts of lay scepticism, dissent and heresy drawn from across these centuries, focusing in particular but not exclusively on the challenges and encounters faced by bishops. Did other churchmen, in particular bishops, also follow Augustine in using individual incidents to establish their own visions for what constituted orthodoxy and orthopraxy by establishing what it was not?

Resistance to ecclesiastical authority, cynicism and incredulity are all common traits of early medieval descriptions of encounters between churchmen and the laity. Popular heresy, by contrast, represents a new phenomenon. There are no reports of widespread popular heresy in the medieval west between the seventh century and the end of the tenth. R. I. Moore and others interpret its re-emergence in the eleventh century as testament, in part at least, to the success of the Church's early medieval programme of pastoral care.[4] The enthusiasm of some lay Christians, as a consequence, brought them into conflict with the ecclesiastical hierarchy. Heresies, and the ways in which churchmen reported them, thus have the potential to provide us with insight into lay as well as clerical perspectives on the nature of the relationship between the Church and its people.

The processes whereby ecclesiastics defined and established who should be regarded as orthodox and who not have much, therefore, to tell us about the success of the pastoral project in this period. They show us the ways in which churchmen sought to impose their views both upon other clerics and the laity. At the same time, they allow us to follow how churchmen responded to lay thoughts and concerns. This chapter traces these processes in three related arenas: the episcopal administration of public penance and excommunication; reports of lay scepticism; and reports of popular heresy. In each circumstance bishops served as judges of right from wrong, orthodoxy from heresy. Their role on such occasions contributed to the construction of their portraits as office holders. They might be described routinely dealing with those who contravened the Church's rules through penance and using excommunication against those who obstreperously ignored their authority. The imposition of such sentences helped to bolster their often fragile authority by defining who was in and who outside the Church, an important matter in a world in which membership of the Church and society was theoretically co-terminus. They also used such sentences to set out what it meant to be a full member of the Church: describing those outside it allowed them to explain what was required of those inside. Tales of lay scepticism performed a similar didactic function. Their authors often used such tales, on the one hand, to depict how Christians should behave and, on the other, to portray particular churchmen as defenders of orthodoxy. Finally, investigation of the reasons why churchmen chose to report examples of heresy and to focus on the details they did similarly allows us to ask how far such accounts had such a purpose. Investigating this material allows us to ask how far the clergy owed the development of their pastoral vision for the Church to the 'feverish restlessness' of lay challengers to their authority?

Excommunication and penance

Bishops used the rites of penance and excommunication to discipline those individuals who contradicted the Church's precepts. They alone had authority to administer those for public penance and excommunication, and there is plenty of evidence to suggest they did so routinely. The evidence for these rites therefore demonstrates the sorts of opposition bishops could routinely expect to encounter to their temporal as well as sacerdotal authority. The liturgies used on such occasions provided a framework for these episcopal encounters with opponents which would have been familiar to other churchmen.

Excommunication – exclusion both from all Christian rites and from any form of social contact with all other Christians – has a long history stretching back to the New Testament. But records of the liturgical formula recited by the bishop when he sentenced someone to excommunication are only recorded from the tenth century.[5] In fact the first text to survive dates from 6 July 900, when twelve bishops assembled in Rheims cathedral to excommunicate the murderers of Fulk, the previous archbishop of Rheims, with the words:

> *In the name of the Lord and by the power of the Holy Spirit, as well as by the authority divinely conferred on bishops by blessed Peter, first of the apostles, we separate these same ones from the bosom of Holy Mother Church, and we condemn them with the anathema of a perpetual curse so that their recovery cannot ever be effected by man nor [may they have] any conversation with Christians.*[6]

Records of these formulas quickly proliferated over the course of the next three centuries, alongside other accounts of excommunication, pointing to its popularity as a favoured weapon in the episcopate's spiritual armoury. For only bishops had the authority to excommunicate, inherited, as the formula declared, from St Peter to whom Christ had given the power to bind and to loose sinners from the consequences of their actions.

Bishops used excommunication in a great variety of situations: against lay men, as at Rheims where the murderers were named as three men of Count Baldwin of Flanders – Winemar, Euverard and Ratrid – and in 1073 when Pope Alexander II excommunicated various counsellors of King Henry IV for encouraging him to support a simoniacal candidate for the archbishopric of Milan; and against other clerics, as in 1008 when

Archbishop Arnulph of Milan excommunicated Bishop Odelric of Asti for accepting the see during the lifetime of his predecessor, or in 1166 when Thomas Becket, Archbishop of Canterbury, excommunicated Gilbert Foliot, Bishop of London.[7] As these cases suggest, it tended to be used in high profile political cases to defend the authority of individual bishops, albeit sometimes in the name of wider principles. It occurs in many less high profile cases as well, as suggested by the wording of many liturgical formulae which refer to disputes over land. The proliferation of such formulae testify to the popularity of this practice which advertised bishops' authority over other men through their ability to prohibit access to Christian communion, confession and burial, and thus the probability of salvation. But bishops only invoked it as a weapon of last resort, when other means had failed, in order to try to bring the other side to the negotiating table: in this they were often successful. In 1008, for example, Archbishop Arnulf lifted the sentence against Bishop Odelric of Asti after he did penance for his disobedience but Odelric retained possession of his see.[8] The imposition of excommunication is thus testimony to the vulnerability and relative weakness of episcopal power, rather than a sign of its strength.

The successful realisation of the sentence of excommunication required the co-operation of the entire Christian community. This is made clear in liturgical rites such as that in Regino's early tenth-century handbook of canon law. The bishop declared it in a solemn and public ceremony which took place within the Mass. He delivered the sentence after the reading of the Gospel 'with clerics and people' in attendance. The formal statement was then read and approved by both the clerics *and* the people who should say 'Amen, Fiat' and 'Anathema sit'. Then the bishop, together with twelve priests, threw down their lighted candles and trampled them with their feet, just as the excommunicant's chances of salvation is extinguished by their recalcitrant behaviour.[9] Church law made provision for publicising the sentence to churches both within the diocese and in those of its neighbours, for it could only be effective as a punishment if imposed universally.[10] It would not work if excommunicants could escape the consequences by moving to another diocese. Canon law also enjoined excommunication on all those who had contact with excommunicants. In harnessing the co-operation of the people and the clergy, both in the congregation and throughout the diocese, into the working of the rite the bishops sought to enforce their authority through communal action.

The role of the wider community becomes even clearer in the rite for the reconciliation of penitent excommunicants. For excommunication is always intended to bring resolution to a conflict, and the liturgy provided for such an occasion. One rite for the reconciliation of excommunicants from eleventh-century England emphasised the importance of lay intercessors in presenting penitent excommunicants to the bishop and thus anticipates a world of negotiation and settlement.[11] But rites which circulated in east and west Frankia at the same time made no such provision, preferring to emphasise the bishop's authority, perhaps because of its vulnerability; we know that in a couple of tenth-century cases the king of the west Franks intervened to get sentences overturned. King Louis, for example, intervened at the request of Count Ragenold in 953 to prevent a sentence of excommunication being declared against him at a synod in Rheims.[12] Leading members of the laity, like Ragenold, seem to have regarded the most powerful weapon in the episcopal armoury as one which was negotiable. The evidence for excommunication in this period is thus evidence for episcopal insecurity, rather than authority.

There is, however, plentiful evidence for actual examples of excommunication which, when combined with the liturgical evidence, suggest that the imposition of the sentence provides a useful occasion to preach to the assembled clerical and lay audience about the implications of excommunication, and thus affords a means by which bishops could instruct their lay flock as to how they should be expected to behave. The relative absence of positive statements about how Christians should behave has already been noted in Chapter 5; the texts of liturgical formulae suggest that excommunication provided a further opportunity for bishops to define the rites that all Christians should attend and undergo by stating those from which excommunicants were excluded. For example, one popular formula found in both canon law collections and pontificals of the period enjoined that excommunicants should be excluded from normal social interaction with other Christians, and from the Mass, Holy Communion, and Christian burial in consecrated ground unless they sought to be reconciled at their own volition:

> *Let no Christian say* Ave *to them. Let no priest presume to celebrate mass or give communion. 'Let them be buried in an ass's grave' [Jer. 22.19] and let them be on a dung heap on top of the face of the earth. And just as these lights thrown down from our hands are extinguished today, so*

> *may their lights be extinguished in eternity, unless haply they come to their senses and make satisfaction to the church of God which they wounded by emendation and proper penance.*[13]

Excommunication thus provided an opportunity for the episcopate to set out correct Christian behaviour. As it was extremely unlikely that those being excommunicated would be present to hear the sentence, this spelling out of what constituted orthopraxy was for the benefit of the assembled congregation. Indeed excommunicants are sometimes cast as 'other' in the formulae, cast out of the Church unless they accepted and submitted to its authority and gave up their claims. In the words of one such text, composed in the late tenth-century Catalan diocese of Elne (965 × 977), the world is divided into Christians, who 'restrain themselves from the poisonous filth of sins' and those who, despite acknowledging themselves to be Christians

> *are not [Christian] but are [instead] of the synagogue of Satan . . . because deserting the justice of God, and fixing upon their own will, they are not subject to the justice of God, but plundering the goods of holy churches, as if most inhuman wolves, they do not hesitate to turn over their bodies and souls to the Devil.*[14]

Such occasions provided bishops with an opportunity to set up their own vision of how the world should be, by establishing what it should not be. They are at once testimony to episcopal claims to spiritual authority and domination, and the fragility of such assertions. Yet they also provided opportunities for bishops to project an ideal of ecclesiastical unity of clergy and people, relying as they did on the co-operation of the *populus* to enforce the sentence. The challenges to Christian unity presented by contumacious recalcitrants unwilling to accept episcopal rule thus allowed the development by certain churchmen of their vision for the Christian life.

Excommunication served as a weapon of last resort for bishops to bring those who consciously and persistently contravened ecclesiastical authority to submission and penance. But despite its increasing popularity, it still constituted a relatively rare event reserved for exceptional cases. Penance was more common. Penance allowed individuals to atone for the inevitable sinfulness of their earthly life through confession, the performance of penitential acts which enabled them to demonstrate their repentance, and through good works to help ensure their salvation in the life to come. It was thus a preventative act which protected Christians from the inevitable consequences of their mortal life.[15]

The liturgical collections compiled between 900 and 1200 distinguished between public penance and penance 'in the usual way'.[16] The bishop imposed the former in a public ceremony on Ash Wednesday, and concluded with the penitents being expelled from the church building and the ecclesiastical community for the duration of Lent before they were formally and publicly reconciled in another rite on Maundy Thursday. Penance 'in the usual way' could be administered by a priest at any time. The rite for public penance, by linking expulsion from the physical building to that from the metaphysical community, is part of a new trend within Christianity which, as we shall see later in this chapter, attributed increasing significance to church buildings as holy spaces.

There is, however, considerable variety in the different forms of individual rites recorded in different places, and different times, across these three centuries, suggesting that the practice of penance constituted a widespread and living tradition, subject to minor variations in custom in different places.[17] Scholars have attempted to distinguish formal public penance from that for penance 'in the usual way'; the former was supposedly reserved for public sins or *scandala* which had offended the public weal in some way, the latter for sins, however heinous, committed in the private domain. This binary distinction reflects the neat divisions of canon law rather than the reality of a much messier practice in which penance 'in the usual way' might be used for public sins.[18]

What all rites for entry into penance emphasise is the importance of the penitent's confession. The priest or bishop administering the rite should hear the penitent's confession and award the penance appropriate to their person, circumstances and the nature of the sin, taking into account, in the words of the tenth-century Romano-German Pontifical, 'the quality of both the sins and the man'.[19] Before doing so the priest should catechise the penitent about the orthodoxy of his belief:

> *Do you believe in God the Father, the Son and the Holy Spirit?* The penitent replies, *I believe.*
>
> *Do you believe that three persons, the Father, the Son and the Holy Spirit, are one God?* He replies, *I do.*

Do you believe that you will arise in this flesh in which you are now, and receive [sentence at the Last Judgement] according to what you have done, both good and evil? He replies, *I do.*

Do you want to forgive the sins of those who have sinned against you, as the Lord says, 'If you will not forgive men their sins, neither will your Father forgive your sins.' If he wishes to forgive them, receive his confession and indicate to him his penance. If he does not want to, do not receive his confession.[20]

This particular text is taken from the rite for the imposition of penance on Ash Wednesday recorded in the mid-tenth-century Romano-German pontifical, but this interrogation circulated very widely in manuscripts of the ninth, tenth and eleventh centuries. The wording of these questions deliberately echoes that of the Creed and the Our Father, the two texts which all Christians were expected to know, and which godparents were expected to teach their godchildren.[21] Formal confession thus afforded priests an opportunity to instruct penitents in orthodoxy. Just as excommunication allowed bishops to define what constituted the norms of Christian life by specifying that the recalcitrant should be excluded from them, penance provided a means for inculcating the norms of orthodox belief amongst individual Christians.

Scepticism and authority

Accounts of lay scepticism drew on the same rhetoric of Christian community and orthodox belief and practice as that used in penitential rites. Modern scholars who have drawn attention to the existence of medieval lay scepticism have focused, for the most part, on the period in the run-up to and immediately after the Fourth Lateran Council (1215), suggesting that it should be interpreted as a consequence of the success of the 'pastoral' revolution in which churchmen sought to educate the laity in the fundamental tenets of the faith.[22] But, as we have already seen, churchmen throughout the years 900 to 1200 kept up an interest in promoting pastoral care to the laity; recent work by scholars of early medieval penance, for example, has suggested that bishops sought anxiously to train priests in penance, and that the practice of confession and penance was widespread in the tenth and eleventh centuries, offering plentiful opportunities to inculcate orthodox belief in the laity.[23] Therefore can the examples of lay scepticism and opposition we encounter regularly in narratives composed in the three centuries before Lateran IV be similarly explained as a consequence of the success of pastoral care in this period? Or is opposition to attempts by the clergy to impose their authority over the lives of lay communities a constant of these accounts, and not a just a consequence of the thirteenth-century pastoral agenda? Popular resentment and cynicism about the powers of particular saints, and the efficacy of particular rites, is a common feature of such reports, but it is worth thinking about the particular circumstances in which particular writers recorded individual anecdotes in order to understand the different roles which such stories played in the thought world of their monastic and clerical authors.

Refuting lay scepticism, for example, is the overt purpose of one account in Book IV of the 'Miracles of Sainte Foy', composed for her shrine at Conques in south-western France in the second half of the eleventh century. It tells of a peasant who jeered at a jerry-built wooden church dedicated to the saint erected by a monk called Deusdet in Sardan in the Bazadais in Gascony. Peasants, we are told, walked past this rickety structure frequently en route to cut down the forest to establish new fields for cultivation, and when they did so they usually 'bowed humbly in honour of the holy place'. But one peasant mocked the others saying 'I think you would be as likely to get salvation from a doghouse'. The vengeful saint did not tolerate his impiety: he was thrown to the ground, and lost his mind, whereupon the others carried him into the church, and prayed for him, keeping vigil, until he was cured by Sainte Foy. The miracle concludes 'And after they had seen this, all who lived around there began to give the place more reverence, and they believed without a doubt that Sainte Foy's power flourished there'. The author used this account not only to emphasise the power of the saint, but also to emphasise that it was the dedication of the church which made it holy, rather than its appearance. He likened the cynical peasant to

> *those heretics who do not understand the mystery of spiritual grace, so they deny the water in the baptismal font is able to change its natural properties and assert that it always stays exactly the same. They need to know and understand that there are two aspects to the sacrament of baptism – the water in the baptismal font and sanctification – and it is*

> *when they are conjoined that the sacrament is imbued with power. And in the same way, out of a material building and a spiritual sacrament one body is made in the edifice of holy Mother Church.*[24]

A generation or so earlier the abbot of Cluny, Peter the Venerable, had mounted a similar defence of baptism and church buildings against the criticisms of the heretic, Peter of Bruis, that salvation was by faith alone, and therefore infant baptism was unnecessary, as were consecrated churches because the Church was not a material construction but rather the spiritual community of the faithful. Peter the Venerable argued that just as baptism reflected the community of the faithful, because godparents made vows on behalf of unknowing infants, so physical buildings acted as the material representation of the congregation of believers.[25] The author of the Sainte Foy miracula anticipated his sociological arguments suggesting that they are part of a more general trend in Latin thought in the central Middle Ages in which the physical church building and its surrounding territory became identified with the Christian community.[26] This tale is, therefore, not so much evidence for popular heresy in eleventh-century Gascony but rather for the way in which an anecdote told within the monastic community at Conques about how one obstreperous peasant got his comeuppance was placed by the *miracula*'s clerical author within the context of contemporary debates about the material church. For, as Dominique Iogna-Prat has shown, the Latin Church Fathers had been remarkably reluctant to regard the sites of churches as holy; the defence of churches as consecrated spaces was something which had to be worked out between the ninth and thirteenth centuries in various *fora*.[27] The tale only became worth writing down because it allowed the author to defend church buildings. The peasant's scepticism in other words served a wider polemical purpose.

Elsewhere authors reported cynical laymen challenging the Church's authority in other ways. Such tales served didactic as well as polemical purposes, and probably resonated with lay and clerical audiences very differently. The *Deeds of the Bishops of Cambrai*, for example, records a story told to Bishop Gerard I of Cambrai (1012–51) by Bishop Adalbold of Utrecht (1010–26). It describes how it had been the custom in one parish within the Utrecht diocese for hardly anyone to take the Eucharist at Easter, so one year the priest took extra care to admonish the common people that such heavenly food is both restorative and will help them to gain heavenly lives. Whilst they hesitated, however, the village chief (*maior*) said he preferred beer to the Eucharist, and led the resistance, getting drunk in the tavern instead of attending Mass; but divine retribution led the *maior* to fall from his horse, breaking his neck. He was buried with the honour befitting his position in the local cemetery. The bishop was absent at the imperial court at the time but when the case was reported to him, he ordered that the dead man be treated as an excommunicant and disinterred. No one, however, dared to implement the sentence in the face of opposition from the *maior*'s powerful kindred; when the bishop returned from court he therefore went to the village and ordered that the body be disinterred, after fifty days, and dragged from the grave with a rope tied around its feet, before being reburied away from the community in unconsecrated ground; within a mile the corpse vomited up the beer as if he had recently drunk it,

> *Because, as the lord bishop always said, for which reason I have written it, it should not be hidden from future generations that the faithful are killed through merit, the unfaithful shaken with terror.*[28]

The tale seems to have been one of Bishop Gerard's favourite anecdotes, and clearly told to boost episcopal authority: no one, however powerful, escapes the consequences of excommunication. But it also had another purpose: to promote the practice of regular communion at Easter by spelling out the consequences for those who did not take part. Although the report in the *Deeds* is clearly aimed at the clerics at the bishop's court, it could also have been used in synodal instruction to parish priests to provide encouragement to their efforts to administer annual communion to their lay flocks.

Another story with a similar moral is recounted in the next chapter of the *Deeds*. Albert, count of Vermandois, had entered a monastery on what he thought was his deathbed in order to atone for the scandalous sins he had committed in his lifetime, but he had then recovered, and reneged on his vows. On his actual deathbed he dared to take the *viaticum* without making a last confession, and the host placed in his mouth burned away his tongue. All his vices and sins for which he had not done penance, or shown contrition, corrupted his tongue. The story's overt moral is that one should always be frightened of the wickedness one had committed, and give thanks for merit.[29] Presumably this story circulated amongst the clerical communities of northern France in part to inculcate good practice. But Theo Riches, in a detailed study of this section of the *Deeds*, has demonstrated how its author chose to include both these tales as part of a complex account in which he sought to emphasise the importance of Bishop Gerard's authority by demonstrating the effectiveness of spiritual weapons.[30] For, in reality, as we shall see when we come to accounts of heresy in the diocese, the authority of the bishop of Arras-Cambrai was fragile and contested by both powerful monasteries like that of St Vaast in Arras and secular castellans like Walter in Cambrai. Stories like these which demonstrated the awesome force of the sacerdotal ministry helped to support the bishop's claims to spiritual lordship in such circumstances.

The author of the *Deeds* was not alone is using the figures of sceptical lay men to demonstrate the orthodoxy and authority of church services and saints, and of the clergy who serve them. But the authors of such texts wrote for clerical communities, and only indirectly for the lay communities they served. The inclusion of some of these stories, such as the attribution of the tale of the drunken *maior* to the bishop of Utrecht, conjures up a world of clerical gossip amongst bishops at the imperial court, at which such tales might be exchanged amongst those seeking assurance about the effectiveness of clerical authority in an uncertain and hostile world. Such accounts thus formed an important basis upon which to secure ideals of clerical authority, and thus clerical identity, but for them to resonate, and their morals to be understood, they needed to be grounded in the realities of day-to-day pastoral care. They can be used as evidence that religious scepticism was widespread, but only because recalcitrance and cynicism are necessary corollaries of flattering portraits of clerical authority: orthodoxy is essential to a portrait of a good bishop, and in order to demonstrate his orthodoxy he has to be seen to judge right from wrong. This aspect of his office acquired renewed significance when confronted with a seemingly new challenge to his authority from those who refused to accept the Church's teachings on correct Christian belief and practice: heresy.

Heresy and orthodoxy

The emergence of an apparently new phenomenon in the early eleventh century, that of popular heretical movements, has to be placed alongside this ideal of the bishop as judge and arbiter of orthodoxy.[31] Between *c.*1015 and *c.*1052 members of the higher clergy identified various groups of lay men and women in north-eastern France, Flanders, Aquitaine, northern Italy and Lotharingia as following various practices and beliefs which they deemed heretical. After fading away as an issue in the second half of the eleventh century, groups of dissenters reappeared in the Low Countries, French Alps and Provence in the early twelfth century, and further groups of heretics are reported in northern France, Flanders, the Rhineland, southern France, and northern and central Italy across the course of the twelfth century. These reports are independent of each other: churchmen writing in Burgundy, Flanders, Aquitaine, northern Italy and the Empire recorded incidents in the first of half of the eleventh century. It was the first time since late Antiquity that churchmen had confronted such challenges to their interpretation of orthodoxy from groups of the populace, and it bothered them, as it has done modern scholars who have sought to explain the reoccurrence of popular heresy in various ways.[32]

Faced with a new problem, medieval writers looked to earlier authors, in particular the Church Fathers, for guidance. Their reliance on earlier authorities, in particular Augustine of Hippo's treatise against heresies, which included detailed descriptions of heretical beliefs, has led to doubts about the authenticity of their descriptions of these medieval groups. Guibert of Nogent, for example, included in his account of the beliefs and practices of one particular group, discovered and tried by the bishop of Soissons in the early twelfth century, the comment 'If one rereads the list of heresies compiled by Augustine one realises that this one is most like that of the Manichaeans'.[33] It has been argued on stylistic grounds that Guibert added the long list of charges of sexual abandon, infanticide and cannibalism which preceded this remark to his original account somewhat later, in order to reinforce the validity of the episcopal court's verdict.[34] Guibert is merely one of several medieval writers to use the Manichaean label; they may have been attracted to it because Augustine had himself been a Manichee before he became a Christian, and therefore left a detailed account.[35] The Manichaeans of Late Antiquity were dualist heretics who taught the existence of not one God, but rather two principles, that of light and darkness. Light ruled the spiritual world, darkness the material world; particles of light were trapped in man, and man was thus locked in a struggle to escape the material world for the spiritual world. The Manichees thus taught abhorrence of sexual congress and the eating of meat, as they sought to escape from the material world of the devil; they also had their own initiation rites. Yet it is impossible to dismiss the Manichaean label invoked by medieval writers to describe these heretical groups as meaningless. Adhemar of Chabannes, writing in Limoges in the early eleventh century, not only described the groups of popular heretics he encountered as Manicheans in his *Chronicon*, but also went to the trouble of writing a series of sermons against various different aspects of dualist teaching. He took the threat to orthodoxy they posed very seriously.[36]

Historians who take what medieval writers wrote seriously have sought to explain the re-emergence of groups seemingly espousing the tenets of dualist heresies in the medieval west by looking to the east.[37] There, a century earlier, in the tenth century, Byzantine churchmen had uncovered a dualist heresy in the Byzantine-ruled Balkans which they called Bogomilism. Some modern scholars argue that reports of western heresy share many similarities with the tenets attributed to the Bogomils by their Byzantine opponents. Others, however, have argued that popular heresy was 'home-grown', and that these groups emerged owing to internal reasons within the Latin West; that the rapid social changes of the eleventh century and the concerns which fuelled the demand for sacerdotal reform, which supported the growth of monasticism, and valued the adoption of an apostolic lifestyle, could and did lead to accusations of heresy amongst both progressives and conservatives.[38] The attempts to treat these myriad outbreaks collectively and thus provide a global explanation for the emergence of heresy has inevitably led to widespread criticism. Recent research has demonstrated the need to treat each particular incident in its own context, rather than as the result of mission, or as a symptom of overarching social or religious change. Yet such an approach means that it is easy to lose sight of the collective challenge which churchmen represented these groups as mounting to those clerics who defined themselves as orthodox. The archdiocese of Rheims, for example, is described by several authors as a hotbed for various different and seemingly independent heretical groups throughout this period: some eleven incidents of heresy are reported as having occurred in the archdiocese of Rheims between *c.*1000 and 1183.[39] By investigating some of the incidents which occurred within a single archdiocese across the eleventh and twelfth centuries, we will be able to consider the role which heresy played in shaping clerical orthodoxy, and the extent to which it represented attempts by localised groups to challenge or expand upon the message of orthodox Churchmen and reformers.[40] We will thus be able to test the hypothesis that heresy is not a figment of the clerical imagination, but rather a label applied in different circumstances to a series of different challenges to established clerical authority.

The earliest challenge to be reported in this period came from a common man (*plebeius*) called Leutard. The monastic chronicler Rodulphus Glaber reports how around the year 1000 Leutard was working in the field one day when he had a dream in which a swarm of bees entered his body through his genitals and exited through his mouth, having 'ordered him to do things impossible for human kind'.[41] As a consequence he returned home, separated from his wife 'by pretended reference to evangelic precept', and then, entering his local church, broke the crucifix. He then started to preach that it was unnecessary to pay tithes, citing Holy Scripture. He also argued that the Old Testament should not 'be believed in everything'. As a consequence he gained widespread support amongst the common people (*vulgus*). He was therefore brought for trial before his local bishop, Gebuin of Châlons-sur-Marne, who through careful examination was able to demonstrate that 'his teachings were not just incorrect but stuffed with great and damnable error'. He consequently lost his popular support and later committed suicide.

Rodulphus Glaber wrote his account over a quarter of a century after the events he describes as part of his *Five Books of Histories.* He structured his work around the millennia of Christ's birth and passion; coming at the end of Book II, Leutard is described as one of a series of problems which threatened the world around the year 1000. Glaber's account of Leutard's teachings owes very little to earlier descriptions of heretical belief; rather his report suggests Leutard anticipated features found in later accounts of eleventh- and twelfth-century popular heresy. He portrays Leutard as an autodidact, whose message is derived from the New Testament; he is represented as the first in a long line in the central Middle Ages of evangelical preachers who sought to enact, and preach, the apostolic life. He divorced his wife in accordance with the Gospel, presumably a reference to Christ's injunction that everyone who forsakes their home, their family and their land for him will inherit an everlasting life (Matthew 19.29). He also criticised one obvious, and relatively new, manifestation of clerical authority, the payment of tithes. Leutard's movement is therefore to be interpreted within a social context as a protest against a reassertive and demanding institutional Church.

But Leutard also attacked the image of Christ on the cross in his local church. His attack occurred in the context of increased devotion to the crucified Christ within the monasteries of tenth- and eleventh-century northern Europe, manifest in theology, prayer and also art.[42] Rachel Fulton has suggested that historians have been misled by the focus of later medieval piety on the humanity and suffering of Christ on the cross, and that contemporaries of Leutard viewed the crucifix rather as an image of justice, of Christ on the Day of Judgement whose suffering will act as a reproach for those who have refused to acknowledge their debt to him and to render what is due to him. Her interpretation suggests that Leutard's attack on the crucifix is therefore part and parcel of his protest against the payment of tithes, and hints at a conservative lay reaction to a new aspect to the doctrine of Christian judgement.[43] Nor was he alone: men in the Périgord are reported as pretending to return to the apostolic life, condemning the eating of meat, rejecting the Eucharist, criticising those who worship the cross or the effigy of the Lord on the grounds that to do so was idolatrous, and also as attacking the Church's right to receive alms.[44] Guy Lobrichon has placed the Périgord report within the context of debates about the nature of monasticism, defending Cluniac reforms against their critics who espoused the *vita apostolica* but failed to live up to it. Leutard's case might be read in a similar way. However, it can also be placed in a wider and more popular context, for in 1012x1015 Gebuin's successor, Bishop Roger I, held a synod to deal with Leutard's supporters.[45] Whilst this council should be read as a bid by Roger I to be seen as the defender of orthodoxy it also suggests that Leutard's movement attracted widespread support.

The see of Châlons-sur-Marne came to be seen by neighbouring bishops as a centre for popular heresy in this period. The heretics tried by Bishop Gerard I of Arras-Cambrai in Arras in January 1025 came from there, and some twenty years later the bishop of Châlon-sur-Marne sought the advice of the bishop of Liège about the heretical teachings of some country folk in his diocese. Certain aspects of Leutard's teachings, namely his attempts to emulate the apostolic life of the Gospels, and to reject various aspects of Church tradition on the grounds that they were not grounded in Biblical traditions, are found in reports of these two later groups, although there are also significant differences. In January 1025 in the city of Arras Bishop Gerard discovered, and tried in the diocesan synod, a group of heretics who said that they had been taught their beliefs by a preacher from Italy called Gundulf who had instructed them 'in the precepts of the Gospels and the apostles and would accept no other scripture than but this to which they adhere in word and deed'. Gerard accused them of abhorring baptism and the Eucharist, denying the efficacy of penance and confession, the authority of the Church, the legitimacy of matrimony, and holding that nobody after the time of the apostles and martyrs ought to be venerated. After he had preached a lengthy sermon, intended to refute their teaching on these and other points, the heretics admitted their error, and signed a formal profession of faith.[46] For heresy is only a fault of those who contumaciously resist the authority of both ecclesiastical tradition and that of the ecclesiastical hierarchy charged with upholding it. For those following beliefs which depart from orthodoxy to be deemed heretics, rather than as having fallen into an error of misunderstanding, they have to choose to persist in their error once it has been explained to them; if instead they chose to recant their error and accept the truth of orthodox doctrines, then there was, according to church law, no penalty. Consequently Gerard freed these heretics without further punishment.

The source for the Arras synod is very different to that for Leutard; this very detailed and lengthy account, known as the *Acta*, together with a letter from Gerard to a neighbouring bishop R. defending his actions, survives in a single late twelfth-century manuscript.[47] There is little reason, however, to doubt its authenticity as it is written in the style of the author of the initial section of the *Deeds of the Bishops of Cambrai*, which we have already seen is a text composed in the mid-eleventh century as an account of Bishop Gerard I's episcopate. Like the *Deeds*, the *Acta* present Gerard as a stalwart defender and promoter of orthodoxy. In the 20,000-word sermon attributed to him, Gerard ascribed to the heretics the belief that Christ was not made flesh, that they reject the fundamental rites of the Christian Church – baptism, penance, the Eucharist, the need for a physical church, for sacred altars, incense, bells, holy orders, Christian burial, marriage, confession to the saints, psalmody, and veneration of the Lord's cross. He ended with a disquisition on false justice. His remit is much wider than the doctrines which the heretics avowed at the end of their trial, when they admitted merely to challenging the necessity of baptism, particularly infant baptism, rejecting the Eucharist, the validity and necessity of confession and penance, the authority of the Church and the legitimacy of marriage. In particular his defence of the sacrality of the physical church, and of the need for Christian burial, seems to have its origins in contemporary ecclesiastical concerns rather than the issues raised by this particular group.[48] Gerard thus used the opportunity afforded by this chance to circulate his sermon to set out a clear statement of his own views about the institutional Church: for him, like Augustine, heresy provided a jumping-off point for his own rhetoric. It allowed him to set out his pastoral convictions about the role the Church should play within the local community.

Gerard's audience was probably not so much his neighbouring bishops but rather those closer to home. The see of Arras-Cambrai crossed a political border. Although located in the west Frankish archdiocese of Rheims, it straddled two kingdoms; the town of Arras was in the county of Flanders in the kingdom of the west Franks, that of Cambrai in the Empire. Consequently the bishop faced various challenges to his authority from both ecclesiastical and secular rivals, particularly in west Frankish Arras. Here the great ninth-century monastery of St Vaast dominated the town; a number of private chapels had also been erected there without episcopal permission which represented a considerable challenge to episcopal authority.[49] This background explains why in the *Acta* Gerard dealt in such detail with the heretics' claim to the right to worship in their homes and private mansions, rather than in church. He argued that the Eucharist is a public act, and therefore should be celebrated in a public place – a church.[50] He also defended burial in consecrated ground; this was not just a money-making scam as it separated the dead from this world whilst they awaited the Last Judgement. In church law only bishops could consecrate churches and graveyards. Here, Gerard's concern with the church and graveyard as consecrated spaces which was, as we have seen above, a relatively new doctrine in the eleventh century, are joined to his defence of his fragile authority within his own diocese. He magnified for his own reasons an issue which, on the basis of the doctrines the heretics are reported to have specifically avowed, seems to have been of very little concern to them. His arguments against heresy, although addressed to another bishop, allowed him to set out his aspirations for episcopal authority and Christian practice within his own diocese.

Much less is known about the heretics who became of such concern to Bishop Roger II of Châlons-sur-Marne some twenty years later that he sought the advice of the bishop of Liège who recommended their excommunication. The heretics are described in Wazo of Liège's reply as

Manichaeans, and given Manichaean attributes, with their own initiation ceremony, meeting in secret for 'filthy acts', abhorring marriage, and avoiding the eating of meat. This case is only known because the letter is cited in the laudatory portrait of Bishop Wazo given in the *Deeds of the Bishops of Liège*, in which Wazo is depicted as a source of wisdom and advice not only within his diocese, but also to neighbouring bishops. In this world, heresy's function is merely to demonstrate that Wazo is a good bishop. It is impossible for us now to determine whether this heresy truly was dualist, or whether the author of the *Deeds* merely drew on literary convention when citing these Manichaean attributes.

There is only one further case of heresy reported in the archdiocese in the following sixty years: that of a local priest, Ramhirdus of Schere in *c.*1077. The bishop of Cambrai accused him of heresy for preaching that simoniacal and unchaste priests should not celebrate mass. Although his message attracted widespread support, he was burnt to death, perhaps even by the bishop's own servants.[51] This case attracted papal condemnation by Gregory VII. It represents a considerable change from the pattern of heretical outbursts in the first forty years or so of the century. In earlier cases, charges of heresy have been levelled only against ignorant lay men. Ramhirdus, by contrast, is portrayed as an educated priest. The message of clerical reform came relatively late to Flanders, and Ramhirdus seems to have been ahead of his time in his espousal of it.

This pattern in the province of Rheims is part of a wider one: popular heresy disappeared as an issue for almost half a century after an initial flurry of reports in the first half of the eleventh century. R. I. Moore suggested that the silence which followed may be explained because the sorts of debates and criticisms being labelled heretical in the early eleventh century had, by 1060 become part of a mainstream reformist critique of the sinfulness of the priesthood, led by members of the papal curia. The promotion of the apostolic life based on biblical precept had become respectable.[52] But, as we have already seen, both the critique of the secular life and the move to the apostolic life had deeper roots in the tenth century.[53] Moreover, the antipathy shared by Leutard and the heretics of Arras to the crucifix and material church is not easily explained by reformist tendencies. Both these matters were, as we have already seen, contentious issues amongst contemporary churchmen. When investigating reports of heretical belief in this period we therefore need to acknowledge the rhetorical significance of heresy within contemporary debates about the nature of the Church.

Popular heresy reappeared in the archdiocese of Rheims in the first half of the twelfth century, when Guibert of Nogent recorded an incident which occurred in the diocese of Soissons *c.*1108x1115. Clement, count of Bucy and his brother Evrard were tried for heresy before the bishop. According to Guibert this heresy had started amongst well-educated people before filtering down to uneducated peasants (*rustici*) who claimed to be leading the apostolic life. They rejected sacerdotal authority, going as far as to 'call the mouth of any priest the mouth of Hell', and rejected the Incarnation of Christ as man as a delusion, and also the validity of infant baptism, the sacerdotal Eucharist, the need for burial in consecrated ground, and the validity of marriage. For Guibert, who had been commissioned to interrogate them privately, this group lacked the necessary education to act as religious leaders – they had read the Acts of the Apostles 'but little else' and when asked what they thought about those baptised according to another faith, replied 'For God's sake, do not expect us to search so deeply'.[54] The sorts of questions preoccupying students like Guibert in the schools of higher education in early twelfth-century northern France seem to have passed this group by, perhaps because they really were, as Guibert suggested, uneducated *rustici*. Indeed, such was their apparent orthodoxy in the face of interrogation that Guibert was reduced to recalling Augustine's warning that heretics may sometimes perjure themselves rather than reveal the truth. As his questioning failed to reveal their views to be heretical, Jay Rubenstein has argued that the absence of evidence for heresy may explain why Guibert added a description of lascivious behaviour, lifted from Augustine's description of the Manichees, when revising his original account; he did so in order to reinforce what he recognised to be an otherwise weak argument for the group's heresy.[55] Guibert seems to have uncovered a group of anticlerical but ultimately pious lay men living under the protection of the local count; whether they were *rustici* (peasants) or local lords is unclear. The touchstones for their critique – clerical authority, infant baptism, burial in consecrated ground – seem very similar to those of Leutard's and Gundolf's followers a century earlier.[56] What all these incidents suggests is that groups of laity had a grounding in the New Testament to which they appealed to challenge the established Church's teachings and practices and monopoly of services. Quite how they acquired their knowledge is unclear. It may be that these groups included educated clerics, as we shall see other groups did. It may be that widespread didactic preaching of the sort promoted by Ælfric in early eleventh-century England provided a sufficient grounding of biblical knowledge for these groups. In other words, they are, perhaps, testimony to the efficacy of churchmen's concern with pastoral care in the tenth and eleventh centuries.

Popular heresy did not appear again as an issue in the province of Rheims until the 1130s, although we have reports of other incidents in the nearby dioceses of Utrecht, Liège and Trier, as well as further afield in the French Alps, Provence and Brittany. In that decade the clergy of Liège discovered in the city a group of heretics who were reported to have come from Mont Aimé in the Champagne plain in Rheims.[57] Liège had a tradition of attributing a Frankish origin to heretics; sometime in the early eleventh century, Eckbert, master of the cathedral school of Liège, wrote a poem dedicated to the bishop of Utrecht in which he described how a grave heresy had come from the west, introduced by the evil Franks (*de malis Francigenis*).[58] But the group discovered in the 1130s are described in rather different terms to those used to describe earlier groups. The description we have comes in a letter written by the clerics of Liège to the pope, seeking his advice as to how they should treat the one member of the group to confess and seek forgiveness: should he share the fate of his fellow members and be burnt by the mob? The group is described as 'new', and as being divided into different ranks. It has auditors, who are being initiated into error, and believers who have already been led astray; it has its own laity, priests and other prelates. The description of the group's structure echoes that of another group discovered in Cologne a few years later, in 1143, which was also described as being composed of 'new heretics', to distinguish them from the 'other heretics', with whom they had been arguing.[59] These two different texts, one composed in Cologne, one in Liège in *c.*1135, thus identified a new heretical organisation, one divided into acolytes and the initiated, as appearing in these neighbouring dioceses within a decade of each other. The description of their structure echoes that of Augustine's account of the Manichees, but it also echoes that of the dualist heretics who became known as the Cathars in the Latin West of the late twelfth and thirteenth century. The Liège heretics may, therefore, herald a new development. However, they also had links to existing traditions of anticlericalism. Like earlier heretics, those in Liège denied that sins are remitted in baptism, held the Eucharist to be useless, asserted that episcopal ordination was valueless, that no one receives the Holy Spirit except by good works, condemned marriage, adjudged every oath a crime, but were willing to dissemble and 'join in celebration of our sacraments in order to veil their own iniquity'. They combined existing critiques of the Church with a new, and sophisticated, structure.

It is important to recognise before coming to any conclusions about this group, and what form of heresy they represent, that we only know about this group because the canons of the cathedral of Liège chose to write to Pope L. for advice about how to deal with them.[60] Such a situation is unusual: it would normally have been dealt with by the bishop, as it was in the other cases we have already examined. Uwe Brunn has situated the letter, which is undated, in the context of a contest between the canons and bishop in the mid-1130s.[61] The cathedral chapter accused the bishop of simony, whereupon he appealed to the pope. In an effort to influence the outcome of the case, the canons wrote several letters to the pope in which they sought to present themselves as defenders of orthodoxy and destroyers of heresy. In this letter they present themselves as defenders of a judicial procedure in which the pope has the last word, determining how they should treat a repentant heretic. In showing the area around Liège to be infected with heresy, and the people indignant about this, they wished to demonstrate that the bishop was failing to maintain his duty of pastoral care, and at the same time signal their own diligence and orthodoxy. Real heresy may have provided the meat, but the reason why the case was reported to Rome owed more to local politics. And as before, those making the accusation of heresy wished to present themselves as defenders of orthodoxy.

Heretical groups continued to be identified within the province throughout the remainder of the twelfth century. It is possible to place each of these cases within a local context, and to attribute the reporting of a particular case to local tensions. But collectively these accounts, drawn from different sources, point to a rise in concern about popular heresy amongst both secular and lay authorities in this area. As in earlier cases, anxious local ecclesiastics used their encounters with dissenters to display their orthodoxy and vigilance. In 1153 the bishop of Arras-Cambrai obtained the pope's support in his campaign against an unspecified heresy.[62] It was not wholly successful for in 1162–63 the king of France reported to the pope that the Archbishop of Rheims had discovered on a visit to Arras a group of men known as 'Populicani', who then appealed against his judgement to the pope.[63] The outcome of that particular case is not known but heretical groups continued to be uncovered. An early thirteenth-century report records an encounter in the late 1170s between a clerk of the archbishop of Rheims and a girl in a vineyard in Rheims which led to the arrest of the members of the heretical group.[64] In 1182 four heretics were arrested in Arras, and in 1183 the Archbishop of Rheims and the Count of Flanders met to take action against heresy within Flanders.[65] The continued involvement of the pope in these cases has much to tell us about how the authorities wished to display themselves before both each other and a higher authority as orthodox and active in the fight against heresy.

The reality, however, is much more problematic. Bishops' authority was confined to their dioceses; those accused by the bishop could, relatively easily, avoid persecution by moving into the jurisdiction of a neighbouring bishop. The career of one particular itinerant preacher points to the ineffectualness of episcopal power in this region. Sometime between 1164 and 1167 a priest named Jonas appealed to the bishop of Cambrai against the abbot of Jette who had sought to prevent him from holding the cure of the parish of Neder-Heembeek in Brabant, near Brussels, on the grounds that he had been convicted and excommunicated for heresy.[66] In the course of his trial, letters from the archbishops of Cologne and Trier, and from two successive bishops of Liège came to light, asserting that Jonas had been tried, and anathematised for preaching the heresy of the Catti. They tell us nothing about the content of his teachings, other than it had been deemed heretical, but they date back to 1152. Jonas seems to have had a successful career as a preacher travelling around the dioceses of Cologne and Trier. Although he attracted condemnation he managed to keep one step ahead of the authorities. His case also demonstrates how the charge of heresy could be raised against a single individual by a series of different bishops in different dioceses. Accusations of heresy are not confined just to one-off charges made in the context of particular local political battles between rivals for ecclesiastical authority, as at Arras in 1025 or Liège 110 years later. By the late twelfth century, if not before, popular heresy had become a real issue in a period of both social and religious change. Lay men and women, and local clerics such as Jonas, questioned the nature of church teaching, and sought their own answers in the New Testament. But for clerics of the time, as for Augustine of Hippo some six hundred years earlier, opposition to and criticism of church teaching offered an opportunity to sort out for their own benefit, and those of their audience, the tenets of orthodoxy and orthopraxy. The increase in incidents of reported popular heresy is thus testament to the vibrancy of Christian culture at all levels of society.

Throughout this period the laity and lesser clergy challenged the authority and teachings of the higher clergy in all sorts of ways. Never passive recipients of ecclesiastical instruction, they continuously rebelled against attempts to discipline them. They might do so inadvertently, necessitating penance, or consciously and deliberately, leading to excommunication. But the rites for ecclesiastical discipline fulfilled the needs not only of sinners but of their sacerdotal and episcopal ministers, providing them with occasions to display their role as instructors and adjudicators of ecclesiastical authority. It is not just the 'feverish restlessness' of heretics but rather that of ordinary practising Christians which provided medieval churchmen with opportunities for instruction. Accounts of lay scepticism and heresy need thus to be read against this background. Exponents of orthodoxy required proponents of heterodoxy; they needed occasions when people challenged established beliefs and practices in order to examine, articulate and demonstrate the correctness and validity of their own views. Orthodoxy could only be established with reference to its opposite. Correct practice and belief could only be articulated through ecclesiastical discipline.

Such concerns provide the framework for surviving accounts of lay scepticism, heresy and disbelief. These in turn point to a rich if largely undocumented world of interest (and occasional active lack of interest) in Christianity on the part of the laity. They suggest that ordinary Christians had a more nuanced, and active relationship with the Church than that presumed by the prescriptive pastoral literature composed by leading churchmen, that they reflected upon changes in ecclesiastical practice, and the demands made of them. And that the challenges the laity posed in turn helped reformers to articulate their own views of what constituted Christianity. For churchmen's visions for the Church perhaps rather perversely depended on those of the people.

Notes and references

1 *St Augustine Concerning the City of God Against the Pagans*, trans. H. Bettenson (Harmondsworth, 1972; repr. 1984), 650.

2 S. Reynolds, 'Social Mentalities and the Case of Medieval Scepticism', *TRHS* 6th series, 1 (1991), 21–41 at p. 29. On scepticism, see also J. H. Arnold, *Belief and Unbelief in Medieval Europe* (London, 2005).

3 D. Iogna-Prat, *Order and Exclusion: Cluny and Christendom Face Heresy, Judaism and Islam (1000–1150)*, trans. G. Robert Edwards (Ithaca, NY, 2002); trans. of *Ordonner et exclure* (Paris, 1998) cites Augustine incidentally at p. 148.

4 R. I. Moore, *The Origins of European Dissent* (London, 1977).

5 E. Vodola, *Excommunication in the Middle Ages* (Berkeley, CA, 1986); G. Steele Edwards, 'Ritual Excommunication in Medieval France and England, 900–1200' (Stanford University, unpublished Ph.D. thesis, 1997); W. Hartmann, *Kirche und Kirchenrecht um 900: Die Bedeutung der spätkarolingischen Zeit für Tradition und Innovation im kirchlichen Recht*, MGH Schriften 58 (Hannover, 2008), 276–86.

6 A. Duchesne, ed., *Historiae Francorum Scriptores* (Paris, 1636), II, 586.

7 I. S. Robinson, *Henry IV of Germany, 1056–1106* (Cambridge, 1999), 122–32; S. Hamilton, 'Inquiring into Adultery and Other Wicked Deeds: Episcopal Justice in Tenth- and Early Eleventh-century Italy', *Viator* 41 (2010), 21–43; F. Barlow, *Thomas Becket* (London, 1986; repr. 1997), 184–85; R. Helmholz, 'Excommunication and the Angevin Leap Forward', *Haskins Society Journal* 7 for 1995 (1997), 133–49.

8 Arnulf of Milan, *Liber gestorum recentium*, I.18–19, 141–43.

9 *Regino*, II. 412–17, 438–44; *PRG* I, 308–17; R. E. Reynolds, 'Rites of Separation and Reconciliation in the Early Middle Ages', *Segni e Riti nella Chiesa Altomedievale Occidentale, Spoleto 11–17 aprile 1985*, Settimane di studio del Centro italiano di studi sull'alto medioevo 33 (Spoleto, 1987), 405–33; repr. in idem, *Law and Liturgy in the Latin Church, 5th–12th Centuries* (Ashgate, 1994), no. X.

10 *Regino* II.413, 442–44; Burchard, XI. 3, *PL* 140, 858.

11 S. Hamilton, 'Absoluimus uos uice beati petri apostolorum principis: Episcopal Authority and the Reconciliation of Excommunicants in England and Francia *c.*900–*c.*1150', in P. Fouracre and D. Ganz, eds, *Frankland: The Franks and the World of the Early Middle Ages* (Manchester, 2008), 209–41.

12 Ibid., 220; *Les Annales de Flodoard*, ed. P. Lauer (Paris, 1905), a. 953, 136.

13 Regino II.416, 444; *PRG* I, 313–14.

14 Ed. in G. Steele Edwards, 'Ritual Excommunication in Medieval France and England, 900–1200' (Stanford University, unpublished Ph.D. thesis, 1997), 141–42.

15 S. Hamilton, *The Practice of Penance, 900–1050* (Woodbridge, 2001), esp. 1–24.

16 Ibid.

17 Ibid., 104–72.

18 Ibid., passim.

19 *PRG* XCIX.44–80, II. 14–23 at XCIX.49, II, 15.

20 *PRG* XCIX.50, II. 15–16.

21 See Chapter 5.

22 S. Reynolds, 'Social Mentalities and the Case of Medieval Scepticism', *TRHS*, 6th series 1 (1991), 21–41, esp. p. 32; Arnold, *Belief and Unbelief*; M. Goodich, *Miracles and Wonders: The Development of the Concept of Miracle 1150–1350* (Aldershot, 2007), 47–68.

23 Hamilton, *The Practice of Penance*; R. Meens, 'Penitentials and the Practice of Penance in the Tenth and Eleventh Centuries', *Early Medieval Europe* 14 (2006), 7–21; idem, 'The Frequency and Nature of Early Medieval Penance', in P. Biller and A. J. Minnis, eds. *Handling Sin: Confession in the Middle Ages* (Woodbridge, 1998), 35–61; A. Gaastra, 'Penance and the Law: The Penitential Canons of the Collection in Nine Books', *Early Medieval Europe* 14 (2006), 85–102; idem, 'Between Liturgy and Canon Law'; L. Körntgen, 'Canon Law and the Practice of Penance: Burchard of Worms's Penitential', *Early Medieval Europe* 14 (2006), 103–17; C. R. Cubitt, 'Bishops, Priests and Penance in late Saxon England', *Early Medieval Europe* 14 (2006), 41–63.

24 *The Book of Sainte Foy*, trans. P. Sheingorn (Philadelphia, 1995), IV.21, 212–13. The complex manuscript history of this collection suggests it was disseminated amongst clerical communities in northern France in order to promote the cult more widely outside its core area of support; it was thus composed with a clerical audience in view.

25 Iogna-Prat, *Order and Exclusion*, 148–81.

26 D. Iogna-Prat, *La Maison Dieu. Une histoire monumentale de l'Église au Moyen Age* (Paris, 2006); idem, 'Churches in the Landscape', in T. F. X. Noble and J. M. H. Smith, eds, *The Cambridge History of Christianity: Early Medieval Christianities c.600–c.1100* (Cambridge, 2008), 363–79.

27 Ibid.

28 *Gesta episcoporum Cameracensium*, *MGH SS VII*, III.22, 473; I first came across this tale in T. M. Riches, 'Bishop Gerard I of Cambrai-Arras, the Three

Orders, and the Problem of Human Weakness', in J. S. Ott and A. Trumbore Jones, eds, *The Bishop Reformed: Studies of Episcopal Power and Culture in the Central Middle Ages* (Aldershot, 2007), 122–36 at pp. 131–32.

29 *Gesta episcoporum Cameracensium*, III.23, 473.

30 Riches, 'Bishop Gerard I'.

31 On popular heresy, see the overviews by M. Lambert, *Medieval Heresy: Popular Movements from the Gregorian Reform to the Reformation*, 3rd edn (Oxford, 2002); R. I. Moore, *The Origins of European Dissent* (London, 1977); A. Roach, *The Devil's World: Heresy and Society 1100–1300* (Harlow, 2003); E. Ann Matter, 'Orthodoxy and Deviance', in Noble and Smith, eds, *Early Medieval Christianities c.600–c.1100*, 510–30.

32 T. Head summarises the literature in '"Naming Names": The Nomenclature of Heresy in the Early Eleventh Century', in R. Fulton and B. W. Holsinger, eds, *History in the Comic Mode: Medieval Communities and the Matter of Person* (New York, 2007), 91–100.

33 Guibert, *Monodiae*, III.17, *PL* 156, 951–53; trans. Archambault, *A Monk's Confession*, 196.

34 C. Mews, 'Guibert of Nogent's *Monodiae*, III, 17', *Revue des études Augustiniennes* 33 (1987), 113–27.

35 Moore, *Origins*, 67. For a nuanced overview which makes clear that medieval writers' use of the terms Arian and Manichee was more nuanced than modern scholars have generally suggested, see T. Head, '"Naming Names": The Nomenclature of Heresy in the Early Eleventh Century', in R. Fulton and B. W. Holsinger, eds, *History in the Comic Mode: Medieval Communities and the Matter of Person* (New York, 2007), 91–100.

36 M. Frassetto, 'The Sermons of Adhemar and the Letter of Heribert: New Sources Concerning the Origins of Medieval Heresy', *Revue bénédictine* 109 (1999), 324–40.

37 Ibid., B. Hamilton, 'Wisdom from the East: The Reception by the Cathars of Eastern Dualist Texts', in P. Biller and A. Hudson, eds, *Heresy and Literacy, 1000–1530* (Cambridge, 1994), 38–60; idem, 'Bogomil Influences on Western Heresy', in M. Frassetto, ed., *Heresy and the Persecuting Society in the Middle Ages: Essays on the Work of R. I. Moore* (Leiden, 2006), 93–114; C. Taylor, *Heresy in Medieval France: Dualism in Aquitaine and the Agenais, 1000–1249* (Woodbridge, 2005), 55–132.

38 J. L. Nelson, 'Society, Theodicy and the Origins of Heresy: Towards a Reassessment of the Medieval Evidence', in D. Baker, ed., *Schism, Heresy and Religious Protest*, Studies in Church History 9 (Cambridge, 1972), 65–77; T. Asad, 'Medieval Heresy: An Anthropological View', *Social History* 11 (1986), 345–62; Moore, *Origins*.

39 Leutard preaches in the diocese of Châlons-sur-Marne *c.*1000 (Rodulphus Glaber, *Histories* II.xi, 88–90); heretics tried at the synod of Arras by Bishop Gerard of Arras-Cambrai *c.*1025 (*Acta Synodi Atrebatensis*, *PL* 142, 1271–312); heresy reported in Châlons-sur-Marne *c.*1043–48 (*Gesta Episcoporum Leodiensis*, *MGH SS* VII, 226–28); Ramhirdus, a priest and preacher of Cambrai tried for heresy *c.*1076 (Chronicle of St André de Castres, III.3, *MGH SS* VII, 540; *The Register of Pope Gregory VII: An English Translation*, ed. and trans. H. E. J. Cowdrey (Oxford, 2002), IV.20, 231–32); Count Clement of Bucy and his brother Evrard tried at Soisson *c.*1108–15 (Guibert of Nogent, *Monodiae*, III.17, *PL* 156, 951–53); heretical group from Mont Aimé tried at Liège *c.*1135 (*Epistola ecclesiae Leodiensis ad Lucum papam II*, ed. *PL* 179, 937–38, trans. W. L. Wakefield and A. P. Evans, *Heresies of the High Middle Ages* (New York, 1969), 139–41); heresy discovered at Arras 1153 (Letter of Pope Eugenius III to the clergy and people of Arras, Mansi, *Concilia*, XXI, 689–90); heresy condemned at the council of Rheims 1157 (Mansi, *Concilia*, XXI, 843); a group of heretics tried at Arras 1162–63 (Bouquet, *Receuil des historiens des Gaules et de la France* XV, 790–99; trans. R. I. Moore, *The Birth of European Heresy* (London, 1975; repr. Toronto, 1995), 80–82); Jonas the priest appeals against condemnation for heresy to the bishop of Cambrai 1164x1167 (P. Bonenfant, 'Un clerc cathare en Lotharingie au milieu du XIIe siècle', *Le Moyen Age* 69 (1963), 271–80); heresy in Rheims 1176–80 (Ralph of Coggeshall, *Chronicon Anglicanum*, ed. J. Stevenson, Rolls Series (London, 1875), 121–25; trans. Moore, *Birth*, 86–88); heretics tried by bishop and count in Arras, 1182–83 (Sigebert of Gembloux, *Sigiberti Gemblacensis chronographia: Continuatio Aquicinctina*, ed. L. C. Bethmann, MGH SS VI, 421; trans. Wakefield and Evans, *Heresies*, 256–57).

40 For a more general introduction to northern heresy, see M. C. Barber, 'Northern Catharism', in Frassetto, ed., *Heresy*, 115–37; and for a detailed study of heresy further east, see U. Brunn, *Des Contestataires aux 'Cathares': Discours de réforme et propagande antihérétique dans les pays du Rhin et de la Meuse avant l'Inquisition* (Paris, 2006).

41 Rodulphus Glaber, *Histories* II.xi, 88–90; for a helpful analysis of this passage, see B. Stock, *The Implications of Literacy: Written Language and Models of Interpretation in the Eleventh and Twelfth Centuries* (Princeton, NJ, 1983), 101–06.

42 R. Fulton, *From Judgment to Passion: Devotion to Christ and the Virgin Mary, 800–1200* (New York, 2002).

43 Ibid. 81–87.

44 G. Lobrichon, 'The Chiaroscuro of Heresy: Early Eleventh-century Aquitaine as Seen from Auxerre', in T. Head and R. Landes, *The Peace of God: Social*

Violence and Religious Response in France around 1000 (Ithaca, NY, 1992), 80–103.

45 H. Fichtenau, *Heretics and Scholars in the High Middle Ages 1000–1200*, trans. D. A. Kaiser (University Park, Pennsylvania, 1998), 16.

46 *Acta Synodi Atrebatensis*, *PL* 142, 1271–1312, partially translated Moore, *Birth*, 15–19. On the synod, see M. Frassetto, 'Reaction and Reform: Reception of Heresy in Arras and Aquitaine in the Early Eleventh Century', *Catholic Historical Review* 83 (1997), 385–400; G. Lobrichon, 'Arras, 1025, ou le vrai procès d'une fausse accusation', in M. Zerner, ed., *Inventer l'hérésie? Discours polémiques et pouvoirs avant l'inquisition* (Nice, 1998), 67–85; Fulton, *From Judgment*, 82–87.

47 Lobrichon, 'Arras, 1025', 70–72.

48 M. Lauwers, 'Dicunt vivorum beneficia nichil prodesse defunctis: Histoire d'une thème polémique (XIe–XIIe siècles)', in Zerner, ed. *Inventer l'hérésie?*, 157–92.

49 D. C. van Meter, 'Eschatological Order and the Moral Arguments for Clerical Celibacy in Francia around the Year 1000', in Frassetto, ed., *Medieval Purity*, 149–75 suggests that the monks of St Vaast sought to undermine clerical authority criticising the administration of penance by impure priests, and that Gerard's sermon is a defence of episcopal authority against such challenges.

50 Lobrichon, 'Arras, 1025'; Lauwers, 'Dicunt vivorum beneficia'; Iogna-Prat, *Order and Exclusion*, 158–61.

51 On involvement of bishops' officers, see *Chronicle of St André de Castres*, III.3, *MGH SS* VII, 540. For condemnation of the killing by Pope Gregory VII, see *The Register*, trans. Cowdrey, IV.20, 231–32.

52 Moore, *Origins*, 46–81.

53 See Chapter 3.

54 See n. 33 above.

55 J. Rubenstein, *Guibert of Nogent: Portrait of a Medieval Mind* (New York, 2002), 114–16, 193–95.

56 Lauwers, 'Dicunt vivorum beneficia'.

57 *PL* 179, 937–38; Wakefield and Evans, trans. *Heresies*, 140–41. Brunn, *Des Contestataires*, has redated the letter from *c.*1144 to 1135, 118–24.

58 Brunn, *Des Contestataires*, 118–19.

59 Eberwin of Steinfeld, *Epistola*, trans. Wakefield and Evans, *Heresies*, 127–32.

60 Trans. Wakefield and Evans, *Heresies*, 139–41.

61 Brunn, *Des contestataires*, 112–24.

62 See n. 39 above.

63 Ibid.

64 Ibid.

65 Ibid.

66 P. Bonenfant, 'Un clerc cathare en Lotharingie au milieu du XIIe siècle', *Le Moyen Age* 69 (1963), 271–80. The early eleventh-century manuscript of Pseudo-Isidore, attributed to Archbishop Heribert of Cologne (999–1021), includes a nota next to a passage about the clergy calling themselves heretics: Cologne, Diözesanbibliothek, Cod. 113, fol. 23r (available at http://www.ceec.uni-koeln.de/; accessed 19th August 2012).

chapter 10

Afterword

In November 1215 the largest and most representative of all the ecclesiastical councils held in the medieval west met in the Lateran Palace in Rome, at the invitation of Pope Innocent III. Some 71 archbishops and prelates, 412 bishops and over 900 abbots and priors took part, alongside representatives from several rulers. Their presence reflects the changes which had taken place in Latin Christianity in the preceding three centuries. It had expanded its influence considerably to include regions which in 900 had been ruled by pagans, Moslems and eastern orthodox Christians. Participants came not just from western Christendom's early medieval core in Italy, northern Spain, France, western Germany, the Low Countries and the British Isles, but from Portugal, Poland, Hungary, Dalmatia, Sardinia, Sicily and Cyprus.[1] In the years covered by this book the British Isles, northern France and Flanders had successfully absorbed and Christianised Scandinavian settlers; Poland and Hungary came under Latin Christian control for the first time, and other regions, such as Portugal, parts of central and southern Spain and Sicily in the west, and Dalmatia and Cyprus in the east had been regained from Moslem and Byzantine rule. This council, now known as the Fourth Lateran Council, embodies the way in which the institutional Church had developed from a loose affiliation of regional churches with a pope in Rome to a more united and international organisation under the direction of the papal *curia* over the course of these three centuries.

It is impossible to imagine any early medieval Latin ruler, either ecclesiastical or secular, being able to hold an event on this scale. The presence of so many men from such a diverse range of places is testament to the ways in which the west had changed in the three centuries since the fall of the Carolingian rulers in the late ninth century. Lateran IV thus marks the end of this study, just as Regino of Prüm's *Two Books of Synodical Cases and Ecclesiastical Discipline*, composed in *c.*906, served to denote its start. The contrasts between the worlds in which these two texts were composed are obvious – but they are worth outlining briefly, for they testify to the ways in which the institutional Church and the social, cultural and economic environments in which it operated had changed across these three centuries. Regino composed his collection of canon law at the request of the Archbishop of Trier but dedicated it to the Archbishop of Mainz. Producing a text for use in two neighbouring east Frankish ecclesiastical provinces represents what was politically feasible in the early tenth century. Both were part of the same political realm. Similarly, throughout the tenth century, church councils could be, and were, held at the level of ecclesiastical provinces under an archbishop, and might even go beyond this to be held for the churchmen of an entire kingdom under the leadership of both archbishops and rulers, as they did on occasion in Germany and England. In the eleventh century, papal church councils remained localised to particular regions such as that for northern France held at Rheims under Leo IX in 1049 or that for southern Italy held at Melfi under Urban II in 1089. Whilst papal councils became increasingly international over the course of the twelfth century, the sheer size of Lateran IV signalled a revival of conciliar activity at both diocesan and international level on a scale not seen since the ninth century.

That Innocent III managed to organise such a well-attended council so quickly reflects the various changes which had taken place within the clergy since the fall of the Carolingians. Building on ninth-century writings, secular and regular churchmen in this period became increasingly self-conscious and professional as a group, setting themselves apart from the laity. As we saw in Chapters 3 and 4, the laity played a crucial role both as a rhetorical 'other' which helped shape clerical identity and as patrons who attached value to the services of a pure clergy. Their wishes, as much as those of higher churchmen, lay behind the repeated attempts at clerical reform in this period. When Lateran IV met, it legislated in various ways to govern the behaviour of bishops and local diocesan clergy. It thus embodies this increased self-consciousness of the clergy as a distinct strand within society. Lateran IV also demonstrates how church government had become more centralised. By the early thirteenth century the papal curia had acquired an importance and assumed a role in the government of local churches throughout the west which it simply lacked in the early tenth century. The sparse evidence which survives for the tenth-century popes indicates that they tended to react to requests rather than instigate change on a wide scale. Even in the eleventh century, Gregory VII's ecclesiastical ambitions were restricted by the political opposition he encountered from Henry IV and his supporters, and Urban II's call to crusade owed much of its success in the French-speaking world to the fact that he preached it in person at Clermont in France, rather than remotely through legates. But over the course of the later eleventh and twelfth centuries the clergy of monasteries, canonries and cathedrals from all over the west increasingly appealed to the papal court for settlement of legal disputes, especially between ecclesiastical institutions; the popes thus became effective heads of the western Church for the first time in the central Middle Ages. They developed the governmental machinery to be able to respond to requests from local churches, delegating more authority to local legates, dealing with direct appeals to Rome itself. Innocent III used this structure to organise Lateran IV, asking legates to preach about the council to the clergy of each province of the Church. He did not view it as simply a top-down exercise but rather as an opportunity to deal with local matters collectively: he invited the bishops of each province to suggest matters for consideration at the council.[2]

The improvements in communications between centre and periphery resulted, in part, simply from the increase in the number of ecclesiastical institutions across the medieval west. The presence of so many abbots and priors as well as bishops at the Lateran Palace in November 1215 reflects on the one hand the substantial growth in the number of monastic institutions in this period, fuelled by greater economic prosperity and consequent noble investment, and on the other the fact that many of the newer foundations of the eleventh and twelfth centuries had organised themselves into orders, with their own internal communications systems, which made it much easier for Rome to send out invitations quickly and effectively.

But how far do these changes in clerical institutions obscure underlying continuities in their relationship with the laity? Both the texts which mark the beginning and end of the period considered in this book, Regino's *Two Books* and Lateran IV's canons, seek to separate the clergy from the laity.

Regino divided his canon law collection into two books of texts, first, those pertaining to the discipline of the clergy and, secondly, those for the laity. Lateran IV's canons dealt primarily with clerical discipline, education and behaviour rather than lay behaviour, although they did require the laity to confess their sins and receive the Eucharist at least once a year at Easter.[3] Both texts focus on distinguishing the clergy from the laity through behaviour – no marriage, no drinking, no hunting, no gaming – dress, and law. Both texts emphasised the importance of priests delivering pastoral care to the laity, including Mass, regular confession, and the rites for the sick and the dying. But both also promoted co-operation between laity and clergy for the good of *ecclesia*. Regino designed his to be used by the bishop whilst visiting his diocese; the laity should co-operate to police both clerical and lay behaviour. The bishop should ask questions of the lay jury in order to establish whether pastoral rites were being properly administered in that particular community. The *decani* should police households in order to ensure that they regularly attended religious services and observed feast days. Pope Innocent III similarly intended that the council he assembled in Rome would begin a joint project by laity and clergy to work together to reform the Christian people and at the same time launch a crusade to the Holy Land. For him, internal reform and clerical leadership went hand in hand with expansionary enterprise. Thus in one surviving invitation to the council sent to the archbishop, bishops, abbots and priors of the French province of Vienne he sets out how the council will come together:

> *to root out vices and plant virtues, to correct excesses and reform morals, to eliminate heresies and strengthen faith, to silence discords and establish peace, to crush oppression and cherish liberty, to induce princes and Christian people to come to aid and relief of the holy land, both clergy and laity [for the progress and advantage of the Christian people].*[4]

Innocent III conceived the council not as telling the clergy, and through them the laity, how to behave, but rather as a common enterprise by laity and clergy, princes and people, to co-operate with each other to reform the world for the common good.

In exploring some of the other aspects of associations in this period between Church and people we must remember that these bonds were conducted against a backdrop of economic, social and political change. The early thirteenth-century world was clearly in many ways very different from that of 900 and the changes within the institutional Church reflect this. The clergy had become an even more self-conscious institutional social grouping, one with its own education, own career structures, and its own much better developed legal identity. The structures which allowed the papacy to interfere in the affairs of local churches throughout Christendom had matured. Houses of monks, canons and nuns had increased in both number and size. The world of Lateran IV is much more wealthy, more urban and more cosmopolitan than that of Regino. But the most striking change for ordinary men and women living in the medieval west in these three centuries, whatever their social rank and status, whether free or unfree, must have been the great proliferation in local church buildings. As we saw in Chapter 2, new and existing settlements acquired local churches often for the first time. And existing local churches grew in size, and wooden churches were rebuilt in stone. These manifestations of religious and lordly power within local communities had repercussions for the religious and financial lives of the majority of Christians living in the medieval west. Their existence meant that the local church became the place where Christians were baptised, where they might confess their sins, where they and their relations were buried, and, of course, where they paid their tithes and other dues. Several other studies of lay piety in the eleventh and twelfth centuries have emphasised how monasticism played a very important role in shaping the piety and devotional lives of members of the lay nobility.[5] This book suggests that monasticism only ever comprised one strand in lay devotion, and that the proliferation of local churches on local piety had as significant an impact on the lives of lay Christians.

The richness of monastic archives, particularly in France, provides a painful contrast to the almost total lack of written evidence for the foundation of local churches and for the services inside them. The bias to the monastic is wholly understandable and represents an important element in lay–clerical relations. But this book, by focusing on the prescriptive texts composed by bishops and higher churchmen for the delivery of pastoral services, helps to redress the balance in favour of the local church. It suggests in Chapter 5 that pastoral care continued to be important to higher churchmen throughout this period and that the mushrooming of local churches across the medieval west was accompanied by a real concern amongst the clerical elite to educate and train the local priests who served them. The religious history of the central Middle Ages thus had more in common with that of the ninth century than is sometimes supposed. Higher churchmen continued the attempts of their Carolingian predecessors to promote correct practice and to encourage Christians to participate regularly in Christian services in order to be good Christians. Lateran IV needs to be placed against the backdrop of this continued concern with pastoral care; the pastoral revolution of the thirteenth century therefore had deeper roots than has often been supposed.

Ninth- and tenth-century churchmen developed a model of what constituted lay noble spirituality which was distinct from that enjoined on the clergy.[6] What mattered was public piety, *orthopraxis*: confession, attendance at Mass, almsgiving, protection of the poor. The early tenth-century nobleman, Gerald of Aurillac, contemplated entering a monastery but his monastic biographer Odo of Cluny reports approvingly how others persuaded him against it, 'for the health of the community'.[7] He would do more good by staying in the world to help the community than by withdrawing from it. Odo conforms here to earlier ninth-century writers who suggested that lay nobles should follow a Christian life in order to provide a model to the lesser orders: Louis II even asked his bishops to inquire into the laity's religious practices so as to ensure that the powerful did not set a bad example.[8] This focus on correct and exemplary practice, rather than on belief, continued to dominate clerical thinking in the central Middle Ages. Higher churchmen exerted considerable efforts to develop and revise liturgical texts for baptism, confession and the rites for the dying in order to make liturgies originally composed for cathedrals and monasteries practicable for use in lay churches. They also produced prayer books to support the laity in their private devotions which suggest a similar concern with practice and simple aspirations rather than monastic meditation.

The higher clergy's continued preoccupation with pastoral care in the central Middle Ages is a consequence of their thought world. The sinfulness of clergy and people had led to God's wrath, manifest in the threats besetting the Christian people; only through improvements in Christian behaviour could these threats be averted. The reasons which led Innocent III to focus on ecclesiastical discipline and clerical reform at Lateran IV were very similar to those behind Regino of Prüm's decision to draw up a pragmatic guide to bishops: both wished to defend Christianity, whether in the early thirteenth-century Holy Land or in early tenth-century Lotharingia. Three years after Regino composed his text, Archbishop Heriveus of

Rheims preached a sermon on a similar theme at the Council of Trosly (909) in north-eastern France:

> *You see before you the wrath of the Lord breaking forth . . . There is nothing but towns emptied of their people, monasteries razed to the ground or burnt down, fields have become deserts . . . Everywhere the strong oppress the weak and men are like the fish blindly devouring each other.*

Heriveus's answer, like that of Regino, like that of Innocent III, was to preach the need for change and improvement in the behaviour expected of all Christians, lay and clerical. Both Regino and Heriveus acted against a backdrop of external threats from pagan Viking attack as well as the problems created by the collapse of Carolingian rule. The revival of interest in pastoral care elsewhere in the central medieval west can similarly be attributed to particular local problems and threats. Political instability in northern Italy led Bishop Rather of Verona to focus on reforming clerical behaviour and inculcating priests in the basics of pastoral care in the 960s. Some fifty years later a similar concern to educate the local clergy in the pastoral ministry can be found in eleventh-century Rome and southern Italy; here the production of various pastorally focused liturgical collections and penitentials also needs to be placed against a background of political uncertainty and threat from outsiders, in this case the Saracens. The threat from another set of outsiders, the Scandinavians, provoked similar efforts in southern England at around the same time. In the late tenth and over much of the eleventh centuries English churchmen invested considerable effort in producing texts intended to reform the behaviour of both priests and laymen, including statutes, sermons, penitentials and manuals of liturgical rites written for local churches. Unusually for the medieval west much of their work was recorded in the vernacular, Old English, reflecting the importance they attached to communicating clearly with local priests in order to educate them in the proper conduct of religious services. Political crisis and external threat only provide a partial context for these localised efforts to promote pastoral care. Others can be situated within wider attempts to reform and educate the diocesan clergy. Burchard of Worms, for example, overtly composed his *Decretum* for the education of his diocesan clergy; his is certainly a pragmatic text but the way in which it circulated throughout the cathedral and monastic libraries of Europe over the course of the eleventh century points to its wider usefulness as a systematic guide to church law.

Such attempts to educate the local clergy in pastoral care were, however, never universal but rather highly localised in the years 900 to 1200. Particular dioceses became the focus for pastoral reform at different times. Thus Regino composed his *Libri duo* in the diocese of Trier in the early tenth century, Ælfric and Wulfstan worked in Sherborne and Worcester around 1000, Gerard in Arras-Cambrai in *c.*1025, Burchard in Worms in *c.*1020, and anonymous clerics of S. XII Apostoli in Rome in *c.*1025. The picture looks quite disparate and could be attributed to the lack of centralised leadership within the Church. But, as Robert Brentano demonstrated some forty years ago in his comparison of English and Italian dioceses in the thirteenth century, even at a time of greater centralisation religious developments in different localities were very different; historical differences in political and ecclesiastical structures led to very different experiences in different local dioceses.[9] It is not therefore surprising to find similar patterns in the central Middle Ages. At the same time, we need to recognise that there are some hidden continuities. The preoccupation with pastoral care begun by Ælfric and Archbishop Wulfstan in southern England continued well into the later eleventh century, and Worcester, especially, remained a centre for the production of texts concerned to educate parish priests into the 1060s. Clergy in the provinces of Trier and Mainz similarly displayed a concern with pastoral care throughout the tenth and eleventh centuries. Regino wrote his *Two Books* at the request of the Archbishop of Trier and dedicated it to the archbishop of Mainz. Two decades later, Archbishop Ratbod of Trier set out his pastoral concerns in a set of *capitula*. The collections of liturgical rites now known as the Romano-German Pontifical, which included significant amounts of didactic and pastoral material, emerged in the late tenth-century province of Mainz and quickly spread within it. And Worms, where Burchard composed his *Decretum* in the early eleventh century, seemingly with the aid of other bishops, was situated in the province of Mainz. Lateran IV needs therefore to be set against this backdrop of earlier concerns with pastoral care as well as the more immediate backdrop of pastorally minded theologians in late twelfth-century Paris.

In some ways the thirteenth-century pastoral reformers were much less ambitious than their earlier predecessors in what they required of the laity: canon 21 of Lateran IV demanded that all Christians communicate and make their confession only once a year, whilst Burchard of Worms, repeating ninth-century legislation, required Christians to communicate three times a year.[10] Mary Mansfield described thirteenth-century pragmatism as a retreat from the wilder hopes and dreams of canonists to a more achievable and limited model of lay orthopraxy.[11] But we need also to note the degree of pragmatism shown earlier by some central medieval churchmen. They did not all share the seemingly unrealistic objectives of the Carolingian reformers. For example, Bishop Gerard of Cambrai, Burchard's Flemish near contemporary, scaled back Carolingian demands for regular communion and confession four times a year to a manageable once a year. Ælfric in his Catholic Homilies assumed that the laity would be present for rather fewer feasts than the minimum number enshrined in church law collections from the ninth century onwards. Burchard of Worms recorded a great variety of superstitions, but treated those based on a misunderstanding of Christian doctrine with sympathy, prescribing only a token penance.

This study has not only traced churchmen's continued concern with pastoral care between the ninth and early thirteenth centuries; by focusing on different facets of the relationship between church and people it has highlighted the significant role the laity played in clerical thought and the development of ecclesiastical institutions. The laity fulfilled an important material and rhetorical role for the clergy. The clergy needed the laity in order to articulate their own vision for the Church. This is perhaps clearest in churchmen's descriptions of scepticism and heresy considered in Chapter 9. In these texts we see how leading churchmen followed Augustine in using particular incidents to construct a vision of orthodoxy and even more of orthopraxy by defining how Christians should behave by recounting how they should not. But churchmen also drew evidence for popular enthusiasm to make their case for the success of particular cults. Since the time of the Gospels the crowd had played an important role as witnesses in Christian history; the people had always been crucial to the success of particular manifestations of divine authority. It is therefore not surprising to see churchmen drawing on such themes in their descriptions of saints' cults and pilgrimages, as we saw in Chapters 7 and 8.

But the laity were never passive supporters of the clergy, following where they led. Instead they developed their own movements, as we saw in Chapters 6, 7, 8 and 9. Records of saints' cults, pilgrimages, and heretical outbreaks all point to the importance of lay experience to the development of clerical thought. And the physical remnants of monasteries, local churches and cathedrals all testify to the reality of the material support the laity gave to local churches in this period. As we have seen, the laity initiated and drove their own autonomous forms of devotion. Some of the confraternities attached to local churches and cathedrals testify to the ways in which individual social groups used their local churches as a focus for their own community. The ways in which some lay men and women chose to live voluntary religious lives outside the constraints of formal monasticism, for example, also indicate the success of Christianisation.

It is important that we resist the temptation to view developments in this period teleologically. Some issues recurred again and again throughout the medieval church. The focus in Lateran IV on clerical behaviour, for example, echoes concerns found in Merovingian councils onwards. Clerical reform had been an especial concern of the ninth-century reformers, and continued to be in the tenth, eleventh and twelfth centuries. The increased emphasis upon the significance of the sacraments, in particular the value of the Eucharist, led to the elevation of sacerdotal status in the ninth century and again in the eleventh century. Theodulf of Orleans's ninth-century *capitula*, for example, emphasised the importance of proper behaviour so that priests offered a good example to their lay flocks. The canons of Lateran IV stated that the clergy 'should not practise callings or business of a secular nature, especially those that are dishonourable', and criticised those who preferred lay conversation to celebrating the Mass.[12] But just as churchmen often had recourse to the same body of law to define the clergy as separate at the same time they constructed a separate and complementary ideal of lay spirituality. Some scholars view the increasing evidence for expressions of lay piety in the central Middle Ages as a consequence of the extension of monastic ideas of penance to earthly society, and suggest that this period witnessed the democratisation of monastic ideals.[13] The lay armies of the first crusade, for example, were often recruited by monks from their lay patrons. Pilgrimage is depicted as embodying the monastic ideal of spiritual exile within the world. The popularity of the *vita apostolica* first began in the monasteries of tenth-century Germany and eleventh-century Italy. This apparent monastic bias in our current picture of lay piety may, however, be a trick of the evidential light, a reflection of the surviving archives rather than lived experience. For at the same time as monastic ideals became popular, this book has shown how other churchmen continued to emphasise the importance of orthopraxis, of conforming to a relatively short checklist of Christian behaviour. We also need to acknowledge that we know far more about the twelfth century than we do the tenth or eleventh centuries; the proliferation of miracle collections, pilgrimage guides, liturgical collections, monastic customaries, saints' lives, and canon law, as well as the increase in surviving architectural remains are all testimony to this. But the continuities in genre between the ninth and twelfth centuries are equally marked: prescriptive episcopal texts, liturgical rites, miracle collections, pilgrimage narratives, confraternity statutes, records of informal religious households, and books of private prayer all survive from across the central Middle Ages. Starting in the tenth century rather than the eleventh or twelfth centuries has therefore revealed a different perspective on religious change and highlighted the degree of continuity in clerical ambition and lay experience. The growing evidence for lay religious enthusiasm in the twelfth century may therefore represent not so much the democratisation of monastic ideals as the pushing out of ninth-century ideals to a wider social spectrum.

This study set out to investigate the relationship between church and people in the years between 900 and 1215. Tracing the contours of that association from the perspective of, first, the laity's relationship with and role in developments in the institutional Church, and then their experiences of pastoral care has revealed the complex and varying nature of that relationship. Reforming clergy needed the laity to articulate their own vision for the Church; the laity thus played a number of different but necessary roles within clerical rhetoric. In doing so they recognised the very positive role the laity played in church life. But the people were never mere followers and supporters of clerically led programmes; rather they developed their own initiatives as founders, builders and patrons of local churches, as founders and patrons of local monasteries, as founders and members of confraternities, as supporters of local and international cults. Theirs was a symbiotic relationship but it was one which, as this study demonstrates, should never be viewed through a single interpretative lens.

Notes and references

1 A. Luchaire, 'Un document retrouvé', *Journal des savants* n.s. 3 (1905), 557–68.

2 *PL* 216, col. 825.

3 Lateran IV, c. 21, in N. P. Tanner, ed. and trans., *Decrees of the Ecumenical Councils I: Nicaea I to Lateran V* (London, 1990), 245.

4 Innocent III, *Regestorum* XVI, Ep. 30, *PL* 216, 824.

5 M.-D. Chénu, 'The Evangelical Awakening', in his *Nature, Man and Society in Twelfth-Century Europe: Essays on New Theological Perspectives in the Latin West*, trans. J. Taylor and L. K. Little (Chicago, 1968), 239–69; A. Vauchez, *La spiritualité de moyen-âge occidental VIII–XII siècles* (Paris, 1975); Bull, *Knightly Piety*; Yarrow, *Saints and their Communities.*

6 T. F. X. Noble, 'Secular Sanctity: Forging an Ethos for the Carolingian Nobility', in P. Wormald and J. L. Nelson, eds, *Lay Intellectuals in the Carolingian World* (Cambridge, 2007), 8–36.

7 Ibid., p. 12, citing *Vita Geraldi*, II.2, *PL* 133, cols 670–71.

8 Ibid., p. 13.

9 R. Brentano, *Two Churches: England and Italy in the Thirteenth Century* (Berkeley, CA, 1968)

10 *PL* 140, 577.

11 M. Mansfield, *The Humiliation of Sinners: Public Penance in Thirteenth-century France* (Ithaca, NY, 1995).

12 Lateran IV, cc. 16, 17, ed. Tanner, *Ecumenical Councils*, p. 243.

13 Chénu, 'The Evangelical Awakening'; Vauchez, *La spiritualité.*

Glossary

Abbot/abbess The head of a community of monks or nuns.

Archbishop Bishop with influence over the other bishoprics in an ecclesiastical province.

Aspersorium Sprinkler used to sprinkle holy water during the Mass.

Bishop Possesses theoretical spiritual and disciplinary authority over all the clergy and laity of the diocese derived from the Apostles; only bishops can ordain priests and only they have the right to confer holy orders and consecrate churches and cemeteries.

Capitulary Royal or episcopal decrees covering administrative matters, divided into *capitula*, i.e. chapters.

Canons (legal) Ecclesiastical laws.

Canons regular Secular clergy, usually priests, living in community according to a rule.

Canon law Ecclesiastical law.

Computus Book supporting process for calculating the date of Easter.

Cura animarum Literally 'the cure of souls'; used to mean the delivery of **pastoral care.**

Customary (monastic) From the tenth century onwards texts known as customaries begin to be recorded which supplement monastic Rules. They provided more detailed prescriptions for the way in which the regular life should be observed in a particular house, or group of houses, setting out how the annual round of the liturgy should be observed, together with other details about the running of the community.

Deacon Cleric in rank immediately below priest.

Decretals Papal letters which are regarded as having the force of law.

Diocese Administrative territorial district of the Church controlled by a bishop; all Christians, lay and clerical, within that diocese come under his pastoral and disciplinary authority.

Epacts Used in the calculation of the date of Easter; this term specifically refers to the excess of days in solar year over lunar year.

Exorcism Use of prayer to expel evil spirits.

Last rites The rites administered by a priest to the dying, which included confession, anointing them, and the ***viaticum***.

Lateran Term used to refer to both the cathedral church of Rome, dedicated to St John, and the adjoining Lateran Palace which was the pope's main residence in Rome.

Lay investiture Practice of lay rulers investing an abbot or bishop with ring and staff before their ecclesiastical consecration.

Liber vitae Literally: book of life. A record of the names, both lay and clerical, whom the community should remember in their prayers. They were kept by clerical communities, usually monastic.

Liber memorialis Literally: memorial book. Similar to ***liber vitae***, a record of the names of the souls whom the religious community, usually monastic, would remember in their prayers. Generally kept on or near the high altar.

Local church The church in which some or all pastoral services are delivered to a lay congregation.

Mass The Latin West's name for the Eucharist.

Mother church or minister The church generally served by a clerical community with a monopoly on delivering pastoral care to a large area.

Nicolaitism Term sometimes used by eleventh-century papal reformers promoting clerical chastity to refer to the sin of clerical fornication and marriage; it comes from reference in the early Church to a sect, the Nicolaitans, whose offences included fornication.

Office Eight services of prayer recited by clergy each day.

Opus Dei Literally, the work of God. In monastic writings means the divine office, i.e. the monks' duty to pray.

Pastoral care The administration of those rites thought necessary to Christian salvation, that is those for baptism, penance, the Eucharist and the dying.

Parish church Church for the delivery of pastoral care to inhabitants living within a district or parish.

Parish A subdivision of a diocese; territory over which a priest had responsibility for the cure of souls.

Pieve A church, often rural, in Italy with sole authority to deliver baptism to those living in a wider area; chapels in that area were subordinate to the authority of the clergy of the *pieve*.

Pontifical Liturgical book containing rites restricted to bishop, e.g. ordination into Holy Orders, consecration of churches, etc.

Priest Ordained cleric who has the authority to celebrate Mass, hear confession and administer the last rites.

Province Group of dioceses, usually under the authority of archbishop.

Regular life Life lived according to a rule, i.e. that followed by monks, nuns or canons.

Rubric Directions to be followed included in a liturgical text for a religious service or ritual.

Sacramentary Liturgical book containing the main texts for the Mass.

Secular life Way of life followed by those clergy living in the world and not under a rule.

Simony So-called after the story in the Acts of the Apostles of how Simon Magus tried to buy the gift of the holy spirit from Peter; came to refer in the central Middle Ages to purchase or sale of spiritual matters including clerical office, either actual or promised.

Soulscot Old English term for burial tax paid to minister church.

Synod A formal meeting of the clergy, often of a diocese (diocesan synod) or province (provincial synod).

Viaticum Holy communion given as part of the rites for the dying, from the Latin term for preparation for a journey.

Vita apostolica Literally: apostolic life. Life of Christians who chose to follow Christ's precepts closely, usually characterised by communal living, poverty, charity and focus on imitating Christ through suffering and penance.

Unction Rite whereby the priest anointed the dying with oil.

Bibliography of primary works

Manuscripts

Cambridge, Corpus Christi College, Ms 190 (digital images are available at the Parker Library on the Web: http://parkerweb.stanford.edu/parker/actions/page.do?forward=home; accessed 19th August 2012).

Cambridge, Corpus Christi College, Ms 422 (digital images are available at the Parker Library on the Web: http://parkerweb.stanford.edu/parker/actions/page.do?forward=home; accessed 19th August 2012).

Cologne, Diözesanbibliothek, Cod. 113 (digital images are available at http://www.ceec.uni-koeln.de/; accessed 19th August 2012).

London, British Library, Ms Additional 28188.

Vatican City, Biblioteca Apostolica Vaticana, Ms Archivio S. Pietro, H.58.

Printed sources

Acta Synodi Atrebatensis, *PL* 142, 1271–1312, partially translated Moore, *Birth*, 15–19.

Adelard, *Epistola Adelardi ad Elfegum Archiepiscopum de Vita Sancti Dunstani*, in *Memorials of Saint Dunstan, Archbishop of Canterbury*, ed. W. Stubbs, Rolls Series 63 (London, 1874).

Adhemar of Chabannes, *Ademari Cabannensis Chronicon*, ed. P. Bourgain, with G. Pon and R. Landes, CCCM 129 (Turnhout, 1999); Adémar de Chabannes, *Chronique*, trans. Y. Chauvin and G. Pon (Turnhout, 2003).

Admonitio Synodalis, ed. R. Amiet, 'Une "Admonitio synodalis" de l'époque carolingienne. Étude critique et édition', *Mediaeval Studies* 26 (1964), 12–82.

Ælfric of Eynsham: Fehr, B., ed., *Die Hirtenbriefe Ælfrics in altenglischer und lateinischer Fassung* (Hamburg, 1914).

Ælfric of Eynsham: *Ælfric's Catholic Homilies: The First Series*, ed. P. Clemoes, EETS SS 17 (Oxford, 1997).

Ælfric of Eynsham: *Ælfric's Catholic Homilies: The Second Series*, ed. M. Godden, EETS SS 5 (Oxford, 1979).

Ælfric of Eynsham: *The Homilies of the Anglo-Saxon Church. The First Part, containing the Sermones Catholici or Homilies of Ælfric in the Original Anglo-Saxon with an English Version*, 2 vols, ed. and trans. B. Thorpe (London, 1844; repr. 1971).

Ælfric's Lives of the Saints, Being a Set of Sermons of Saints' Days Formerly Observed by the English Church, ed. and trans. W. Skeat, EETS o.s. 76, 82, 94, 114 (London, 1881–1900).

Aelfric's Pastoral Letter for Wulfsige III, Bishop of Sherborne, no. 40, C&S I.i, 191–226.

Ælred of Rievaulx, *Relatio de standardo*, ed. R. Howlett, *Chronicles of the Reigns of Stephen, Henry I and Richard I*, Rolls Series 82.3 (London, 1886).

Andreas of Strumi, *Vita sancti Arialdi*, ed. F. Baethgen in MGH SS xxx.2 (Leipzig, 1934), 1047–104.

Andreas of Sturmi, *Vita Iohannis Gualberti*, ed. F. Baethgen, *MGH SS* xxx.2, 1080–104.

Anglo-Saxon Charters, ed. and trans. A. J. Robertson (Cambridge, 1939).

Arnulf of Lisieux, *The Letters of Arnulf of Lisieux*, ed. F. Barlow, Camden Society 3r ser. 61 (London, 1939); *The Letter Collections of Arnulf of Lisieux*, trans. C. P. Schriber (Lewiston, NY, 1997).

Arnulf of Milan, *Liber Gestorum Recentium*, ed. C. Zey, MGH SRG 67 (Hannover, 1994).

Atti della causa tre Giovanni Vescovo Bresciano e Gonterio Abate di Leno', in F. A. Zaccaria, *Dell'antichissima Badia di Leno* (Venice, 1767).

Atto of Vercelli, *Capitulare*, *MGH Capitula Episcoporum III*, ed. R. Pokorny (Hannover, 1995), 243–304.

Atto of Vercelli, *De pressuris ecclesiasticis*, *PL* 134, 51–96.

Atto Pistoriensi, *Vita s. Joanis Gualberti*, *PL* 146, 667–706.

Augustine, *De Civitate Dei, St Augustine Concerning the City of God Against the Pagans*, trans. H. Bettenson (Harmondsworth, 1972; repr. 1984).

Bernard of Cluny, *Ordo Cluniacensis par Bernardum saeculi XI. Scriptorem*, ed. M. Herrgott, *Vetus Disciplina Monastica* (Paris, 1726).

Bernerus US, *De Translatione Corporis S. Hunegundis Virginis Apud Viromanduos*, *PL* 137, 59–72.

Bernold of Constance, *Chronicon*, ed. G. Pertz, MGH SS V, 385–467; trans. I. S. Robinson, *Eleventh-century Germany: The Swabian Chronicles* (Manchester, 2008), 245–337.

Bertram, J., *The Chrodegang Rules: The Rules for the Common Life of the Secular Clergy from the Eighth and Ninth Centuries: Critical Texts with Translations and Commentary* (Aldershot, 2005).

Bonizo of Sutri, *Liber de Vita Christiana*, ed. E. Perels (Berlin, 1930; repr. Hildesheim, 1998).

Burchard of Worms, *Decretum PL* 140, 537–1058.

Byrhtferth of Ramsey, *Life of St Oswald*, in Byrhtferth of Ramsey, *The Lives of St Oswald and St Ecgwine*, ed. M. Lapidge (Oxford, 2009).

Cheney, C. R., *English Synodalia* (Oxford, 1968).

Chronicle of St André de Castres, ed. L. C. Bethmann *MGH SS* VII, 526–50.

Coffey, T. F., L. K. Davidson and M. Dunn, eds, *The Miracles of Saint James* (New York, 1996).

Constitutiones Canonicorum Regularium Springirsbacenses-Rodenses, ed. S. Weinfurter, CCCM 48 (Turnhout, 1978).

Constitutiones quae vocantur Ordinis Praemonstratensis, ed. M. L. Colker, CCCM 216 (Turnhout, 2008).

Consuetudines Floriacenses Antiquiores, ed. A. Davril and L. Donnat, CCM 7.3 (Siegburg, 1984).

Councils and Synods with Other Documents Relating to the English Church: 871–1204, ed. D. Whitelock, M. Brett and C.N.L. Brooke, 2 vols (Oxford, 1981).

Davis-Weyer, C., *Early Medieval Art 300–1150* (Englewood Cliffs, NJ, 1971).

De miraculis beatae Mariae Laudunensis, *PL* 156, 961–1018.

Dhuoda, Manuel pour mon fils, ed. P. Riché, trans. B. de Vregille and C. Mondésert, Sources Chrétiennes 225 (Paris, 1975).

Die Bussbücher und die Bussdiscipin der Kirche II: Die Bussbücher und das kanonische Bussverfahren nach handschriftlichen Quellen, ed. H.J. Schmitz (Düsseldorf, 1898).

Drogo of Sint-Winoksbergen, *Life of St Godelieve*, ed. M. Coens, *Analecta Bollandiana* 44 (1926), 103–37; trans. B. L. Venarde, in T. Head, ed., *Medieval Hagiography: An Anthology* (New York, 2001), 359–73.

Duchesne, A., ed., *Historiae Francorum Scriptores* (Paris, 1636).

Egbert of Hersfeld, *Vita Heimeradi*, *AASS Iunii V*, 385–95.

Ekkehard IV, *Casus s. Galli*, *MGH SS* II, 74–147.

English Historical Documents, ed. D. Whitelock (London, 1955).

Epistola ecclesiae Leodiensis ad Lucum papam II, ed. *PL* 179, 937–38, trans. Wakefield and Evans, *Heresies*, 139–41.

Epistolae diversorum ad S. Hugonem Cluniacensis, Ep. 6, *PL* 159, 931–32.

Flodoard, *Les Annales de Flodoard*, ed. P. Lauer (Paris, 1905).

Fulbert of Chartres, *The Letters and Poems of Fulbert of Chartres*, ed. F. Behrends (Oxford, 1976).

Gerald of Wales, *De Rebus a Gestis*, in *Giraldus Cambriensis Opera*, ed. J. S. Brewer, J. F. Dimock and G. F. Warner, 8 vols, Rolls Series 21 (London, 1861–91); H. E. Butler, ed. and trans. *The Autobiography of Giraldus Cambrensis* (London, 1937).

Gerhard, *Vita Oudalrici*, ed. G. Waitz, *MGH SS* IV, 377–428.

Gesta episcoporum Cameracensium, ed. L. C. Bethmann *MGH SS VII*, 393–525.

Gesta Episcoporum Leodiensis, ed. R. Koepke *MGH SS* VII, 134–234.

Gesta Francorum et aliorum Hierosolimitanorum, ed. R. Hill (London, 1962).

Gesta Normannorum Ducum of William of Jumièges, Orderic Vitalis and Robert of Torigni, ed. E. van Houts (Oxford, 1995).

Gilbert Foliot and his Letters, ed. A. Morey and C. N. L. Brooke (Cambridge, 1965).

Gilbert of Limerick, *Gille of Limerick (c.1070–1145): Architect of a Medieval Church*, ed. J. Fleming (Dublin, 2001).

Gonterus, *Vita Gerardi Abbatis Broniensis*, *MGH SS XV.2*, 654–73.

Goscelin of Saint-Bertin, *Historia Translationis Sancti Augustini*, *PL* 155, 13–46.

Goscelin of Saint-Bertin, *The Miracles of St Æthelthryth the Virgin*, in Goscelin of Saint-Bertin, *The Hagiography of the Female Saints of Ely*, ed. R. C. Love (Oxford, 2004).

Gratian, *Decretum*, in *Corpus Iuris Canonici*, ed. E. Friedberg, 2 vols (repr. Graz, 1955) available at http://geschichte.digitale–sammlungen.de/decretum–gratiani/online/angebot.

Grégoire le Grand, *Règle pastorale*, ed. B. Judic, F. Rommel and C. Morel, Sources chrétiennes 381, 382 (Paris, 1992); Gregory the Great, *Pastoral Care*, trans. H. Davis (London, 1950).

Gregory of Catino, *Il Chronicon Farfense*, Fonti per la Storia d'Italia 33, 34 (1903).

Gregory the Great, *XL Homiliarum in Evangelia Libri duo*, *PL* 76, 1075–1312.

Gregory the Great, *Moralia in Job*, *PL* 75–76.

Gregory VII, *Das Register Gregors VII*, ed. E. Caspar, MGH Epistolae selectae II, 2 vols (Hannover, 1920–23); translated in H. E. J. Cowdrey, *The Register of Pope Gregory VII, 1073–1085: An English Translation* (Oxford, 2002).

Guibert of Nogent, *Gesta dei per Francos: The Deeds of God through the Franks*, trans. R. Levine (Woodbridge, 1997).

Guibert of Nogent, *Monodiae*, *PL* 156, 837–962; trans. in *Self and Society in Medieval France: the Memoirs of Abbot Guibert of Nogent*, trans John F. Benton (New York, 1970; repr. Toronto, 1984) and *A Monk's Confession: The Memoirs of Guibert of Nogent*, trans. P. Archambault (University Park, PA, 1995).

Haito von Basel, *Capitula*, *MGH Capitula Episcoporum I*, ed. P. Brommer (Hannover, 1984).

Hartmann, W., ed., 'Neue Text zur bischöflichen Reformgestzgebung aus den Jahren 829/31. Vier Diözesansynoden Halitgars von Cambrai', *Deutsches Archiv für Erforschung des Mittelalters* 35 (1979), 368–94.

Head, T., ed., *Medieval Hagiography: An Anthology* (New York, 2001).

Herbert de Losinga: *The Life, Letters, and Sermons of Bishop Herbert de Losinga*, ed. E. M. Goulburn and Henry Symonds, 2 vols (Oxford, 1878).

Hermann of Tournai, *Liber de restauratione monasterii Sancti Martini Tornacensis*, ed. G. Waitz, MGH SS XIV, 274–317; *The Restoration of the Monastery of Saint Martin of Tournai*, trans L. H. Nelson (Washington, DC, 1996).

Hildemar *Expositio regulae ab Hildemero tradita, et nunc primum typis mandata*, ed. R. Mittermüller (Regensburg, 1880).

Hrabanus Maurus, *Declericorum institutione*, *PL* 107, 293–420.

Hugh of Farfa, *Destructio monasterii Farfensi*, ed. L. Bethmann, *MGH SS* XI.2, 530–44.

Hugh of Flavigny, *Chronicon*, ed. G. H. Pertz, *MGH SS* VIII, 288–502.

Hugo Francigena, *Tractatus de Conversione Pontii de Laracio et exordia Salvaniensis monasterii vera narratio*, ed. in B. M. Kienzle, 'The Works of Hugo Francigena: Tractatus de Conversione Pontii de Laracio et exordii Salvaniensis monasterii vera narratio, epistolae (Dijon, Bibliothèque municipale, Ms 611', *Sacris Erudiri* 34 (1994), 273–311; translated eadem, 'The Tract on the Conversion of Pons of Léras and the True Account of the Beginning of the Monastery at Silvanès', in T. Head, ed., *Medieval Hagiography: An Anthology* (New York, 2001), 499–512.

Humbert of Silva Candida, *Libri III Adversus Simoniacos*, ed. F. Thaner, *MGH Libelli de Lite imperatorum et pontificum saeculis XI et XII*, I (Hannover, 1891, repr. 1956).

Jean de Saint-Arnoul, *La vie de Jean, abbé de Gorze*, ed. M. Parisse (Paris, 1999).

John of Ford, *Wulfric of Haselbury*, ed. M. Bell, Somerset Record Society 47 (1933).

John of Salerno, *Vita Odonis*, *PL* 133, 43–85; trans. G. Sitwell, *St Odo of Cluny* (London, 1958).

le Grand, L. *Statuts dehotels-Dieu et de léproseries: Recueil de textes du XIIe au XIVe siècle* (Paris, 1901).

L'Estoire des Engleis, ed. A. Bell, Anglo-Norman Text Society, 1960.

Lanfranc, H. Clover and M. Gibson (eds), *The Letters of Lanfranc, Archbishop of Canterbury* (Oxford, 1979).

Lanfranc, *The Monastic Constitutions of Lanfranc*, ed. D. Knowles and C. N. L. Brooke (Oxford, 2002).

Langefeld, B., ed., *The Old English Version of the Enlarged Rule of Chrodegang: Edited Together with the Latin Text and an English Translation*, Texte und Untersuchungen zur englischen Philologie, 26 (Frankfurt am Main, 2003).

Lantfred, *Translatio et miracula s. Swithuni*, in M. Lapidge, *The Cult of St Swithun* (Oxford, 2003), 217–333.

Lapidge, M., *The Cult of St Swithun* (Oxford, 2003).

Le Pontifical Romano-Germanique du dixième siècle, ed. C. Vogel and R. Elze, 3 vols (Vatican City, 1963, 1972).

Les Miracles de Notre-Dame de Rocamodour au XIIe siècle, ed. and trans. E. Albe, rev. J. Rocacher (Toulouse, 1996); trans. in M. Bull, *The Miracles of Our Lady of Rocamadour: Analysis and Translation* (Woodbridge, 1999).

Les miracles de Saint Benoit, ed. E. de Certain (Paris, 1858).

Liber Miraculorum Sancte Fidis, ed. A. Bouillet (Paris, 1897); English trans. *The Book of Sainte Foy*, trans. P. Sheingorn (Philadelphia, 1995).

Liber sancti Gileberti, ed. R. Foreville and G. Keir (Oxford, 1987).

Liber Sancti Jacobi: Codex Calixtinus, ed. W. Muir Whitehill *et al.*, 3 vols (Santiago, 1944).

Liber Tramitis Aevi Odilonis Abbatis, ed. P. Dinter, CCM X (Siegburg, 1980).

Mansi, J. D., *Sacrorum conciliorum nova et amplissima collection*, 59 vols (Venice, 1759–98; repr. Graz, 1960).

Meersseman, G. G., *Dossier de l'ordre de la pénitence au XIIIe siècle*, Spicilegium Friburgense 7 (Freiburg, 1961).

Meersseman, G. G., *Ordo fraternitatis: confraternite e pietàdei laici nel medioevo* (Rome, 1977).

MGH Capitula Episcoporum I, ed. P. Brommer (Hannover, 1984).

MGH Capitula Episcoporum II, ed. R. Pokorny, M. Stratmann, W.-D. Runge (Hannover, 1995).

MGH Capitula Episcoporum III, ed. R. Pokorny (Hannover, 1995).

MGH Capitularia Regum Francorum, ed. A. Boretius and V. Krause, 2 vols (Hannover, 1883–1897).

MGH Concilia III: Concilia aevi Karolini 843–59, ed. W. Hartmann (Hannover, 1984).

MGH Concilia VI: Concilia aevi Saxonici I: 916–60, ed. E.-D. Hehl and H. Fuhrmann (Hannover, 1987).

MGH Constitutiones et acta publica imperatorum et regum 911–1197, I, ed. L. Weiland (Hannover, 1893).

MGH Diplomatum regum et imperatorum Germaniae III: Henri II et Arduini Diplomata (Hannover, 1900–1903).

MGH Leges III. Concilia II: Concilia Aevi Karolini, ed. A. Werminghoff (Hannover, 1906).

MGH Libelli de Lite Imperatorum et Pontificum saeculis XI et XII, ed. E. Dümmler *et al.*, 3 vols (Hannover, 1891–97).

MGH Ordines de celebrando concilio, ed. H. Schneider (Hannover, 1996).

Miracula S. Swithuni, in M. Lapidge *et al.*, *The Cult of St Swithun* (Oxford, 2003), 641–97.

Moore, R. I., *The Birth of European Heresy* (London, 1975; repr. Toronto, 1995).

Norbert of Xanten, *Vita Norberti Archiepiscopi Magdeburgensis*, ed. R. Welmans, *MGH SS* XII, 663–706; trans. in *Norbert and Early Norbertine Spirituality*, trans. T. J. Antry, O. Praem, C. Neel (New York, 2007).

Odo of Cluny, *Life of St Gerald of Aurillac*, *PL* 133, 639–704; trans. G. Sitwell, *St Odo of Cluny Being the Life of St Odo of Cluny by John of Salerno and the Life of St Gerald of Aurillac by St Odo* (London, 1958).

Orderic Vitalis, *Historia Ecclesiastica*, ed. M. Chibnall, 6 vols (Oxford, 1969–80).

Otloh of St Emmeram, *Dialogus de tribus quaestionibus*, *PL* 146, 59–134.

Otloh of St Emmeram, *Liber de cursu spirituali*, *PL* 146, 139–242.

Otto of Freising, *The Two Cities: A Chronicle of Universal History to the Year 1146*, trans. C. C. Mierow (New York, 1928).

Paul Bernried, The *Life of Gregory VII*, in *The Papal Reform of the Eleven Century: the Lives of Pope Leo IX and Pope Gregory VII*, trans. I. S. Robinson (Manchester, 2004), 262–364.

Peregrinationes tres: Saewulf, Iohannes Wirziburgensis, Theodericus, ed. R. B. C. Huygens with J. H. Pryor, CCCM 139 (Turnhut, 1994); for English translation, see J. Wilkinson, J. Hill and W. F. Ryan, trans, *Jerusalem Pilgrimage 1099–1185*, Hakluyt Society 2nd series 167 (London, 1988).

Peter Damian, *Die Briefe des Petrus Damiani*, ed. K. Reindel, 4 vols, MGH (Munich, 1983–1993); *Peter Damian, Letters*, trans. O. J. Blum, 5 vols (Washington, DC, 1990–2004).

Peter Damian, *Vita Beati Romualdi*, ed. G. Tabacco, Fonti per la storia d'Italia 94 (Rome, 1957).

Pontal, O., *Les statuts synodaux Français du XIIIe siècle I: Les Statuts de Paris et le synodal de l'ouest* (Paris, 1971).

R. Somerville, ed., *The Councils of Urban II*, vol. 1: *Decreta Claromontensia* (Amsterdam, 1972).

Ralph of Coggeshall, *Chronicon Anglicanum*, ed. J. Stevenson, Rolls Series (London, 1875).

Raoul of Saint-Sépulchre, *Vita Lietberti episcopi Cameracensis*, ed. A. Hofmeister, *MGH SS* XXX.2, 838–66.

Rather of Verona, *The Complete Works of Rather of Verona*, trans. P. L. D. Reid (Binghamton, NY, 1991).

Rather of Verona, *Die Briefe des Bischofs Rather von Verona*, ed. F. Weigle, MGH Die Briefe der deutschen Kaiserzeit I (Weimar, 1949).

Rather of Verona, *Opera Minora*, ed. P. L. D. Reid, CCCM 46 (Turnhout, 1976).

Rather of Verona, *Praeloquiorum libri VI and Other Works*, ed. P. L. Reid, F. Dolbeau, B. Bischoff and C. Leonardi, CCCM 46A (Turnhout, 1984).

Regino of Prüm, *History and Politics in Late Carolingian and Ottonian Europe: The Chronicle of Regino of Prüm and Adalbert of Magdeburg*, trans. and annotated by S. MacLean (Manchester, 2009).

Regino of Prüm, *Libri duo de Synodalibus Causis et Disciplinis Ecclesiasticis*, ed. F. G. A. Wasserschleben, rev. and ed. W. Hartmann, *Das Sendhandbuch des Regino von Prüm* (Darmstadt, 2004).

Regularis Concordia Anglicae nationis monachorum sanctimonialiumque, ed. T. Symons (London, 1953).

Richard of Hexham, *De gestis regis Stephani*, ed. R. Howlett, *Chronicles of the Reigns of Stephen, Henry II and Richard I*, Roll Series 82.3 (London, 1886).

Robert of Abrissel, *Les deux vies de Robert D'Arbrissel fondateur de Fontevraud : légendes, écrits et témoignages*, ed. J. Dalarun *et al.* (Turnhout, 2006); English trans. *Robert of Arbrissel: A Medieval Religious Life*, ed. B. Venarde (Washington, DC, 2003).

Robert the Monk, *Historia Hierosolymitana*, VII.1, *Recueil des Historiens des Croisades*, 16 vols, Academie des Inscriptions et Belles Lettres (Paris, 1841–1906), Historiens Occidentaux, vol. III, 771–882.

Robertson, J. C., *Materials for the History of Thomas Becket, Archbishop of Canterbury*, Rolls series 67 (London, 1876).

Rodulf of Saint-Trond, *Gesta abbatum Trudonensium*, ed. R. Koepke, *MGH SS* X, 227–72.

Rodulfus Glaber, *Historiarum Libri Quinque*, ed. and trans. J. France (Oxford, 1989).

Roger of Cambrai, *Precepta Synodalia*, ed. J. Avril, 'Les *Precepta synodalia* de Roger de Cambrai', *Bulletin of Medieval Canon Law*, New series 2 (1972), 7–15.

Ruotger, *Vita Brunonis*, *MGH SS* IV, 252–75.

Sacramentario del vescovo Warmondo di Ivrea: fine secolo X: Ivrea, Biblioteca capitolare, MS 31 LXXXVI (Pavone Canavese) (Turin, 1990).

Sacramentarium Fuldense saeculi X. Cod. Theol. 231 der K. Universitätsbibliothek zu Göttingen, ed. G. Richter and A. Schönfelder, repr. Henry Bradshaw Society 101 (London, 1972–77).

Saints and Cities in Medieval Italy, ed. and trans. D. Webb (Manchester, 2007).

Scriftboc, Oxford, Bodleian Library, Junius 121, ed. and trans. A. Frantzen, *The Anglo-Saxon Penitentials: A Cultural Database* (http://www.anglo-saxon.net/penance/index.html; accessed 19th August 2012).

Shinners, J., ed., *Medieval Popular Religion 1000–1500: A Reader* (Peterborough, Ontario, 1997).

Sigebert of Gembloux, *Sigiberti Gemblacensis chronographia: Continuatio Aquicinctina*, ed. L. C. Bethmann, *MGH SS* VI, 421; trans. Wakefield and Evans, *Heresies*, 256–57.

Somerville, R. and B. Brasington, trans, *Prefaces to Canon Law Books in Latin Christianity: Selected Translations 500–1245* (New Haven, CT and London, 1998).

Somerville, R., with S. Kuttner, *Pope Urban II, the Collectio Britannica and the Council of Melfi (1089)* (Oxford, 1996).

Statuta Petri Venerabilis, *Consuetudines Benedictinae Variae (saec. XI–saec. XIV)*, ed. G. Constable *et al*, CCM VI (Siegburg, 1975).

Storms, G. ed., *Anglo-Saxon Magic* (The Hague, 1948).

Suger, *Abbot Suger on the Abbey Church of St Denis and its Art Treasures*, ed. and trans. Erwin Panofsky (Princeton, NJ, 1946).

The Anglo-Saxon Chronicle: A Collaborative Edition V: Ms C, ed. K. O'Brien O'Keeffe (Cambridge, 2001).

The Anglo-Saxon Chronicles, trans. M. Swanton (London, 1996).

The Blickling Homilies, ed. and trans. R. J. Kelly (London, 2003).

The Canterbury Benedictional, ed. R. M. Woolley, Henry Bradshaw Society 51 (London, 1917).

The Cartulary of Montier-en-Der 666–1129, ed. C. B. Bouchard (Toronto, 2004).

The Decrees of the Ecumenical Councils, ed. and trans N. P. Tanner and G. Alberigo, 2 vols (London, 1990).

The Letters of Peter the Venerable, ed. G. Constable, 2 vols (Cambridge, MA, 1967).

The Life of St Æthelwold, ed. and trans. M. Lapidge and M. Winterbottom (Oxford, 1991).

The Missal in Latin and English Being the Text of the Missale Romanum with English Rubrics and a New Translation (London, 1949).

The Miracle of St Maximinus, trans. T. Head in T. Head, *Medieval Hagiography: An Anthology* (New York, 2001), 287–92.

The Miracles of Our Lady of Rocamadour: Analysis and Translation, trans. M. Bull (Woodbridge, 1999).

The Register of Eudes of Rouen, trans. S. M. Brown and ed. J. F. O'Sullivan (New York, 1964).

The Rule of Benedict: A Guide to Christian Living, ed. and trans. G. Holzherr (Dublin, 1994).

Theodulf, *Capitula* I in *MGH Capitula Episcoporum I*, ed. P. Brommer (Hannover, 1984); English trans. *Carolingian Civilization. A Reader*, ed. P. E. Dutton, 2nd edn (Peterborough, 2004).

Thietmar of Merseburg, *Chronicon*, ed. R. Holtzmann, *MGH SRG* n.s. 9 (Berlin, 1935); trans. *Ottonian Germany: The Chronicon of Thietmar of Merseburg*, trans. D. A. Warner (Manchester, 2001).

Thorpe, B., *Diplomatarium Anglicum Aevi Saxonici* (London, 1865).

Twelfth-century Homilies in MS. Bodley 343. Part I, Text and Translation, ed. A. Belfour, Early English Text Society 0S 137 (London, 1909).

Twelfth-century Statutes from the Cistercian General Chapter, ed. C. Waddell, (Brecht, 2002).

Udalrich of Cluny, *Antiquiores Consuetudines Cluniacensis, PL* 149, 635–778.

Visio Tnugdali, The Vision of Tnugdal, ed. and trans. J.-M. Picard, with introduction by Y. de Pontfarcy (Dublin, 1989).

Vita Adelheidis Abbatissae Vilicensis auctore Bertha, ed. O. Holder-Egger, *MGH SS* 15.2, 754–63; English translation: M. Bergen Dick, *Mater Spiritualis: The Life of Adelheid of Vilich* (Toronto, 1994).

Vita altera S. Ottones, *AASS Julii I*, 425–56.

Vita Altmanni episcopi Pataviensis, ed. W. Wattenbach, *MGH SS* XII, 226–43.

Vita Burchardi Episcopi Wormatiensis, ed. G. H. Waitz, *MGH SS* IV, 829–46; *The Life of Burchard Bishop of Worms, 1025*, trans. by W. North, available at http://www.fordham.edu/halsall/source/1025burchard-vita.asp (accessed 19th August 2012).

Vita et Miracula S. Kenelmi, in *Three Eleventh-Century Anglo-Latin Saints' Lives: Vita S. Birini, Vita et Miracula S. Kenelmi and Vita S. Rumwoldi*, ed. R. Love (Oxford, 1996), 50–73.

Vita Mathilda Antiquior, in *Die Lebensbeschreibungen der Königin Mathilde*, ed. B. Schütte, *MGH SRG* 66 (Hannover, 1994), 107–42; trans. in S. Gilsdorf, *Queenship and Sanctity: The Lives of Mathilda and the Epitaph of Adelheid* (Washington, DC, 2004), 71–87.

Vita Mathildis Posterior, *Die Lebensbeschreibungen der Königin Mathilde*, ed. B. Schütte, *MGH SRG* 66 (Hannover, 1994), 143–202; trans. in S. Gilsdorf, *Queenship and Sanctity: The Lives of Mathilda and the Epitaph of Adelheid* (Washington, DC, 2004), 88–127.

Vita Raimondo Palmario, Acta Sanctorum Iulii VI, 645–57; trans. D. Webb, *Saints and Cities in Medieval Italy* (Manchester, 2007), 65–92.

Vita S. Bobonis, Acta sanctorum, Mai V, 184–91.

Vita S. Conrado seu Cunone, AASS Junii I, 126–34.

Vita S. Gerlaci, AASS Januarii I, 306–20.

Vita S. Theodorici II, AASS Januarii II, 788–90.

Vita S. Ubaldi, AASS Maii III, 628–39.

Vita S. Udalrici, AASS Julii II, 97–125.

Waddell, C., *Cistercian Lay Brothers: Twelfth-century Usages with Related Texts*, Commentarii Cistercienses Studia et Documenta X (Cîteaux, 2000).

Wakefield, W. L., and A. P. Evans, trans., *Heresies of the High Middle Ages* (New York, 1969).

Walahfrid Strabo, *Libellus de exordiis et incrementis quarundam in observationibus ecclesiasticis rerum*, ed. V. Krause, *MGH Capit.* II (Hannover, 1897), trans. A. L. Harting-Correa, *Walahfrid Strabo, Libellus de exordiis et incrementis quarundam in observationibus ecclesiasticis rerum: A Translation and Liturgical Commentary* (Leiden, 1996).

Walter Daniel, *The Life of Ailred of Rievaulx by Walter Daniel*, ed. and trans. M. Powicke (London, 1950; repr. Oxford, 1978).

Walter Map, *De Nugis Curialium*, ed. M. R. James, R. A. B. Mynors and C. N. L. Brooke (Oxford, 1983).

Waltharius and Ruodlieb, ed. and trans. D. M. Katz (New York, 1984).

Widukind of Corvey, *Rerum gestarum Saxonicarum libri tres*, ed. H. E. Lohmann and P. Hirsch, *MGH SRG* 60 (Hannover, 1935).

William of Malmesbury, *Gesta Regum Anglorum*, ed. and trans. R. A. B. Mynors, R. M. Thomson and M. Winterbottom, 2 vols (Oxford, 1998–99).

William of Malmesbury, *Vita Dunstani*, ed. M. Winterbottom and R. M. Thomson, *William of Malmesbury, Saints' Lives* (Oxford, 2002), 166–302.

William of Malmesbury, *Vita Wulfstani*, ed. M. Winterbottom and R. M. Thomson, *William of Malmesbury, Saints' Lives* (Oxford, 2002), 8–154.

Wilson, D. M., *The Bayeux Tapestry* (London, 1985).

Wulfstan of Winchester, *Narratio metrica de S. Swithuno*, in M. Lapidge, *The Cult of St Swithun* (Oxford, 2003), 335–551.

Wulfstan, *Sermo lupi ad anglos*, ed. D. Whitelock, 3rd edn (London, 1963).

Wulfstan, *The Homilies of Wulfstan*, ed. D. Bethurum (Oxford, 1957).

Bibliography of secondary works

Abou-el Haj, B., 'The Audiences for the Medieval Cult of Saints', *Gesta* 30 (1991), 3–15.

Addleshaw, G. W. O., *The Development of the Parochial System from Charlemagne (768–814) to Urban II (1088–1099),* Borthwick Papers 6 (London, 1954).

Aird, W., *St Cuthbert and the Normans* (Woodbridge, 1998).

Andrews, F., *The Early Humiliati* (Cambridge, 1999).

Andrieu, M., 'Le sacre épiscopal d'après Hincmar de Reims', *Revue d'histoire écclesiastique* 48 (1953), 22–73.

Angenendt, A., *Geschichte der Religiosität im Mittelalter* (Darmstadt, 1997).

Anton, H. H., *Fürstenspiegel und Herrscherethos in der Karolingerzeit* (Bonn, 1968).

Arnold, B. *Count and Bishop in Medieval Germany: A Study of Regional Power 1100–1350* (Philadelphia, 1991).

Arnold, J. H., *Belief and Unbelief in Medieval Europe* (London, 2005).

Arnold, J. C., 'Arcadia Becomes Jerusalem: Angelic Caverns and Shrine Conversion at Monte Gargano', *Speculum* 75 (2000), 567–88.

Arnoux, M., *Des clercs au service de la réforme: Études et documents sur les chanoines réguliers de la province de Rouen* (Turnhout, 2000).

Asad, T., 'Medieval Heresy: An Anthropological View', *Social History* 11 (1986), 345–62.

Ashley, K. M. and P. Sheingorn, *Writing Faith: Text, Sign and History in the Miracles of Sainte Foy* (Chicago, 1999).

Aubrun, M., *La Paroisse en France, des origines au XVe siècle* (Paris, 1986).

Aubrun, M., *L'ancien diocèse de Limoges des origines au milieu du XIe siècle* (Clermont-Ferrand, 1981).

Aurell, M., *Les noces du comte: mariage et pouvoir en Catalogne (785–1213)* (Paris, 1995).

Austin, G., 'Bishops and Religious Law 900–1050', in J. Ott and A. Trumbore Jones, eds, *The Bishop Reformed: Studies of Episcopal Power and Culture in the Central Middle Ages* (Aldershot, 2007), 40–57.

Austin, G., 'Jurisprudence in the Service of Pastoral Care: The Decretum of Burchard of Worms', *Speculum* 79 (2004), 929–59.

Austin, G., *Shaping Church Law Around the Year 1000: The Decretum of Burchard of Worms* (Ashgate, 2009).

Avery, M., *The Exultet Rolls of South Italy*, 2 vols (Princeton, NJ, 1936).

Avril, F. and J.-R. Gaborit, 'L'*Itinerarium Bernardi monachi* et les pèlerinages d'Italie du Sud pendant le haut moyen-age,' *Melanges d'archéologie et d'histoire* 79 (1967), 269–98.

Avril, J., 'L'Évolution du synode diocésain principalement dans la France du nord du Xe au XIIe siécle', in P. A. Linehan, ed., *Proceedings of the Seventh International Congress of Medieval Canon Law* (Vatican City, 1988), 305–25.

Avril, J., 'La Paroisse medievale: bilan et perspectives d'après quelques travaux récents', *Revue d'histoire de l'Eglise de France* 54 (1988), 91–113.

Avril, J., 'Recherches sur la politique paroissiale des établissements monastiques et canoniaux (XIe et XIIIe s.), *Revue Mabillon* 59 (1980), 453–517.

Avril, J., 'Remarques sur un aspect de la vie paroissale: La pratique de la confession et de la communion du Xe au XIVe siècle', in *L'Encadrement religiux des fidèles au Moyen-Age et pastorale- la dévotion. Actes du 109e congrès national des sociétés savantes, Dijon 1984. Section d'histoire médiévale et de philologie I* (Paris, 1985), 345–63.

Avril, J., 'La "paroisse" dans la France de l'an Mil', in M. Parisse, and X. Barral i Altet, eds, *Le roi de France et son royaume, autour de l'an Mil* (Picard, 1992), 203–18.

Bachrach, B. S., 'The Pilgrimages of Fulk Nerra, Count of the Angevins 987–1040', in T. F. X. Noble and J. J. Contreni, eds, *Religion, Culture and Society in the Middle Ages: Studies in Honour of Richard E. Sullivan* (Kalamazoo, MI, 1987), 205–217.

Bainbridge, V. R., *Gilds in the Medieval Countryside: Social and Religious Change in Cambridgeshire c.1350–1558* (Woodbridge, 1996).

Baker, N. and R. Holt, 'The Origins of Urban Parish Boundaries', in *The Church in the Medieval Town*, ed. T. R. Slater and G. Rosser (Aldershot, 1998), 209–35.

Barber, M. C., 'Northern Catharism', in Frassetto, ed., *Heresy*, 115–37.

Barlow, F., *The English Church 1000–1066: A History of the Later Anglo-Saxon Church* (London, 1979).

Barlow, F., *Thomas Becket* (London, 1986; repr. 1997).

Barnes Jr, Carl F., 'Cult of the Carts', *Dictionary of Art*, ed. J. Turner (London, 1996), 8: 257–59.

Barrow, 'The Clergy in English Dioceses, *c.*900–*c.*1050', in F. Tinti, ed., *Pastoral Care in Late Anglo-Saxon England* (Woodbridge, 2005), 17–26.

Barrow, J. 'Review Article: Chrodegang, His rule and Its successors', *Early Medieval Europe* 14 (2006), 201–12.

Barrow, J., 'Ideas and Applications of Reform', in T. F. X. Noble and J. M. H. Smith, eds, *The Cambridge History of Christianity III: Early Medieval Christianities c.600–c.1100* (Cambridge, 2008), 345–62.

Barrow, J., 'The Clergy in the Diocese of Hereford in the Eleventh and Twelfth Centuries', *Anglo-Norman Studies XXVI: Proceedings of the Battle Conference 2003* (Woodbridge, 2004), 37–53.

Barrow, J., 'The Ideology of the Tenth-century English Benedictine "Reform"', in P. Skinner, ed., *Challenging the Boundaries of Medieval History: The Legacy of Timothy Reuter* (Turnhout, 2009), 141–54.

Barrow, J., 'Urban Cemetery Location in the High Middle Ages', in S. Bassett, ed., *Death in Towns: Urban Responses to the Dying and the Dead, 100–1600* (Leicester, 1992), 78–100.

Barthélemy, D., 'Le Paix de Dieu dans son contexte', *Cahiers de civilisation médiévale* 40 (1997), 3–35.

Barthelémy, D., *The Serf, the Knight and the Historian*, trans. G. Robert Edwards (Ithaca, NY, 2009).

Barthélemy, D., 'Le Mutation féodale, a-t-elle eu lieu?', *Annales* 47 (1992), 767–77.

Bartlett, R., *England under the Norman and Angevin Kings 1075–1225* (Oxford, 2000).

Bartlett, R., *The Making of Europe: Conquest, Colonisation and Cultural Change 950–1350* (London, 1993).

Bautier, R-H., 'L'Hérésie d'Orléans et le muvement intellectuel au début du XIe siècle. Documents et hypothèses', *Enseignement et vie intellectuelle* (Paris, 1975), 63–88.

Becquet, J., 'Le clergé Limousin au XII siècle', in *L'Encadrement religieux*, 311–15.

Bedingfield, M. B., *The Dramatic Liturgy of Anglo-Saxon England* (Woodbridge, 2002).

Bell, D.N., 'Ailred of Rievaulx', *ODNB*.

Bergman, R., *The Salerno Ivories: Ars Sacra from Medieval Amalfi* (Cambridge, MA, 1980).

Berkhofer, R. F., 'Abbatial Authority Over Lay Agents', in idem, A. Cooper and A. J. Kosto, eds, *The Experience of Power in Medieval Europe, 950–1350* (Aldershot, 2005), 43–57.

Berlière, U., 'L'Exercice du ministère paroissial par les moines du XIIe au XVIIIe siècle', *Revue Bénédictine* 39 (1927), 340–64.

Berlière, U., 'Les pèlerinages judiciares au moyen âge', *Revue bénédictine* 7 (1890), 520–26.

Bernhardt, J. W., *Itinerant Kingship and Royal Monasteries in Early Medieval Germany c.936–1075* (Cambridge, 1993).

Bijsterveld, A.-J., 'Looking for Common Ground: From Monastic Fraternitas to Lay Confraternity in the Southern Low Countries in the Tenth to Twelfth Centuries', in E. Jamroziak and J. Burton, eds, *Religious and Laity in Western Europe 1000–1400* (Turnhout, 2006), 287–314.

Birch, D., *Pilgrimage to Rome in the Middle Ages: Continuity and Change* (Woodbridge, 1998).

Birkett, H., 'The Pastoral Application of the Lateran IV Reforms in the Northern Province, 1215–1348', *Northern History* 43 (2006), 199–219.

Bischoff, G. and B.-M. Tock, eds, *Léon IX et son temps* (Turnhout, 2006).

Blair, J., 'A Handlist of Anglo-Saxon Saints', in Thacker and Sharpe, eds, *Local Saints*, 495–565.

Blair, J., 'A Saint for Every Minster? Local Cults in Anglo-Saxon England', in Thacker and Sharpe, eds, *Local Saints*, 455–94.

Blair, J., 'Bishopstone, its Minster and its Saint: The Evidence of Drogo's *Historia translationis sanctae Lewinnae*', in G. Thomas, *The Later Anglo-Saxon Settlement at Bishopstone: A Downland Manor in the Making*, Council for British Archaeology Research Report 163 (York, 2010), 22–26.

Blair, J., 'Debate: Ecclesiastical Organization and Pastoral Care in Anglo-Saxon England', *Early Medieval Europe* 4 (1995), 193–212.

Blair, J., 'Local Churches in Domesday Book and Before', in J. C. Holt, ed., *Domesday Studies* (Woodbridge, 1987), 265–78.

Blair, J., 'Minster Churches in the Landscape', in D. Hooke, ed., *Anglo-Saxon Settlements* (Oxford, 1988), 35–58.

Blair, J., 'Secular Minster Churches in Domesday Book', in P. H. Sawyer, ed., *Domesday Book: A Reassessment* (London, 1985), 104–42.

Blair, J., *Anglo-Saxon Oxfordshire* (Oxford, 1994).

Blair, J., ed., *Minsters and Parish Churches: the Local Church in Transition, 950–1200* (Oxford, 1988).

Blair, J., *The Church in Anglo-Saxon Society* (Oxford, 2005).

Blanc, C., 'Les pratiques de piété des laïcs dans les pays du Bas-Rhône aux XIe et XIIe siècles', *Annales du Midi* 72 (1960), 137–47.

Blumenthal, U.-R., *The Investiture Controversy: Church and Monarchy from the Ninth to the Twelfth Century* (Philadelphia, 1991).

Boddington, A., *Raunds Furnells: The Anglo-Saxon Church and Churchyard* (London, 1996).

Böhringer, L., 'Der Kaiser und die Stiftsdamen. Die Gründung des Frauenstifts Vilich im Spannungsfeld von religiösem Leben und adliger Welt', *Bonner Geschichtsblätter* 53 (2004), 57–77.

Bolton, B., *The Medieval Reformation* (London, 1983).

Bolton, B. M., 'A Show with Meaning: Innocent III's Approach to the Fourth Lateran Council 1215', *Medieval History* 1 (1991), 53–67.

Bonenfant, P., 'Un clerc cathare en Lotharingie au milieu du XIIe siècle', *Le Moyen Age* 69 (1963), 271–80.

Bouchard, C. '*"Those of My Blood": Constructing Noble Families in Medieval Francia* (Philadelphia, 2001).

Bouchard, C. B., 'The Geographical, Social and Ecclesiastical Origins of the Bishops of Auxerre and Sens in the Central Middle Ages', *Church History* 46 (1977), 277–95.

Bouchard, C. B., *Sword, Miter, and Cloister: Nobility and the Church in Burgundy, 980–1198* (Ithaca, NY, 1987).

Bouchard, C. B., 'Consanguinity and Noble Marriages in the Tenth and Eleventh Centuries', *Speculum* 56 (1981), 268–87.

Boussard, J., 'Les évêques en Neustrie avant la réforme Grégorienne (950–1050 environ)', *Journal des Savants*, Juillet–Septembre 1970: 161–96.

Bowman, J. A., 'Councils, Memory and Mills: The Early Development of the Peace of God in Catalonia', *Early Medieval Europe* 8 (1999), 99–129.

Boyd, C. E., *Tithes and Parishes in Medieval Italy: The Historical Roots of a Modern Problem* (Ithaca, NY, 1952).

Boynton, S. and I. Cochelin, *From Dead of Night to End of Day: The Medieval Customs of Cluny/Du Coeur de la nuit à la fin du jour. Les coutume clunisiennes au moyen âge* (Turnhout, 2005).

Boynton, S. *Shaping a Monastic Identity: Liturgy and History at the Imperial Abbey of Farfa, 1000–1125* (Ithaca, NY, 2006).

Brett, M., *The English Church under Henry I* (Oxford, 1975).

Brink, S., 'The Formation of the Scandinavian Parish, with Some Remarks Regarding the English Impact on the Process', in J. Hill and M. Swan, eds, *The Community, the Family, and the Saint: Patterns of Power in Early Medieval Europe* (Turnhout, 1998), 19–44.

Brooke, C. N. L., 'The Missionary at Home: the Church in the Towns, 1000–1250', in G. J. Cuming, ed., *The Mission of the Church and the Propagation of the Faith*, Studies in Church History 6 (Oxford, 1970), 59–83.

Brown, P., *The Cult of Saints: Its Rise and Function in Latin Christianity* (London, 1981).

Bruce, S. G., 'An Abbot Between Two Cultures: Maiolus Of Cluny Considers the Muslims of La Garde-Freinet', *Early Medieval Europe* 15 (2007), 426–40.

Brühl, C., 'Die Sozialstruktur des deutschen episkopats im 11. und 12 Jahrhundert', *Le Istituzioni ecclesiastiche della 'Societas Christiana' dei secoli XI–XII. Diocesi, pievi e parrocchie. Atti della sesta Settimana internazionale di studio Milano*, 1–7 settembre 1974, Miscellanea del centro di studi medioevali 8 (Milan, 1978), 42–56.

Brundage, J. A., *Law, Sex and Christian Society in Medieval Europe* (Chicago, 1987).

Brunn, U., *Des Contestataires aux 'Cathares'. Discours de réforme et propagande antihérétique dans les pays du Rhin et de la Meuse avant l'Inquisition* (Paris, 2006).

Budny, M., *Insular, Anglo-Saxon and Early Anglo-Norman Manuscript Art at Corpus Christi College, Cambridge: An Illustrated Catalogue* (Kalamazoo, MI, 1997).

Bührer-Thierry, G., *Évêques et pouvoir dans le royaume de Germanie. Les Églises de Bavière et de Souabe, 876–973* (Paris, 1997).

Bull, M., 'The Confraternity of La Sauve-Majeure: A Foreshadowing of the Military Order', in M. Barber, ed., *The Military Orders: Fighting For the Faith and Caring for the Sick* (Aldershot, 1994), 313–19.

Bull, M., *Knightly Piety and the Lay Response to the First Crusade: The Limousin and Gascony c.970–c.1130* (Oxford, 1993).

Bullough, D., 'The Carolingian Liturgical Experience', in R. N. Swanson, ed., *Continuity and Change In Christian Worship*, Studies in Church History 35 (Woodbridge, 1999), 29–64.

Cambridge, E. and D. Rollason, 'Debate: The Pastoral Organization of the Anglo-Saxon Church: A Review of the 'Minster Hypothesis', *Early Medieval Europe* 4 (1995), 87–104.

Campbell, J., 'The Church in Anglo-Saxon Towns', in D. Baker, ed., *The Church in Town and Countryside*, Studies in Church History 16 (1979), 119–35.

Carozzi, C., 'La vie de Saint Bobon: un modèle clunisien de sainteté laïque', in M. Lauwers, ed., *Guerriers et moines. Conversion et sainteté aristocratiques dans l'occident médiéval (IXe–XIIe siècle)* (Antibes, 2002), 467–91.

Cattaneo, E., 'La partecipazione dei laici alla liturgia', in *I laici nella 'societas cristiana' dei secoli XI e XII: atti della terza settimana internazionale di studio Mendola, 21–27 agosto 1965*, Miscellanea del centro di studi medioevali, Milan 5 (1965), 396–427.

Chélini, J., *L'Aube du moyen âge: naissance de la chrétienté occidentale* , 2nd edn (Paris, 1997).

Cheney, M. G., *Roger, Bishop of Worcester 1164–1179* (Oxford, 1980).

Chenu, M.-D., 'The Evangelical Awakening', in his *Nature, Man and Society in the Twelfth Century: Essays on New Theological Perspectives in the Latin West*, trans. J. Taylor and L. K. Little (Chicago, 1968), 239–69.

Claussen, M., 'Review of J. Bertram, *The Chrodegang Rules*', *The Medieval Review*, 6 August 2006, https://scholarworks.iu.edu/dspace/handle/2022/6209 (accessed 13 August 2010).

Constable, G., 'Monastic Possession of Churches and "Spiritualia" in the Age of Reform', in *Il Monachesimo e la riforma ecclesiastica (1049–1112): atti della quarta settimana internazionale di studio Mendola, 23–29 agosto 1968*, Miscellanea 6 (1971), 304–31.

Constable, G., 'Introduction: Beards in History', in *Apologiae duae. Gozechini epistola ad Walcherum. Burchardi ut videtur abbatis Bellevallis, Apologia de barbis*, ed. R. B. C. Huygens, CCCM LXII (Turnhout, 1985).

Constable, G., 'Monasteries, Rural Churches and the Cura Animarum in the Early Middle Ages' in *Cristianizzazione ed organizzazione ecclesiastica delle campagne nell'alto medioevo: espansione e resistenze*, Settimane 28 (1982), 349–89.

Constable, G., 'Renewal and Reform in Religious Life: Concepts and Realities', in R. Benson and G. Constable with C. D. Lanham, eds, *Renaissance and Renewal in the Twelfth Century* (Oxford, 1982), 37–67.

Constable, G., *Monastic Tithes: From their Origins to the Twelfth Century* (Cambridge, 1964).

Constable, G., *The Reformation of the Twelfth Century* (Cambridge, 1996).

Constable, G., *Three Studies in Medieval Religious and Social Thought* (Cambridge, 1995).

Constable, G., '*Famuli* and *Conversi* at Cluny: A Note on Statute 24 of Peter the Venerable', *Revue bénédictine* 83 (1973), 326–50.

Constable, G., 'The Treatise "Hortatur Nos" and Accompanying Canonical Works on the Performance of Pastoral Work by Monks', in his *Religious Life and Thought (11th–12th Centuries)* (London, 1979), no. 9.

Contreni, J. J., 'From Polis to Parish' in T. F. X. Noble and J. J. Contreni, eds, *Religion, Culture and Society in the Middle Ages: Studies in Honour of Richard E. Sullivan* (Kalamazoo, MI, 1987), 155–64.

Cooper, T. A. 'The Homilies of a Pragmatic Archbishop's Handbook in Context: Cotton Tiberius A.iii', *Anglo-Norman Studies* 28 (2006), 47–64.

Cooper, T. A., 'Lay Piety, Confessional Directives and the Compiler's Method in Late Anglo-Saxon England', *Haskins Society Journal* 16 (2006), 46–61.

Coornaert, E., 'Les ghildes médiévales (Ve–XIVe siècles: definition et évolution', *Revue historique* 199 (1948), 22–55, 208–43.

Corbet, P., *Autour de Burchard de Worms: L'Église allemande et les interdits de parenté (IXème–XIIème siècle)* (Frankfurt am Main, 2001).

Corbet, P., *Les saints ottoniens* (Sigmaringen, 1986).

Coué, S., *Hagiographie im Kontext. Schreibanlass und Funktion von Bischofsviten aus dem 11. und vom Anfang des 12. Jahrhunderts* (Berlin, 1997).

Coulet, N., *Les Visites pastorales*, Typologie des sources du moyen âge occidental 23 (Turnhout, 1977).

Cowdrey, H. E. J., 'Pope Gregory VII and the Chastity of the Clergy', in Frassetto, ed., *Medieval Purity and Piety*, 269–302.

Cowdrey, H. E. J., 'The Papacy, the Patarenes and the Church of Milan', *TRHS* 5th ser. 18 (1968), 25–48.

Cowdrey, H. E. J., *Lanfranc: Scholar, Monk and Archbishop* (Oxford, 2003).

Cowdrey, H. E. J., *Pope Gregory VII, 1073–1085* (Oxford, 1998).

Cox, J. Charles, *Sanctuaries and Sanctuary Seekers* (London, 1911).

Cragoe, C. Davidson, 'The Custom of the English Church: Parish Church Maintenance in England before 1300', *Journal of Medieval History* 30 (2010), 20–38.

Cramer, P., *Baptism and Change in the Early Middle Ages* (Cambridge, 1993).

Crawford, S., *Childhood in Anglo-Saxon England* (Stroud, 1999).

Crick, J. C. and E. van Houts, eds, *A Social History of England, 900–1200* (Cambridge, 2011).

Crouch, D., 'The Troubled Deathbeds of Henry I's Servants: Death, Confession and Secular Conduct in the Twelfth Century', *Albion: A Quarterly Journal Concerned with British Studies* 34 (2002), 24–36.

Cubitt, C., 'Images of St Peter: The Clergy and the Religious Life in Anglo-Saxon England', in *The Christian Tradition in Anglo-Saxon England: Approaches to Current Scholarship and Teaching*, ed. P. Cavill (Cambridge, 2004), 41–54.

Cubitt, C., 'Bishops, Priests and Penance in late Saxon England', *Early Medieval Europe* 14 (2006), 41–63.

Cushing, K., *Reform and the Papacy in the Eleventh Century: Spirituality and Social Change* (Manchester, 2005).

Cushing, K., 'Events that Led to Sainthood: Sanctity and Reformers in the Eleventh Century', in R. Gameson and H. Leyser, eds, *Belief and Culture in the Middle Ages: Studies presented to Henry Mayr-Harting* (Oxford, 2001), 187–96.

D'Avray, D. L., 'Method in the Study of Medieval Sermons', in N. Bériou and D. L. D'Avray, eds, *Modern Questions about Medieval Sermons. Essays on Marriage, Death, History and Sanctity* (Spoleto, 1994), 3–29.

D'Avray, D. L., *The Preaching of the Friars: Sermons Diffused from Paris before 1300* (Oxford, 1985).

D'Avray, D. L., *Medieval Marriage: Symbolism and Society* (Oxford, 2005).

Dalarun, J., *Robert of Arbrissel: Sex, Sin and Salvation in the Middle Ages*, trans. B. L. Venarde (Washington, DC, 2006).

Daniell, C., 'Conquest, Crime and Theology in the Burial Record, 1066–1200', in Lucy and Reynolds, *Burial*, 241–54.

Davidson, C. F., 'Written in Stone: Architecture, Liturgy and the Laity in English Parish Churches, *c.*1125–*c.*1250' (University of London Ph.D. thesis, 1998).

Davies, W., 'Priests and Rural Communities in East Brittany in the Ninth Century', *Études celtiques* 20 (1983), 177–97.

Davies, W., '"Protected Space" in Britain and Ireland in the Middle Ages', in B. E. Crawford, ed., *Scotland in Dark Age Britain* (Aberdeen, 1996), 1–19.

Davies, W., *Acts of Giving: Individual, Community and Church in Tenth-Century Christian Spain* (Oxford, 2007).

de Jong, M., 'Carolingian Monasticism: The Power of Prayer', *NCMH* II, 622–53.

de Jong, M., *The Penitential State. Authority and Atonement in the Age of Louis the Pious, 814–840* (Cambridge, 2009).

de Jong, M., 'Growing Up in a Carolingian Monastery: Magister Hildemar and his Oblates', *Journal of Medieval History* 9 (1983), 99–128.

de Jong, M., 'Pollution, Penance and Sanctity: Ekkehard's *Life* of Iso of St Gall', in J. Hill and M. Swan, eds, *The Community, the Family and the Saint: Patterns of Power in Early Medieval Europe* (Turnhout, 1998), 145–58.

de Jong, M., *In Samuel's Image: Child Oblation in the Early Medieval West* (Leiden, 1996).

de Miramon, C., 'Embrasser l'état monastique à l'âge adulte (1050–1200): étude sur la conversion tardive', *Annales. Histoire, Sciences Sociales* 54 (1999), 825–49.

Defries, D. J., 'Drogo of Saint-Winnoc and the Innocent Martyrdom of Godeliph of Gistel', *Mediaeval Studies* 70 (2008), 29–65.

Defries, D., 'The Making of a Minor Saint in Drogo of Saint-Winnoc's *Historia translationis. s. Lewinnae*', *Early Medieval Europe* 16 (2008), 423–44.

Deleeuw, P. A. 'The Changing Face of the Village Parish I: The Parish in the Early Middle Ages', in J. A. Raftis, ed., *Pathways to Medieval Peasants* (Toronto, 1981), 311–322.

Desportes, P., 'Les sociétiés confraternelles de curés en France du Nord au bas Moyen Âge', in *L'Encadrement religieux*, 295–309.

Devailly, G., 'Le Clergé régulier de le ministère paroissal', *Cahiers d'histoire* 20 (1975), 259–77.

Dey, H. W., 'Diaconiae, Xenodochia, Hospitalia and Monasteries: 'Social Security' and the Meaning of Monasticism in Early Medieval Rome', *Early Medieval Europe* 16 (2008), 398–422.

Dickson, G. 'Medieval Christian Crowds and the Origins of Crowd Psychology', *Revue d'histoire ecclésiastique* 95 (2000), 54–75.

Dickson, G., 'Religious Enthusiasm in the Medieval West and the Second Conversion of Europe', in his *Religious Enthusiasm in the Medieval West: Revivals, Crusades, Saints* (Aldershot, 2000), I.

Dillard, H., *Daughters of the Reconquest: Women in Castilian Town Society 1100–1300* (Cambridge, 1984).

Drake, C. S., *The Romanesque Fonts of Northern Europe and Scandinavia* (Woodbridge, 2001).

Driscoll, M. S., 'Death, Dying, and Burial: Liturgical Considerations from the Early Middle Ages', *The Jurist* 59 (1999), 229–48.

Duby, G., 'Le budget de Cluny entre 1080 et 1155', in *Hommes et structures du Moyen Age* (Paris, 1973).

Duby, G., *Medieval Marriage: Two Models from Twelfth-century France*, trans. E. Foster (Baltimore, 1978).

Duby, G., *The Knight, The Lady and the Priest: The Making of Modern Marriage in Medieval France*, trans. B. Bray (Harmondsworth, 1985).

Duffy, E., *Marking the Hours: English People and their Prayers 1240–1570* (New Haven, CT, 2006).

Duffy, *The Stripping of the Altars: Traditional Religion in England 1400–1580* (New Haven, CT, 1992).

Eade, J., and M. J. Sallnow, eds, *Contesting the Sacred: the Anthropology of Christian Pilgrimage*, 2nd edn (Urbana and Chicago, IL, 2000).

Edgington, S., 'The First Crusade: Reviewing the Evidence', in Phillips, ed., *The First Crusade*, 57–77.

Egger, C., 'La regole seguite dai canonici regolari nei secoli XI e XII', in *La vita commune del clero nei secoli xi e xii: atti della settimana di studio, Mendola, settembre 1959*, Miscellanea del centro di studi medioevali, Milan 3 (1962), II, 9–12.

Elkins, S., *Holy Women of Twelfth-century England* (Chapel Hill, NC, 1988).

Elliott, D., 'The Priest's Wife: Female Erasure and the Gregorian Reform', in C. Hoffmann Berman, ed., *Medieval Religion: New Approaches* (London, 2004), 123–55.

Felten, F. G., *Äbte und Laienäbte im Frankenreich* (Stuttgart, 1980).

Fernie, E., *The Architecture of Norman England* (Oxford, 2000).

Fernie, E., *The Architecture of the Anglo-Saxons* (London, 1983).

Ferrari, M. C., 'From Pilgrim's Guide to Living Relic: Symeon of Trier and his Biographer Eberwin', in M. W. Herren, C. J. McDonough and R. G. Arthur, eds, *Latin Culture in the Eleventh Century: Proceedings of the Third International Conference of Medieval Latin Studies*, Cambridge, September 9–12, 1998, 2 vols, Publications of the Journal of Medieval Latin 5 (Turnhout, 2002), I, 325–43.

Fichtenau, H., *Living in the Tenth Century: Mentalities and Social Orders*, trans. P. J. Geary (Chicago, 1991).

Fichtenau, H., *Heretics and Scholars in the High Middle Ages 1000–1200*, trans. D. A. Kaiser (University Park, PA, 1998).

Fixot, M. and E. Zadora-Rio, *L'Église, le terroir* (Paris, 1989).

Fleming, R., 'The New Wealth, The New Rich and the New Political Style in Late Anglo-Saxon England', *Anglo-Norman Studies* 23 (2001), 1–22.

Fletcher, R. A., *Saint James's Catapult: The Life and Times of Diego Gelmirez of Santiago de Compostela* (Oxford, 1984).

Fliche, A., *La Réforme grégorienne et la Reconquête chrétienne (1057–1125)* (Paris, 1950).

Flint, V. I. J., *The Rise of Magic in Early Medieval Europe* (Oxford, 1993).

Foot, S., *Veiled Women II: Female Religious Communities in England, 871–1066* (Aldershot, 2000).

Foote, D., *Lordship, Reform, and the Development of Civil Society in Medieval Italy: the Bishopric of Orvieto, 1100–1250* (Notre Dame, IN, 2004).

France, J., 'Patronage and the Appeal of the First Crusade', in J. Phillips, ed., *The First Crusade: Origins and Impact* (Manchester, 1997), 5–20.

Frassetto, M., 'Reaction and Reform: Reception of Heresy in Arras and Aquitaine in the Early Eleventh Century', *Catholic Historical Review* 83 (1997), 385–400.

Frassetto, M., 'The Sermons of Adhemar and the Letter of Heribert: New Sources Concerning the Origins of Medieval Heresy', *Revue bénédictine* 109 (1999), 324–40.

Frassetto, M., ed., *Heresy and the Persecuting Society in the Middle Ages: Essays on the Work of R. I. Moore* (London, 2006).

Frassetto, M., ed., *Medieval Purity and Piety: Essays on Medieval Clerical Celibacy and Religious Reform* (New York, 1998).

Frauenknecht, E., *Die Verteidigung der Priesterehe in der Reformzeit* (Hannover, 1997).

French, K., G. G. Gibbs and B. A. Kümin, eds, *The Parish in English Life 1400–1600* (Manchester, 1997).

French, K., *The People of the Parish: Community Life in a Late Medieval Diocese* (Philadelphia, 2001).

Gaastra, A., 'Between Liturgy and Canon Law: A Study of Books of Confession and Penance in Eleventh- and Twelfth-century Italy' (unpublished Ph.D. thesis, University of Utrecht, 2007).

Gaastra, A., 'Penance and the Law: The Penitential Canons of the *Collection in Nine Books*', *Early Medieval Europe* 14 (2006), 85–102.

Gajano, S. B., 'Storia e tradizione vallombrosane', *Bullettino dell'istituto storico italiano per il medio evo e Archivio Muratoriano* 76 (1964), 99–215.

Gatch, M. McC., 'Miracles in Architectural Settings: Christ Church, Canterbury and St Clement's, Sandwich in the Old English Vision of Leofric', *Anglo-Saxon England* 22 (1993), 227–52.

Gatch, M. McC., 'Piety and Liturgy in the Old English Vision of Leofric', in M. Korhammer, ed., *Words, Texts and Manuscripts* (Cambridge, 1992), 159–79.

Gaudemet, J., 'La paroisse au moyen âge: état des questions', *Revue d'histoire de l'église de France* 59 (1973), 5–21.

Geary, P., *Phantoms of Remembrance: Memory and Oblivion at the End of the First Millennium* (Princeton, NJ, 1994).

Gem, R., 'The English Parish Church in the Eleventh and Early Twelfth Centuries: A Great Rebuilding?', in J. Blair, ed., *Minsters and Parish Churches: The Local Church in Transition, 950–1200* (Oxford, 1988), 21–30.

Giandrea, M. F., *Episcopal Culture in Late Anglo-Saxon England* (Woodbridge, 2007).

Gilsdorf, S., ed., *The Bishop: Power and Piety at the First Millennium* (Münster, 2004).

Gittos, H., 'Is there any Evidence for the Liturgy of Parish Churches in Late Anglo-Saxon England? The Red Book of Darley and the Status of Old English', in F. Tinti, ed., *Pastoral Care in Late Anglo-Saxon England* (Woodbridge, 2005), 63–82.

Gittos, H., 'Creating the Sacred: Anglo-Saxon Rites for Consecrating Cemeteries', in S. Lucy and A. Reynolds, eds, *Burial in Early Medieval England and Wales*, Society for Medieval Archaeology Monograph Series 17 (London, 2002), 195–208.

Godden, M., *Ælfric's Catholic Homilies: Introduction, Commentary and Glossary*, EETS SS 18 (Oxford, 2000).

Goldberg, E. J., 'Regina nitens sanctissimae Hemma: Queen Emma (872–76), Bishop Witgar of Augsburg and the Witgar-Belt', in B. Weiler and S. MacLean, eds, *Representations of Power in Medieval Germany 800–1500* (Turnhout, 2006), 57–95.

Goodich, M., *Miracles and Wonders: The Development of the Concept of Miracle 1150–1350* (Aldershot, 2007).

Gorecki, P., *Parishes, Tithes and Society in Earlier Medieval Poland c.1100–1250*, Transactions for the American Philosophical Society 83.2 (Philadelphia, 1993).

Graham, T., 'The Old English Liturgical Directions in Corpus Christi College, Cambridge MS 422', *Anglia* 111 (1993), 439–46.

Guillotel, H., 'Du role des cimètieres en Bretagne dans le renouveau du XIe et de la première moitié du xiie siècle', *Memoires de la sociétè d'histoire et d'archéologie de Bretagne* 52 (1972–74), 5–26.

Haggenmüller, R., 'Zur Rezeption der Beda und Egbert zugeschriebenen Bussbücher', in H. Mordek, ed., *Aus Archiven und Bibliotheken. Festschrift für Raymund Kottje zum 65. Geburtstag* (Frankfurt a. M., 1992), 149–69.

Hall, D., 'The Sanctuary of St Cuthbert', in G. Bonner, D. Rollason and C. Stancliffe, eds, *St Cuthbert, His Cult and His Community to AD1200* (Woodbridge, 1989), 425–36.

Hall, T. N., 'Wulfstan's Latin Sermons', in M. Townend, ed., *Wulfstan, Archbishop of York: The Proceedings of the Second Alcuin Conference* (Turnhout, 2004), 94–139.

Hamilton, B., *Religion in the Medieval West* (London, 1986).

Hamilton, B., 'Wisdom from the East: The Reception by the Cathars of Eastern Dualist Texts', in P. Biller and A. Hudson, eds, *Heresy and Literacy, 1000–1530* (Cambridge, 1994), 38–60.

Hamilton, B., 'Bogomil Influences on Western Heresy', in M. Frassetto, ed., *Heresy and the Persecuting Society in the Middle Ages: Essays on the Work of R. I. Moore* (Leiden, 2006), 93–114.

Hamilton, B., 'The Impact of Crusader Jerusalem on Western Christendom', *Catholic Historical Review* 80 (1994), 695–713.

Hamilton, B., 'The Monastic Revival in Tenth-Century Rome', *Studia Monastica* 4 (1962), 35–68.

Hamilton, S., 'Absoluimus uos uice beati petri apostolorum principis: Episcopal Authority and the Reconciliation of Excommunicants in England and Francia c.900–c.1150', in P. Fouracre and D. Ganz, eds, *Frankland: The Franks and the World of the Early Middle Ages* (Manchester, 2008), 209–41.

Hamilton, S., 'Doing Penance', in M. Rubin, ed., *Medieval Christianity in Practice* (Princeton, NJ, 2009), 135–43.

Hamilton, S., 'Inquiring into Adultery and Other Wicked Deeds: Episcopal Justice in Tenth- and Early Eleventh-Century Italy', *Viator* 41 (2010), 21–43.

Hamilton, S., '"Most Illustrious King of Kings": Evidence for Ottonian Kingship in the Otto III Prayerbook (Munich, Bayerische Staatsbibliothek, Clm 30111', *Journal of Medieval History* 27 (2001), 257–88.

Hamilton, S., 'Otto III's Penance: A Case Study of Unity and Diversity in the Eleventh-Century Church', in R. N. Swanson, ed., *Unity and Diversity in the Church*, Studies in Church History 32 (Oxford, 1996), 83–94.

Hamilton, S., 'Pastoral Care in Early Eleventh-century Rome', *Dutch Review of Church History* 84 (2004), 37–56.

Hamilton, S., 'Rites of Passage and Pastoral Care', in J. Crick and E. van Houts, eds, *A Social History of Britain 900–1200* (Cambridge, 2011), 290–308.

Hamilton, S., 'The Rituale: The Evolution of a New Liturgical Book', in R. N. Swanson, ed., *The Church and the Book*, Studies in Church History 38 (Woodbridge, 2004), 74–86.

Hamilton, S., *The Practice of Penance, 900–1050* (Woodbridge, 2001).

Hammer, C. I., *A Large-scale Slave Society of the Early Middle Ages: Slaves and their Families in Early Medieval Bavaria* (Aldershot, 2002).

Hammer, C. I., 'Country Churches, Clerical Inventories and the Carolingian Renaissance in Bavaria', *Church History* 49 (1980), 5–17.

Harmening, D., *Superstitio. Überlieferungs-und theoriegeschichtliche Untersuchungen zur kirchlich-theologischen Aberglaubensliteratur des Mittelalters* (Berlin, 1979).

Harmening, D., *Superstitio. Überlieferungs-und theoriegeschichtliche Untersuchungen zur kirchlich-theologischen Aberglaubensliteratur des Mittelalters* (Berlin, 1979).

Harper-Bill, C., 'The Struggle for Benefices in Twelfth-century East Anglia', in R. Allen Brown, ed., *Anglo-Norman Studies XI; Proceedings of the Battle Conference 1988* (Woodbridge, 1989), 113–32.

Hartmann, W., 'I vescovo com giudice', *Rivista di storia della chiesa in Italia* 40 (1986), 320–41.

Hartmann, W., *Die Synoden der karolingerzeit im Frankenreich und in Italien* (Paderborn, 1989).

Hartmann, W., ed., *Bischof Burchard von Worms 1000–1025* (Mainz, 2000).

Hartmann, W., ed., *Recht und Gericht in Kirche und Welt um 900*, Schriften des Historischen Kollegs Kolloquien 69 (Munich, 2007).

Hartmann, W., *Kirche und Kirchenrecht um 900. Die Bedeutung der spätkarolingischen Zeit für Tradition und Innovation im kirchlichen Recht*, MGH Schriften 58 (Hannover, 2008).

Head, T. and R. Landes, ed., *The Peace of God: Social Violence and Religious Response in France around the Year 1000*, (Ithaca, NY, 1992).

Head, T., '"Naming Names": The Nomenclature of Heresy in the Early Eleventh Century', in R. Fulton and B. W. Holsinger, eds, *History in the Comic Mode: Medieval Communities and the Matter of Person* (New York, 2007), 91–100.

Head, T., 'Peace and Power in France around the Year 1000', *Essays in Medieval Studies* 23 (2006), 1–17.

Head, T., 'The Judgement of God: Andrew of Fleury's Account of the Peace League of Bourges', in Head and Landes, *The Peace of God*, 219–38.

Head, T., 'The Development of the Peace of God in Aquitaine (970–1005)', *Speculum* 74 (1999), 656–86.

Head, T., *Hagiography and the Cult of the Saints: the Diocese of Orlèans 800–1200* (Cambridge, 1990).

Healy, P., *The Chronicle of Hugh of Flavigny* (Aldershot, 2006).

Héfèle, C. J., *Histoire des conciles d'après les documents originaux* (Paris, 1911).

Helmholz, R., 'Excommunication and the Angevin Leap Forward', *Haskins Society Journal* 7 for 1995 (1997), 133–49.

Helmholz, R. H., 'Marriage Contracts in Medieval England' in Reynolds and Witte, *To Have and to Hold*, 260–86.

Hen, Y., 'Review Article: Liturgy and Religious Culture in Late Anglo-Saxon England', *Early Medieval Europe* 17 (2009), 329–42.

Hiley, D., *Gregorian Chant* (Cambridge, 2009).

Hoffmann, H., and R. Pokorny, *Das Dekret des Bischofs Burchard von Worms: Textstufen frühe Verbreitung Vorlagen*, MGH Hilfsmittel 12 (Hannover, 1991).

Hohler, C., 'A Note on the Jacobus', *Journal of Warburg and Courtauld Institutes* 35 (1972), 31–80.

Horden, P., 'The Confraternities of Byzantium', in W. J. Sheils and D. Wood, eds, *Voluntary Religion*, Studies in Church History 23 (Oxford, 1986), 25–45.

Howard-Johnston, J., and P. A. Hayward, eds, *The Cult of Saints in Late Antiquity and the Early Middle Ages* (Oxford, 1999).

Hubert, J., 'La place faite aux laïcs dans les églises monastiques et dans les cathedrales aux XIe et XIIe siècles', *I laici nella 'Societas Christiana' dei secoli XI e XII*, Settimana Mendola 3 (Milan, 1968).

Huyghebaert, N., *Les documents necrologiques*, Typologie des sources du Moyen Âge 4 (Turnhout, 1972).

Hull, P. and R. Sharpe, 'Peter of Cornwall and Launceston', *Cornish Studies* 13 (1986), 5–53.

Imbart de la Tour, P., *Les origines religieuses de la France: les paroisses rurales du 4e au 11e siècle* (Paris, 1900).

Iogan-Prat, D. 'Churches in the Landscape', in T. F. X. Noble and J. M. H. Smith, eds, *The Cambridge History of Christianity: Early Medieval Christianities c.600–c.1100* (Cambridge, 2008), 363–79.

Iogna-Prat, D. *La Maison Dieu. Une histoire monumentale de l'Église au Moyen Age* (Paris, 2006).

Iogna-Prat, D., *Order and Exclusion: Cluny and Christendom Face Heresy, Judaism and Islam (1000–1150)*, trans. G. Robert Edwards (Ithaca, NY, 2002); trans. of *Ordonner et exclure* (Paris, 1998).

Istituzioni ecclesiastiche della 'Societas christiana' dei secoli 11–12: diocesi, pievi et parrocchie: atti della 6a Settimana internazionale di studio, Milano, 1–7 settembre 1974, Miscellanea del centro di studi medioevali 8, (Milan, 1977).

Istituzioni monastiche e istituzioni canonicali in Occidente (1123–1215): atti della settima Settimana internazionale di studio Mendola, 28 agosto–3 settembre 1977, Miscellanea del centro di studi medioevali, 9 (Milan, 1980).

Jamroziak, E. and J. Burton, eds, *Religious and Laity in Western Europe 1000–1400: Interaction, Negotiation and Power* (Turnhout, 2006).

Jamroziak, E., *Rievaulx Abbey and its Social Context, 1132–1300: Memory, Locality and Networks* (Turnhout, 2005).

Jestice, P. G., 'The Gorzian Reform and the Light under the Bushel', *Viator* 24 (1993), 51–78.

Jestice, P. G., *Wayward Monks and the Religious Revolution of the Eleventh Century* (Leiden, 1997).

Johnson, C., 'Marriage Agreements from Twelfth-century Southern France', in Reynolds and Witte, *To Have and to Hold*, 260–86.

Jolly, K., *Popular Religion in Late Anglo-Saxon England: Elf Charms in Context* (Chapel Hill, NC, 1996).

Kaiser, R., 'Quêtes itinerantes avec des reliques pour financer la construction des églises (XIe–XIIe siècles)', *Le moyen âge* 101 (1995), 205–25.

Kamen, H., *The Phoenix and the Flame: Catalonia and the Counter Reformation* (New Haven, CT, 1993).

Kemp, B. 'Some Aspects of the *Parochia* of Leominster in the Twelfth Century', in Blair, ed., *Minsters and Parish Churches*, 83–95.

Kemp, B., 'Archdeacons and Parish Churches in England in the Twelfth Century', in G. Garnett and J. Hudson, eds, *Law and Government in Medieval England and Normandy: Essays in Honour of Sir James Holt* (Cambridge, 1994), 341–64.

Kerff, F., 'Libri paenitentiales und kirchliche Strafgerichtsbarkeit bis zum Decretum Gratiani. Ein Diskussionsvorschlag', *Zeitschrift der Savigny-Stiftung für Rechtsgeschichte. Kanonistische Abteilung* 75 (1989), 23–57.

Kershaw, P. J. E., 'Eberhard of Friuli, a Carolingian Lay Intellectual', in P. Wormald and J. L. Nelson, eds, *Lay Intellectuals in the Carolingian World* (Cambridge, 2007), 77–105.

Kéry, L., *Canonical Collections of the Early Middle Ages (c.400–1140). A Bibliographical Guide to the Manuscripts and Literature* (Washington, DC, 1999).

King, V., 'St Oswald's Tenants', in N. Brooks and C. Cubitt, ed., *St Oswald of Worcester: Life and Influence* (London, 1996), 100–16.

Kingsley Porter, A., *Medieval Architecture: Its Origins and Development with Lists of Monuments and Bibliographies*, 2 vols (1909; repr. New York, 1969).

Körntgen, L. 'Canon Law and the Practice of Penance: Burchard of Worms's Penitential', *Early Medieval Europe* 14 (2006), 103–17.

Körntgen, L., 'Fortschreibung frühmittelalterlicher Busspraxis. Burchards "Liber Corrector" und seine Quellen', in W. Hartmann, ed., *Bischof Burchard von Worms, 1000–1025* (2000), 199–226.

Körntgen, L., *Studien zu den Quellen der frühmittelalterlichen Bussbücher* (Sigmaringen, 1993).

Kottje, R., 'Busse oder Strafe? Zur "Iustitia" in den "Libri Paenitentiales"', in *La Giustizia nell'alto medioevo (secoli V–VIII)*, Settimane 42 (Spoleto, 1995), 443–474.

Koziol, G., 'Monks, Feuds and the Making of Peace in Eleventh-century Flanders', in Head and Landes, eds, *The Peace of God*, 239–58.

Krautheimer, R., *Rome: Profile of a City, 312–1308* (Princeton, NJ, 2000).

Kümin, B., *The Shaping of a Community: The Rise and Reformation of the English Parish c. 1400–1560* (Aldershot, 1995).

Kupper, J.-L., *Liège et l'Église imperiale XIe–XIIe siècles* (Paris, 1981).

La vita commune del clero nei secoli xi e xii: atti della Settimana di studio, Mendola, settembre 1959, Miscellanea del centro di studi medioevali, Milan 3 (1962).

Ladner, G. B., 'Gregory the Great and Gregory VII: A Comparison of their Concepts of Renewal', *Viator* 4 (1973), 1–31.

Ladner, G. B., *The Idea of Reform: Its Impact on Christian Thought and Action in the Age of the Fathers* (Cambridge, MA, 1959).

Lambert, M., *Medieval Heresy: Popular Movements from the Gregorian Reform to the Reformation*, 3rd edn (Oxford, 2002).

Lapidge, M., 'Dunstan [St Dunstan], d. 988, archbishop of Canterbury', *ODNB*.

Lapidge, M., 'Surviving Booklists from Anglo-Saxon England', in M. Lapidge, and H. Gneuss, eds, *Learning and Literature in Anglo-Saxon England: Studies Presented to Peter Clemoes on the Occasion of his Sixty-Fifth Birthday* (Cambridge, 1985), 33–89, no. VI.

Laudage, J., *Priesterbild und Reformpapsttum im 11. Jahrhundert* (Cologne, 1984).

Lauwers, M., 'Dicunt vivorum beneficia nichil prodesse defunctis. Histoire d'une thème polémique (XIe–XIIe siècles)', in Zerner, ed. *Inventer l'hérésie?*, 157–92.

Lauwers, M., *La mémoire des ancêtres, le souci des morts: Morts, rites et société au moyen âge (diocèse de Liège, Xe–XIIIe siècles)* (Paris, 1997).

Lauwers, M., *Naissance du cimitière. Lieux sacrés et terre des morts dans l'Occident médiéval* (Paris, 2005).

Lawrence, C. H., *Medieval Monasticism: Forms of Religious Life in Western Europe in the Middle Ages*, 2nd edn (London, 1989).

le Blévec, D., 'Fondations et oeuvres charitables au Moyen Âge', in J. Dufour and H. Platelle, eds, *Fondations et oeuvres charitables au moyen âge* (Paris, 1999), 7–21.

Lea, H. C., *History of Sacerdotal Celibacy in the Christian Church*, 4th edn (London, 1932).

Lennard, R., *Rural England 1086–1135: A Study of Social and Agrarian Conditions* (Oxford 1959).

Leyser, K. J., *Rule and Conflict in an Early Medieval Society* (Bloomington, IN, 1979).

Leyser, C., 'Episcopal Office in the Italy of Liudprand of Cremona c.890–c.970', *English Historical Review* 125 (2010), 795–817.

Licence, T., *The Rise of Hermits and Recluses: England and Western Europe 970–1220* (Oxford, 2011).

Lipton, S., 'Images in the World: Reading the Crucifixion', in M. Rubin, ed., *Medieval Christianity in Practice* (Princeton, NJ, 2009), 173–85.

Lipton, S., 'The Sweet Lean of His Head: Writing about Looking at the Crucifix in the High Middle Ages', *Speculum* 80 (2005), 1172–208.

Little, L. K., *Religious Poverty and the Profit Economy in Medieval Europe* (London, 1978).

Lobrichon, G., 'Arras, 1025, ou le vrai procès d'une fausse accusation', in M. Zerner, ed., *Inventer l'hérésie? Discours polémiques et pouvoirs avant l'inquisition* (Nice, 1998), 67–85.

Lobrichon, G., 'The Chiaroscuro of Heresy: Early Eleventh-century Aquitaine as Seen from Auxerre', in T. Head and R. Landes, *The Peace of God: Social Violence and Religious Response in France around 1000* (Ithaca, NY, 1992), 80–103.

Lötter, F., 'Ein kanonistisches Handbuch über die Amtspflichten des Pfarrklerus als gemeinsame Vorlage für den Sermo synodalis "Fratres presbyteri" und Reginos Werk "De Synodalibus Causis"', *Zeitschrift der Savigny-Stiftung für Rechtsgeschichte: Kanonistische Abteilung* 62 (1976), 1–57.

Loud, G. A., *Church and Society in the Norman Principality of Capua, 1058–1197* (Oxford, 1985).

Luchaire, A., 'Un document retrouvé', *Journal des savants* n.s. 3 (1905), 557–68.

Lucy, S. and A. Reynolds, eds, *Burial in Early Medieval England and Wales* (London, 2002).

Lynch, J. H., *Godparents and Kinship in Early Medieval Europe* (Princeton, NJ, 1986).

Lynch, J. H., 'Baptismal Sponsorship and Monks and Nuns, 500–1000', *American Benedictine Review* 31 (1980), 108–29.

Lynch, J. H., *Simoniacal Entry into Religious Life from 1000 to 1260* (Columbus, OH, 1976).

MacLean, S., *Kingship and Politics in the Later Ninth Century: Charles the Fat and the End of the Carolingian Empire* (Cambridge, 2003).

Macy, G., *The Hidden History of Women's Ordination: Female Clergy in the Medieval West* (Oxford, 2008).

Magnou-Nortier, E., *La société laïque et l'église dans la province ecclésiastique de Narbonne (zone cispyrénéenne) de la fin du VIIIe à la fin du XIe siècle* (Toulouse, 1974).

Martindale, J., 'Peace and War in the Early Eleventh-century Aquitaine', in C. Harper-Bill and R. Harvey, eds, *Medieval Knighthood IV: Papers from the Fifth Strawberry Hill Conference* (Woodbridge, 1992), 147–176.

Mason, E., *St Wulfstan of Worcester, c.1008–1095* (Oxford, 1990).

Mason, E., 'The Role of the English Parishioner 1100–1500', *Journal of Ecclesiastical History* 27 (1976), 17–29.

Matter, E. A., 'Orthodoxy and Deviance', in Noble and Smith, eds, *Early Medieval Christianities c.600–c.1100*, 510–30.

Matthew, H. C. G. and B. Harrison, eds, *Oxford Dictionary of National Biography: From the Earliest Times to the Year 2000* (Oxford, 2004).

Mayr-Harting, H., 'Functions of a Twelfth-century Shrine', in Mayr-Harting, H. and R. I. Moore, eds, *Studies in Medieval History Presented to R. H. C. Davis* (London, 1985).

McCune, J., 'Rethinking the Pseudo–Eligius Sermon Collection', *Early Medieval Europe* 16.4 (2008), 445–76.

McKitterick, R., *The Frankish Church and the Carolingian Reforms, 789–895* (London, 1977).

McKitterick. R., ed., *New Cambridge Medieval History II c.700–900* (Cambridge, 1995).

McLaughlin, M., *Consorting with Saints. Prayer for the Dead in Early Medieval France* (Ithaca, 1994).

McLaughlin, M., *Sex, Gender, and Episcopal Authority in an Age of Reform, 1000–1122* (Oxford, 2010).

Meens, R., 'Penitentials and the Practice of Penance in the Tenth and Eleventh Centuries', *Early Medieval Europe* 14 (2006), 7–21.

Meens, R., 'Sanctuary, Penance and Dispute Settlement under Charlemagne: The Conflict between Alcuin and Theodulf of Orléans over a Sinful Cleric', *Speculum* 82 (2007), 277–300.

Meens, Rob, 'The Frequency and Nature of Early Medieval Penance', in P. Biller and A. J. Minnis, eds, *Handling Sin: Confession in the Middle Ages* (Woodbridge, 1998), 35–61.

Méhu, D., *Paix et communautés autour de l'abbaye de Cluny Xe–XVe siècle* (Lyons, 2001).

Mews, C., 'Guibert of Nogent's *Monodiae*, III, 17', *Revue des études Augustiniennes* 33 (1987), 113–27.

Michaud-Quantin, P., 'Les methodes de la pastorale du XIIIe au XVe siècle', *Miscellanea Medievalia* 7 (1970), 76–91.

Michaud-Quantin, P., *Universitas. Expressions du mouvement communautaire dans le moyen-age latin* (Paris, 1970).

Mierau, H. J., *Vita communis und Pfarrseelsorge. Studien zu den Diözesen Salzburg und Passau im Hoch-und Spätmittelalter* (Köln, 1997).

Miller, E. and J. Hatcher, *Medieval England: Rural Society and Economic Change 1086–1384* (London, 1978).

Miller, M. C., *The Formation of a Medieval Church. Ecclesiastical Change in Verona, 950–1150* (Ithaca, NY, 1993).

Miller, M., 'Religion Makes a Difference: Clerical and Lay Cultures in the Courts of Northern Italy, 1000–1130', *American Historical Review* 105 (2000), 1095–1300.

Miller, M., 'Clerical Identity and Reform: Notarial Descriptions of the Secular Clergy in the Po Valley, 750–1200', in M. Frassetto, ed., *Medieval Purity and Piety: Essays on Medieval Clerical Celibacy and Religious Reform* (New York, 1998), 305–35.

Miller, M., 'Toward a New Periodization of Ecclesiastical History', in S. K. Cohn and S. A. Epstein, eds, *Portraits of Medieval and Renaissance Living: Essays in Memory of David Herlihy* (Ann Arbor, MI, 1996), 233–44.

Miller, M. C., *Power and the Holy in the Age of the Investiture Conflict: A Brief History with Documents* (Boston, 2005).

Miller, M. C., *The Bishop's Palace: Architecture and Authority in Medieval Italy* (Ithaca, NY, 2000).

Mills, R., 'The Signification of the Tonsure', in P. H. Cullum and K. J. Lewis, eds, *Holiness and Masculinity in the Middle Ages* (Cardiff, 2004), 109–26.

Misonne, D., 'Gérard de Brogne: moine et réformateur (d. 959)', *Revue bénédictine* 111 (2001), 25–49.

Moore, R. I., 'Between Sanctity And Superstition: Saints and Their Miracles in the Age of Revolution' in M. Rubin, ed., *The Work of Jacques Le Goff and the Challenges of Medieval History* (Woodbridge, 1997), 55–67.

Moore, R. I., 'Family, Community and Cult on the Eve of the Gregorian Reform', *TRHS* 5th ser. 30 (1980), 49–69.

Moore, R. I., *The First European Revolution c.970–1215* (Oxford, 2000).

Moore, R. I., *The Origins of European Dissent* (London, 1977).

Morison, P. R., 'The Miraculous and French Society c.950–1100' (unpublished D.Phil. thesis, University of Oxford, 1983).

Morris, C., *The Papal Monarchy: The Western Church from 1050 to 1250* (Oxford, 1989).

Morris, C. and P. Roberts, eds, *Pilgrimage: The English Experience from Becket to Bunyan* (Cambridge, 2002).

Morris, R., 'Baptismal Places 600–800', in I. Wood and N. Lund, eds, *People and Places in Northern Europe 500–1600: Essays in Honour of Peter Hayes Sawyer* (Woodbridge, 1991), 15–24.

Morris, R., *Churches in the Landscape* (London, 1989).

Morris, R., *The Church in British Archaeology*, Council for British Archaeology Research Report 47 (London, 1983).

Muir, B. J., 'The Early Insular Prayer Book Tradition and the Development of the Book of Hours', in M. M. Manion and B. J. Muir, eds, *The Art of the Book: Its Place in Medieval Worship* (Exeter, 1998), 9–19.

Murray, A., *Reason and Society in the Middle Ages* (Oxford, 1978).

Nanni, L., *La Parrocchia studiata nei documenti lucchesi dei secoli viii–xiii* (Rome, 1948).

Nelson, Janet L., 'Church Properties and the Propertied Church: Donors, the Clergy and the Church in Medieval Western Europe from the Fourth Century to the Twelfth: The *Proprietary Church in the Medieval West.* By Susan Wood', *English Historical Review* 124 (2009), 355–74.

Nelson, Janet L., 'Making Ends Meet: Wealth and Poverty in the Carolingian Church', in W. Sheils and D. Wood, *The Church and Wealth*, Studies in Church History 24 (Oxford, 1987), 25–36; repr. in eadem, *The Frankish World, c.750–c.900* (London, 1996), 145–53.

Nelson, Janet L., review of T. Head and R. Landes, ed., *The Peace of God* in *Speculum* 69 (1994), 163–69.

Nelson, Janet L., 'Society, Theodicy and the Origins of Heresy: Towards a Reassessment of the Medieval Evidence', in D. Baker, ed., *Schism, Heresy and Religious Protest*, Studies in Church History 9 (Cambridge, 1972), 65–77.

Nightingale, J., *Monasteries and their Patrons in the Gorze Reform: Lotharingia c.850–1000* (Oxford, 2001).

Niles, J. D., 'The Æcerbot Ritual in Context', in J. D. Niles, ed., *Old English Literature in Context* (Cambridge, 1980), 44–56.

Nip, R., 'Godelieve of Gistel and Ida of Boulogne', in A. Mulder-Bakker, ed., *Sanctity and Motherhood: Essays on Holy Mothers in the Middle Ages* (New York, 1995), 191–223.

Noble, T. F. X. and J. M. H. Smith, eds, *The Cambridge History of Christianity III: Early Medieval Christianities c.600–c.1100* (Cambridge, 2008).

Noble, T. F. X., 'Secular Sanctity: Forging an Ethos for the Carolingian Nobility', in P. Wormald and J. L. Nelson, eds, *Lay Intellectuals in the Carolingian World* (Cambridge, 2007), 8–36.

Ortenberg, V., 'Archbishop Sigeric's Journey to Rome in 990', *Anglo-Saxon England*, 19 (1990), 197–246.

Oswald, F., L. Schaefer, H. R. Sennhauser, *Vorromanische Kirchenbauten. Katalog der Denkmäler bis zum Ausgang der Ottonen*, 2nd edn (Munich, 1991).

Ott, J. S. and A. Trumbore Jones, eds, *The Bishop Reformed: Studies of Episcopal Power and Culture in the Central Middle Ages* (Aldershot, 2007).

Ott, J. S., '"Both Mary and Martha": Bishop Lietbert of Cambrai and the Construction of Episcopal Sanctity in a Border Diocese around 1100', in Ott and Trumbore Jones, *The Bishop Reformed*, 137–60.

Padel, O. J., 'Local Saints and Place-names in Cornwall', in Thacker and Sharpe, eds, *Local Saints*, 303–60.

Page, R. I., 'Old English Liturgical Rubrics in Corpus Christi College, Cambridge MS 422', *Anglia* 96 (1978), 149–58.

Palliser, D. M., 'Review Article: The "Minster Hypothesis": A Case Study', *Early Medieval Europe* 5 (1996), 207–14.

Parisse, M., 'Princes laïques et/ou moines, les évêques du Xe siècle', *Il Secolo di ferro: mito e realtà del secolo X*, Settimane di studio del centro italiano di studi sull'alto medioevo, Spoleto 38, 2 vols (Spoleto, 1991) I. 449–513.

Partner, N., 'Henry of Huntingdon: Clerical Celibacy and the Writing of History', *Church History* 42 (1973), 462–75.

Patzold, S., 'L'épiscopat du haut Moyen Âge du point de vue de la médiévistique allemande', *Cahiers de civilisation médiévale Xe–XIIe siècles* 48 (2005), 341–58.

Paxton, F. S., *Christianizing Death: The Creation of a Ritual Process in Early Medieval Europe* (Ithaca, NY, 1990).

Perrel, J., 'Une révolution populaire au moyen âge: le mouvement des Capuchonnés du Puy, 1182–84', *Cahiers de la Haute-Loire* (1977), 61–79.

Pestell, T., 'Using Material Culture to Define Holy Space: The Bromholm Project', in A. Spicer and S. Hamilton, eds, *Defining the Holy: Sacred Space in Medieval and Early Modern Europe* (Aldershot, 2005), 161–86.

Peters, E., 'The Death of the Subdean: Ecclesiastical Order and Disorder in Eleventh-century Francia', in B. S. Bachrach and D. Nicholas, eds, *Law, Custom and the Social Fabric in Medieval Europe: Essays in Honour of Bryce Lyon* (Kalamazoo, MI, 1990), 51–71.

Phillips, J., ed., *The First Crusade: Origins and Impact* (Manchester, 1997).

Platelle, H., 'La violence et ses remèdes en Flandre au XIe siècle', *Sacris Erudiri: Jaarboek voor Godsdienstwetenschappen* 20 (1971), 101–73.

Platelle, H., *La justice seigneuriale de l'Abbaye de Saint Amand: son organisation judiciare, sa procédure et sa compétence du XIe au XVIe siècle* (Louvain, 1965).

Poly, J.-P. and E. Bournazel, *La mutation féodale, Xe–XIIe siècles* (Paris 1980), trans. Caroline Higgitt as *The Feudal Transformation, 900–1200* (New York, 1991).

Pontal, O., *Les statuts synodaux*, Typologie des sources du Moyen Âge occidental 11 (Turnhout, 1975).

Postles, D., 'Lamps, Lights and Layfolk', *Journal of Medieval History* 25 (1999), 97–114.

Pringle, D., *The Churches of the Crusader Kingdom of Jerusalem: A Corpus*, 4 vols (Cambridge, 1993–2009).

Prinz, F., *Klerus und Krieg im früheren Mittelalter* (Stuttgart, 1971).

Ramseyer, V., *The Transformation of a Religious Landscape: Medieval Southern Italy, 850–1150* (Ithaca, NY, 2006).

Rasche, U., 'The Early Phase of Appropriation of Parish Churches in Medieval England', *Journal of Medieval History* 26 (2000), 213–27.

Reilly, D. J., *The Art of Reform in Eleventh-century Flanders: Gerard of Cambrai, Richard of Saint-Vanne and the Saint-Vaast Bible* (Leiden, 2006).

Resnick, I. M., 'Litterati, Spirituales, and Lay Christians according to Otloh of Saint Emmeram', *Church History* 55 (1986), 165–78.

Reuter, T., 'The "Imperial Church System" of the Ottonian and Salian Rulers: A Reconsideration', *Journal of Ecclesiastical History* 33 (1982), 347–74.

Reuter, T., 'Ein Europa der Bischöfe. Das Zeitalter Burchards von Worms', in W. Hartmann, ed., *Bischof Burchard von Worms 1000–1025* (Mainz, 2000), 1–28.

Reuter, T., 'Pastorale pedum ante pedes apostolici posuit: Dis- and Reinvestiture in the Era of the Investiture Contest', in R. Gameson and H. Leyser, eds, *Belief and Culture in the Middle Ages* (Oxford, 2001), 197–210.

Reuter, T., *Medieval Polities and Modern Mentalities*, ed. J. L. Nelson (Cambridge, 2006).

Reynolds, P. L. and J. Witte, eds, *To Have and To Hold: Marrying and its Documentation in Western Christendom, 400–1600* (Cambridge, 2007).

Reynolds, P. L., 'Dotal Charters in the Frankish Tradition', in P. L. Reynolds and J. Witte, eds, *To Have and To Hold: Marrying and its Documentation in Western Christendom, 400–1600* (Cambridge, 2007), 114–64.

Reynolds, P. L., *Marriage in the Western Church: The Christianization of Marriage during the Patristic and Early Medieval Periods* (Leiden, 1994; repr. 2001).

Reynolds, R. E., 'Rites of Separation and Reconciliation in the Early Middle Ages', *Segni e Riti nella Chiesa Altomedievale Occidentale, Spoleto 11–17 aprile 1985*, Settimane di studio del Centro italiano di studi sull'alto medioevo 33 (Spoleto, 1987), 405–33; repr. in R. E. Reynolds, *Law and Liturgy in the Latin Church, 5th–12th Centuries* (Ashgate, 1994), no. X.

Reynolds, S., 'Social Mentalities and the Case of Medieval Scepticism', *TRHS*, 6th series 1 (1991), 21–41.

Reynolds, S., *Kingdoms and Communities in Western Europe 900–1300* (Oxford, 1984).

Riches, T., 'Bishop Gerard I of Cambrai (1012–51) and the Representation of Authority in the *Gesta episcoporum cameracensium*' (Ph.D. thesis, King's College, London, University of London, 2006).

Riches, T. M., 'Bishop Gerard I of Cambrai-Arras, the Three Orders, and the Problem of Human Weakness', in J. S. Ott and A. Trumbore Jones, eds,

The Bishop Reformed: Studies of Episcopal Power and Culture in the Central Middle Ages (Aldershot, 2007), 122–36.

Richter, M., *Giraldus Cambrensis: The Growth of a Welsh Nation*, 2nd edn (Aberystwyth, 1976).

Riley–Smith, J., *The First Crusaders, 1095–1131* (Cambridge, 1997).

Ritzer, K., *Le Mariage dans les Églises chrétiennes du Ier au XIe* siècle (Paris, 1970) (French translation of 1962 German original).

Roach, A., *The Devil's World: Heresy and Society 1100–1300* (Harlow, 2003).

Robinson, I. S., *Henry IV of Germany 1056–1106* (Cambridge, 1999).

Rodwell, W. and K. Rodwell, *Rivenhall: Investigations of a Villa, Church and Village*, 2 vols, Council for British Archaeology Research Reports 55, 80 (London, 1985–93).

Rodwell, W. and K. Rodwell, 'St Peter's Church, Barton-upon-Humber', *Antiquaries Journal* 62 (1982), 283–315.

Roest, B., 'Church and Laity in the Later Middle Ages: A Short Essay on Models and Perspectives in Medieval Religious History', *Theoretische Geschiedenis* 25 (1998), 78–87.

Rollason, D., A. J. Piper, M. Harvey, L. Rollason, eds, *The Durham Liber Vitae and its Context* (Woodbridge, 2004).

Rosenwein, B., *Negotiating Space: Power, Restraint, and Privileges of Immunity in Early Medieval Europe* (Manchester, 1999).

Rosenwein, B. H., *To Be the Neighbor of Saint Peter: The Social Meaning of Cluny's Property 909–1049* (Ithaca, NY, 1989).

Rosser, G., 'Communities of Parish and Guild in the Late Middle Ages', in S. J. Wright, ed., *Parish, Church and People: Local Studies in Lay Religion 1350–1750* (London, 1988), 29–55.

Rosser, G., 'Going to the Fraternal Feast: Commensality and Social Relations in Late Medieval England', *Journal of British Studies* 33 (1994), 430–46.

Rotondo-McCord, J., '*Locum Sepulturae Meae . . . Elegi*: Property, Graves and Sacral Power in Eleventh-century Germany', *Viator* 26 (1995), 77–106.

Rubenstein, J., *Guibert of Nogent: Portrait of a Medieval Mind* (New York, 2002).

Rubin, M. and W. Simon, eds, *The Cambridge History of Christianity IV: Christianity in Western Europe c.1100–1500* (Cambridge, 2009).

Runciman, S., 'The Pilgrimages to Palestine before 1095', in K. M. Setton (gen. ed.), *A History of the Crusades, I: The First Hundred Years*, ed. Marshall W. Baldwin (Madison, Milwaukee and London, 1969), 68–78.

Salch, C.-L. and D. Fèvre, 'Réseau paroissial et implantations castrales du IXe au XIIIe siècle en Vivarais', *L'Encadrement religieux des fidèles au Moyen Age et jusqu'au Concile de Trente. Actes du 109e Congrès national des sociétés savants, Dijon, 1984: Section d'histoire médiévale et de philologie* (Paris, 1985), 47–66.

Schein, S., *Gateway to the Heavenly City: Crusader Jerusalem and the Catholic West (1099–1187)* (Aldershot, 2005).

Schroll, A., *Benedictine Monasticism as Reflected in the Warnefrid-Hildemar Commentaries on the Rule* (New York, 1941).

Semmler, J., 'Zehntgebot und Pfarrtermination in karolingischer Zeit', in H. Mordek, ed., *Aus Kirche und Reich: Festschrift für Friedrich Kempf* (Sigmaringen, 1983), 33–44.

Sergi, G., 'The Kingdom of Italy', in T. Reuter, ed., *New Cambridge Medieval History III: c.900–c.1024* (Cambridge, 1999), 346–71.

Sheehan, M. M., 'Choice of Marriage Partner in the Middle Ages: Development and Mode of Application of a Theory of Marriage', *Studies in Medieval and Renaissance History* 1 (1978), 1–33; repr. in C. Neel, ed., *Medieval Families: Perspectives on Marriage, Household and Children* (Toronto, 2004), 157–91.

Siegwart, J., *Die Chorherren-und Chorfrauengemeinschaften in der deutschsprachigen Schweiz von 6. Jahrhundert bis 1160 mit einem Überblick über die deutsche Kanonikerreform des 10. und 11. Jahrhunderts* (Freiburg, 1962).

Sigal, P.-A., 'Les Voyages des reliques aux onzième et douzième siècles,' in *Voyage, quête, pélerinage dans la litterature et la civilisation médiévale* (Paris, 1976), 75–103.

Smith, J. M. H., '"Emending Evil Ways and Praising God's Omnipotence": Einhard and the Uses of Roman Martyrs', in K. Mills and A. Grafton, eds, *Conversion in Late Antiquity and the Early Middle Ages: Seeing and Believing* (Rochester, NY, 2003), 189–223.

Smith, J. M. H., 'Religion and Lay Society', in R. McKitterick, ed., *New Cambridge Medieval History c.700–c.900* (Cambridge, 1995), 654–78.

Smith, J. M. H., 'Oral and Written: Saints, Miracles and Relics in Brittany, c.850–1250', *Speculum* 65 (1990), 309–43.

Smith, J. M. H., 'Old Saints, New Cults: Roman Relics in Carolingian Francia', in J. M. H. Smith, ed., *Early Medieval Rome and the Christian West: Essays in Honour of Donald A. Bullough* (Leiden, 2000), 317–39.

Smith, J. M. H., 'Saints and Their Cults', in Noble and Smith, eds, *The Cambridge History of Christianity: Early Medieval Christianities c.600–c.1100*, 581–605.

Smith, M. F., R. Fleming and P. Halpin, 'Court and Piety in Late Anglo-Saxon England', *Catholic Historical Review* 87 (2001), 569–602.

Somerville, R. with S. Kuttner, *Pope Urban II, the Collectio Britannica and the Council of Melfi (1089)* (Oxford, 1996).

Somerville, R., 'The Council of Clermont (1095) and Latin Christian Society', *Archivum Historiae Pontificiae* 12 (1974), 55–90.

Sot, M., *Un historien et son Église. Flodoard de Reims* (Paris, 1993).

Southern, R. W., *The Making of the Middle Ages* (London, 1953).

Spinks, B. D., *Early and Medieval Rituals and Theologies of Baptism: From the New Testament to the Council of Trent* (Aldershot, 2006), 109–33.

Steele Edwards, G., 'Ritual Excommunication in Medieval France and England, 900–1200' (Stanford University, unpublished Ph.D. thesis, 1997).

Stevenson, K., *Nuptial Blessing: A Study of Christian Marriage Rites*, Alcuin Club Collections 64 (London, 1982).

Stock, B., *The Implications of Literacy: Written Language and Models of Interpretation in the Eleventh and Twelfth Centuries* (Princeton, NJ, 1983).

Stocker, D. and P. Everson, *Summoning St Michael: Early Romanesque Towers in Lincolnshire* (Oxford, 2006).

Stocker, D., 'Monuments and Merchants: Irregularities in the Distribution of Stone Sculpture in Lincolnshire and Yorkshire in the Tenth Century', in D. M. Hadley and J. D. Richards, eds, *Cultures in Contact: Scandinavian Settlement in England in the Ninth and Tenth Centuries* (Turnhout, 2000), 179–212.

Stopani, R., *La via francigena in Toscana*, 2nd edn (Florence, 1984).

Stutz, U., 'The Proprietary Church as an Element of Medieval German Ecclesiastical Law', trans. G. Barraclough, *Mediaeval Germany 911–1250* (Oxford, 1938), II. 35–70.

Swanson, R., *Religion and Devotion in Europe c.1215–c.1515* (Cambridge, 1995).

Symes, C., 'The Lordship of Jongleurs', in R. F. Berkhofer, A. Cooper and A. J. Kosto, eds, *The Experience of Power in Medieval Europe 950–1350: Essays in Honour of T. N. Bisson* (Aldershot, 2005), 237–52.

Tatlock, J. S. P., 'The English Journey of the Laon Canons', *Speculum* 8 (1933), 454–65.

Taylor, C. K., *Heresy in Medieval France: Dualism in Aquitaine and the Agenais, 1000–1249* (Woodbridge, 2005).

Taylor, H. M. and J. Taylor, *Anglo-Saxon Architecture,* 3 vols (Cambridge, 1965–78).

Tellenbach, G., trans. T. Reuter, *The Church in Western Europe from the Tenth to the Early Twelfth Century* (Cambridge, 1993).

Thacker, A. and R. Sharpe, eds, *Local Saints and Local Churches in the Early Medieval West* (Oxford, 2002).

Thesaurus of Old English: http://libra.englang.arts.gla.ac.uk/oethesaurus/aboutoe.html (accessed 21 January 2011).

Thibodeaux, J. D., 'Man of the Church or Man of the Village? Gender and Parish Clergy in Medieval Normandy', *Gender and History* 18 (2006), 380–99.

Thibodeaux, J. D., ed., *Negotiating Clerical Identities: Priests, Monks and Masculinity in the Middle Ages* (Houndsmills, 2010).

Thomas, H. M., 'Lay Piety in England from 1066 to 1215', *Anglo-Norman Studies 29* (2006), 179–92.

Thompson, N. M., 'The Carolingian *De Festiuitatibus* and the Blickling Book', in A. J. Kleist, ed., *The Old English Homily: Precedent, Practice and Appropriation* (Turnhout, 2007), 97–119.

Thompson, V., 'Constructing Salvation: A Homiletic and Penitential Context for Late Anglo-Saxon Burial Practice', in S. Lucy and A. Reynolds, eds, *Burial in Early Medieval England and Wales* (London, 2002), 229–40.

Thompson, V., 'The Pastoral Contract in Late Anglo-Saxon England: Priest and Parishioner in Oxford, Bodleian Library, MS Laud Miscellaneous 482', in F. Tinti, ed., *Pastoral Care in Late Anglo-Saxon England* (Woodbridge, 2005), 106–20.

Thompson, V., *Dying and Death in Later Anglo-Saxon England* (Woodbridge, 2004).

Tinti, F. ed., *Pastoral Care in Late Anglo-Saxon England* (Woodbridge, 2005).

Tinti, F., 'The "Costs" of Pastoral Care: Church Dues in Late Anglo-Saxon England', in F. Tinti, ed., *Pastoral Care in Late Anglo-Saxon England* (Woodbridge, 2005), 27–51.

Tinti, F., *Sustaining Belief: The Church of Worcester from c.870–c.1100* (Aldershot, 2010).

Toubert, P., *Les structures du Latium médiéval: le Latium méridional et la Sabine du IXe siècle à la fin du XIIe siècle*, 2 vols (Rome, 1973).

Townend, M. ed., *Wulfstan. Archbishop of York: The Proceedings of the Second Alcuin Conference* (Turnhout, 2004).

Trichet, L., *La Tonsure. Vie et mort d'une pratique ecclésiastique* (Paris, 1990).

Tudor, V., 'Godric of Finchale', *ODNB*.

Upchurch, R. K., 'For Pastoral Care and Political Gain: Ælfric of Eynsham's Preaching on Marital Celibacy', *Traditio* 59 (2004), 40–78.

van Engen, J., 'The Christian Middle Ages', *American Historical Review* 91 (1986), 519–52.

van Meter, D. C., 'Count Baldwin IV, Richard of Saint-Vanne, and the Inception of Monastic Reform in Eleventh-century Flanders', *Revue bénédictine*, 107 (1997), 130–48.

van Meter, D. C., 'Eschatological Order and the Moral Arguments for Clerical Celibacy in Francia Around the Year 1000', in Frassetto, ed., *Medieval Purity*, 149–75.

van Rhijn, C., *Shepherds of the Lord: Priests and Episcopal Statutes in the Carolingian Period* (Turnhout, 2007).

Vauchez, A., ed., *Faire croire: modalités de la diffusion et de la réception des messages religieux du XIIe au XVe siècle*, Collection de l'École française de Rome 51 (Rome, 1981).

Vauchez, A., ed., *The Laity in the Middle Ages: Religious Belief and Devotional Practices*, trans. D. E. Bornstein (Notre Dame, IN, 1993).

Vauchez, A., *La spiritualité de moyen-âge occidental VIII–XII siècles* (Paris, 1975), English trans. by C. Friedlander as *The Spirituality of the Medieval West: The Eighth to the Twelfth Century* (Kalamazoo, MI, 1993).

Venarde, B., *Women's Monasticism and Medieval Society. Nunneries in France and England, 890–1215* (Ithaca, NY, 1997).

Viader, R., *L'Andorre du IXe au XIVe siècle: montagne, féodalité, et communautés* (Toulouse, 2003).

Violante, C., *La Pataria Milanese e la riforma ecclesiastica, i, Le premesse* (Rome, 1955).

Violante, C., 'Les prêts sur gage foncier dans la vie économique et sociale de Milan au xie siècle', *Cahiers de civilisation médiéval* 5 (I962), 147–68, 437–59.

Vodola, E., *Excommunication in the Middle Ages* (Berkeley, CA, 1986).

Vogel, C., 'Le Pèlerinage pénitentiel', *Revue des sciences religieuses* 38 (1964) 113–53; repr in Vogel, C., *En Rémission des péchés: recherches sur les systèmes pénitentiels dans l'église latine*, ed. A. Faivre (Aldershot, 1994), no. VII.

Vogel, C., 'Pratiques superstitieuses au début du XIe siècle d'après le Corrector sive medicus de Buchard, évêque de Worms (965–1025)', *Mélanges E.-R. Labande, Études de civilisation medieval (IXe–XII siècles)* (Poitier, 1974), 751–61, repr. C. Vogel, *En rémission des péchés. Recherches sur les systèmes pénitentiels dans l'Église latine* (Aldershot, 1994), no. X.

Wallace-Hadrill, J. M., *The Frankish Church* (Oxford, 1983).

Walsham, A., *The Reformation of the Landscape: Religion, Identity and Memory in Early Modern Britain and Ireland* (Oxford, 2011).

Ward, B., *Miracles and the Medieval Mind: Theory, Record and Event, 1000–1215* (Aldershot, 1982).

Wareham, A., 'St Oswald's Family and Kin', in N. Brooks and C. Cubitt, eds, *St Oswald of Worcester: Life and Influence* (London, 1996), 46–63.

Warner, P., 'Shared Churchyards, Freemen Church-Builders and the Development of Parishes in Eleventh-century East Anglia', *Landscape History* 8 (1986), 39–52.

Watkins, C. S., *History and the Supernatural in Medieval England* (Cambridge, 2007).

Watson, S. and N. Tanner, 'Least of the Laity: The Minimum Requirements for a Medieval Christian', *Journal of Medieval History* 32:4 (2006), 395–423.

Watts, L., P. Rahtz, A. Okasha, S. A. J. Bradley and J. Higgitt, 'Kirkdale – the Inscriptions', *Medieval Archaeology* 41 (1997), 51–99.

Webb, D., 'Domestic Space and Devotion in the Middle Ages', in A. Spicer and S. Hamilton, eds, *Defining the Holy: Sacred Space in Medieval and Early Modern Europe* (Aldershot, 2006), 27–47.

Webb, D., *Medieval European Pilgrimage* (Houndsmills, 2002).

Webb, D., *Pilgrims and Pilgrimage in the Medieval West* (London and New York, 1999).

Wemple, S. F., *Atto of Vercelli: Church, State and Christian Society in Tenth-century Italy* (Rome, 1979).

West, C., 'The Significance of the Carolingian Advocate', *Early Medieval Europe* 17 (2009), 186–206.

Wilcox, J., 'Ælfric in Dorset and the Landscape of Pastoral Care', in F. Tinti, ed., *Pastoral Care in Late Anglo-Saxon England* (Woodbridge, 2005), 52–62.

Williams, A., 'Swein, earl, d. 1052', *ODNB*.

Williams, A., 'Thegnly Piety and Ecclesiastical Patronage in the Late Old English Kingdom', *Anglo-Norman Studies* 24 (2002), 1–24.

Witters, W., 'Pauvres et pauvreté dans les coutumes monastique du Moyen Age', in M. Mollat, ed., *Études sur l'Historie de la Pauvreté (Moyen Age–XVI siècle)* (Paris, 1974), 177–215.

Wollasch, J., 'Monasticism: The First Wave of Reform', *NCMH* III, 163–85.

Wood, S., *The Proprietary Church in the Medieval West* (Oxford, 2006).

Yarrow, S., *Saints and Their Communities: Miracle Stories in Twelfth-century England* (Oxford, 2006).

Zadora-Rio, E., 'Constructions de châteaux et fondation de paroisses en Anjou aux XIe–XIIe siècles', *Archéologie médiévale* 9 (1979), 115–25.

Zerner, M., ed., *Inventer l'hérésie? Discours polémiques et pouvoirs avant l'inquisition* (Nice, 1998).

Index

Page references to Figures or Tables will be in *italics*; references to Notes will be followed by the letter 'n'.